Drug Action and Drug Resistance in Bacteria

Drug Action and Drug Resistance in Bacteria

1. Macrolide Antibiotics and Lincomycin

Edited by **Susumu Mitsuhashi**

UNIVERSITY PARK PRESS

© UNIVERSITY OF TOKYO PRESS, 1971
UTP No. 3045-67567-5149
Printed in Japan.

Originally published in 1971 by
UNIVERSITY OF TOKYO PRESS

UNIVERSITY PARK PRESS
Baltimore • London • Tokyo
Library of Congress Cataloging in Publication Data
Main entry under title:

Macrolide antibiotics and lincomycin.
(Drug action and drug resistance in bacteria, v. 1)
Includes bibliographies.
1. Drug resistance in micro-organisms. 2. Antibiotics.
3. Staphylococcus. I. Mitsuhashi, Susumu, 1917– ed.
II. Series.
QR177.M3   616.01'4   74-171254
ISBN 0-8391-0642-4

PREFACE

The introduction into medicine of the antibacterial agents, which include both antibiotics and chemotherapeutic agents, caused revolutionary changes in the clinical treatment of certain diseases. Furthermore, biochemical studies on the mode of action of these antibacterial agents progressed in parallel to the almost exponential progress in biochemistry, and included the establishment of *in vitro* systems of protein and nucleic acid synthesis, the use of isotopes, and improvements in the purification of biochemical materials. Thus, antibacterial agents, such as actinomycin D, chloramphenicol, rifampicin, etc., as enzyme inhibitors have become indispensable tools in the study of the role of enzymes in biochemical reactions. However, in spite of the progress being made in discovering the modes of drug action in biochemistry, the information collected from these studies has not always been used to facilitate the introduction of new drugs into chemotherapy.

Parallel to the worldwide use of antibacterial agents, the numbers of multiple-resistant strains have increased in clinical isolates, offering new problems and challenges to both the clinical and genetic research fields. Epidemiological surveys have disclosed the role of episomes, plasmids, and bacteriophages in infective heredity for the wide and rapid spread of multiple resistance. It was surprising to find that the biochemical mechanisms of drug resistance in clinical isolates were mostly different from those of *in vitro*-developed resistance and were common in both the gram-positive and gram-negative bacteria isolated in any country; mechanisms of resistance included phosphorylation, acetylation, adenylylation, β-lactamase activity, etc. Similarly, the wide distribution of mechanisms for the induction for drug resistance in resistant bacteria, *i.e.*, β-lactamase, macrolide resistance, chloramphenicol, acetyltransferase, tetracycline resistance, etc., aroused our interests not only because of the clinical importance but also because of possible genetic and evolutionary significance. Thus, the information and findings of drug resistance in bacteria have become important tools in the study and introduction of new antibacterial agents by concentrating on the mode of action of enzyme inhibition which is responsible for resistance and by modifying known drugs to become more effective toward the emerging resistant strains. The symposium was planned for the purpose of correlating information on both drug action and drug resistance in bacteria, as the mechanisms of drug resistance are not always the reverse of the mechanisms of drug action.

On May 24–25, 1970, the symposium was held at the beautiful lakeside located in the crater of the dead volcano, Mt. Haruna, surrounded by high mountains. Though attendance at this conference was limited because of financial difficulties, we are very pleased to report that all individuals intended to invite to the symposium graciously consented to contribute to this monograph. My purpose in publishing this monograph and a forthcoming series is to provide information and solutions to the problems of bacterial drug resistance from the clinical, genetic or biochemical points of view.

I am deeply indebted to Drs. H. Umezawa, T. Hata, and T. Osono for their encouragement which made the symposium possible. I am also grateful to Dr. M. R. Smith, who kindly read the entire manuscript. I am also indebted to the financial support received from the many pharmaceutical companies without whose assistance the symposium would not have been possible.

Susumu Mitsuhashi

Department of Microbiology
School of Medicine
Gunma University

CONTENTS

II. ACTION AND RESISTANCE IN MACROLIDE ANTIBIOTICS
AND LINCOMYCIN

THE CHEMISTRY AND CONFORMATION OF
ERYTHROMYCIN   T. J. Perun   123

MODE OF ACTION OF ERYTHROMYCIN
                                    J. C. -H. Mao   153

I. EPIDEMIOLOGY OF RESISTANCE TO MACROLIDE ANTIBIOTICS AND LINCOMYCIN

EPIDEMIOLOGICAL STUDY OF ERYTHROMYCIN RESISTANCE IN *STAPHYLOCOCCUS AUREUS* IN JAPAN

Hirokazu OTAYA

Shionogi & Co., Ltd., Osaka, Japan

Seventeen years have passed since erythromycin was commercially used for the first time in Japan in 1953. Since then, other macrolide antibiotics, such as leucomycin (1956), oleandomycin (1958) and spiramycin (1964), have come into use.

The emergence of erythromycin-resistant staphylococci has been noted since 1964. The data shown in Fig. 1 summarize the results on the resistance of staphylococci to erythromycin as reported in Japanese scientific journals between 1955 and 1965. A gradual increase in the rate of resistant strains being isolated is evident. It is also obvious that this increase is connected with the quantity of sales of erythromycin in Japan as shown in Fig. 2. However, as shown in Fig. 1, there is a marked fluctuation among individual test results on the resistance of staphylococci.

Since 1965, we have been running studies continuously on sensitivities to erythromycin and other antibiotics frequently used against pathogenic staphylococci and *Escherichia coli*, which were isolated at general hospitals throughout Japan.

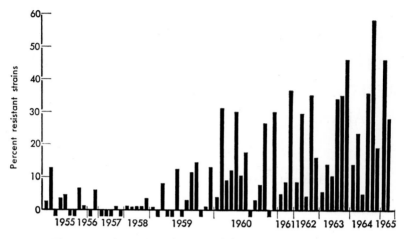

Fig. 1.   Erythromycin-resistant staphylococci reported in journals between 1955 and 1965. One block in the figure is related to one paper.
The height of the blocks on the zero line shows the percentage of resistant strains reported in the papers cited. The block extending below
the zero line, without regard to its length, means no resistant strain.

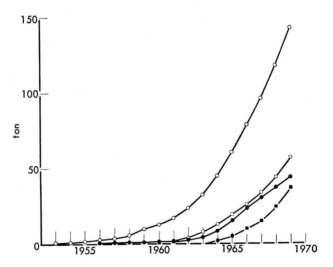

Fig. 2.   Estimated cumulative sales of macrolide antibiotics in
Japan. ○, erythromycin; □, oleandomycin; ●, leucomycin; ■, spiramycin.

Our objective was to investigate the annual trends of bacterial resistance to the antibiotics and sulfonamides frequently used in hospitals. The test results on erythromycin in *Staphylococcus aureus* are as follows.

Materials and methods

1. Bacterial strains
Bacterial isolates and hospitals were selected by a statistical sampling method and bacterial isolates which were sampled in the central clinical laboratories or other equivalent laboratories of hospitals were examined.

Testing method: Isolated strains were propagated in a modified Mueller-Hinton broth medium (37°C, 18 hr). A loopful from each culture was suspended in 5 ml of saline with a 1 mm standard platinum loop. Modified Mueller-Hinton medium was used for culture media. Drug-sensitivity tests were performed using the two-fold agar dilution method with the same media. 1 mm platinum loop. Agar streak method (about 10^4 cells, 37°C, 18 hr).

Mueller-Hinton medium (modified) consisted of:

200.0 ml	beef heart infusion	0.05 g	L-cystine
16.5 g	casamino acids	5.0 μg	biotin
1.5 g	starch	15.0 g	agar
2.0 g	glucose	and distilled water	1,000.0 ml
0.05 g	L-tryptophan		(pH 7.4 ± 0.1).

2. Chemotherapeutic agents tested
Erythromycin (EM), penicillin-G (PC-G), streptomycin (SM), chloramphenicol (CP), tetracycline (TC), kanamycin (KM), cephalothin (CET), cephaloridine (CER), sulfamethoxazole (SIM) and aminobenzyl-penicillin (AB-PC) were used.

3. Period of study (June, 1965 – May, 1969)
Each year was divided into two parts in the annual investigation; and each annual period of investigation started in June and ended in May the following year, as stated:

1965:   June, 1965–May, 1966

TABLE I
Districts, Sampling Hospitals and Number of Strains

District	Population $(\times 10^3)$	No. of hospitals	No. of sampling hospitals	No. of strains		
				S. aureus	E. coli	Total
I Chiba, Tokyo, Kanagawa	18710	568	60	1205	753	1958
II Kyoto, Shiga, Osaka, Hyogo, Nara, Wakayama	16498	594	62	776	489	1265
III Hokkaido, Aomori, Iwate, Miyagi, Akita, Yamagata, Fukushima	14751	340	50	512	257	769
IV Gifu, Shizuoka, Aichi, Mie	11433	274	45	622	320	942
V Tottori, Shimane, Okayama, Hiroshima, Yamaguchi, Tokushima, Kagawa, Ehime, Kochi	11188	324	27	322	169	491
VI Fukuoka, Saga, Nagasaki, Kumamoto, Oita, Miyazaki, Kagoshima	12770	246	37	415	298	713
VII Ibaragi, Tochigi, Gumma, Saitama, Toyama, Niigata, Ishikawa, Fukui, Yamanashi, Nagano	16639	293	64	622	410	1032
Total	101989	2639	345	4474	2696	7170

TABLE II

Number of *S. aureus* (coagulase positive) Strains Classified by Years and Sources

(Period: June, 1965 – May, 1969)

Specimen	1965		1966		1967		1968		Total	
	No. of strains	%	No. of strains	%	No. of strains	%	No. of strains	%	No. of strains	%
Pus	707	71.2	671	71.3	827	67.4	733	71.1	2938	70.1
Pharyngeal mucus	101	10.2	90	9.6	151	12.3	111	10.8	453	10.8
Sputum	80	8.0	63	6.7	92	7.5	113	10.9	348	8.3
Urine	58	5.8	66	7.0	89	7.2	27	2.6	240	5.7
Feces	4	0.4	2	0.2	14	1.1	8	0.8	28	0.7
Blood	11	1.1	12	1.3	8	0.7	7	0.7	38	0.9
Spinal fluid	6	0.6	2	0.2	7	0.6	4	0.4	19	0.5
Punctate	4	0.4	8	0.8	8	0.7	2	0.2	22	0.5
Ascites	2	0.2							2	
Thoracic fluid	7	0.7	7	0.7	5	0.4	4	0.4	23	0.5
Bile	4	0.4	2	0.2	8	0.7	8	0.8	22	0.5
Joint fluid	1	0.1	4	0.4	3	0.2	3	0.3	11	0.3
Washout liquid	2	0.2	1	0.1	1	0.2			4	0.1
Skin piece	3	0.3	1	0.1					4	
etc.	4	0.4	13	1.4	13	1.1	11	1.0	41	1.0
Total	994	100.0	942	100.0	1226	100.0	1031	100.0	4193	100.0

TABLE III
Multiple Correlation Coefficients for the Items Shown in Table I

Items				Level of significance
A—B	C	D	E	$P=0.01$
B—A	C	D	E	//
C—A	B	D	E	//
D—A	B	C	E	//
E—A	B	C	D	//

A: Population. B: Total number of hospitals. C: Number of sampling hospitals.
D: Number of *S. aureus* strains. E: Number of *E. coli* strains.

1966:   June, 1966–May, 1967
1967:   June, 1967–May, 1968
1968:   June, 1968–May, 1969

4. Items for analysis

1) Results of sampling.* 2) Changes of drug sensitivities: a) general tendency,* b) multiple-drug resistance.* 3) Grouping by districts (seven). 4) Grouping by the size of hospitals (expressed in number of beds). 5) Grouping by inpatients and outpatients. 6) Grouping by age. 7) Grouping by the sources of strains.*

Hospitals from which bacterial isolates were collected: among the general hospitals equipped with central clinical laboratories, 10% of the larger hospitals were selected in each prefecture.

Results

1. Districts, sampling hospitals and number of strains (Tables I and II)
2. Correlation analysis of the results of sampling (Table III)
The correlation analysis of the factors involved have made possible the assumption of the drug sensitivities of the isolates submitted to central clinical laboratories of the hospitals in Japan.

General tendency of drug sensitivities

1. Methods of analysis
In analyzing the data from our annual investigations of bacterial

---
* Marked items are reported herein.

drug sensitivities, we compared the average values of the M.I.C. of the total isolates studied to those we have reported on previous (2–4). This comparison was made on the assumption that the levels of sensitivities of the isolates to each drug gave a normal distribution curve, but it was found that this assumption did not fit all the drugs used. We have, therefore, classified the bacterial isolates into groups of high sensitivity, intermediate sensitivity and low sensitivity according to their M.I.C. values in the present investigation. Annual changes of the bacterial drug sensitivities were compared statistically in terms of the frequencies of these three groups. The bacteria studied were those isolated from various specimens. The results are reported here for erythromycin only.

2. Results on erythromycin

A decrease in the high-sensitivity group and an increase in the low-sensitivity group occurred between 1965 and 1966. The intermediate-sensitivity group decreased and the low-sensitivity group increased between 1966 and 1967. An increase in the low-sensitivity group was found between 1967 and 1968, but no change was observed in the other groups in this period. Consequently, a marked decrease in the high-sensitivity group and a decrease in the intermediate-sensitivity group occurred between 1965 and 1968, resulting in a remarkable increase in the low-sensitivity group.

M.I.C. (μg/ml)	No. of strains				Percentage			
Year	'65	'66	'67	'68	'65	'66	'67	'68
0.0125–1.56	819	726	907	714	76.90	72.24	69.24	66.42
3.13 –12.5	56	52	34	23	5.26	5.17	2.60	2.14
25.0–≧100	190	227	369	338	17.84	22.59	28.17	31.44
Year	'65–'66		'65–'67		'65–'68	'66–'67		'66–'68	'67–'68
0.0125–1.56	*		**		**	—		**	—
3.13 –12.5	—		**		**	**		**	—
25.0–≧100	**		**		**	**		**	.

Notes: **, $P=0.01$; *, $P=0.05$; · , $P=0.1$; —, no significance.

Differences in drug sensitivities by the sources of isolation

Since, according to the previous results (2–4), the degrees of drug

TABLE IV
Differences of Erythromycin Sensitivity by the Sources of Isolation in *S. aureus*

Group	M.I.C. (μg/ml)	Urine				Pus				Pharyngeal mucus				Sputum			
		1965	1966	1967	1968	1965	1966	1967	1968	1965	1966	1967	1968	1965	1966	1967	1968
		n=57	n=66	n=87	n=26	n=702	n=668	n=801	n=713	n=97	n=90	n=147	n=57	n=79	n=63	n=93	n=110
A	0.025≧	3.5%				1.5	0.3	0.2		3.1			3.5	3.8			
	0.05	24.6	1.5			20.1	1.5	1.1	0.4	30.9	2.2	2.7	24.6	22.8	3.2	2.2	28.2
	0.1	19.3	34.8	49.4	26.9	38.7	44.3	43.6	24.5	37.1	53.3	48.3	19.3	19.0	44.4	52.7	34.5
	0.2	5.3	34.8	9.2	30.8	10.4	21.3	18.4	36.0	11.3	25.6	27.9	5.3	8.9	19.0	20.4	5.5
	0.39	1.8	1.5	1.1		1.6	0.3	2.4	2.0	1.0			1.8	1.3	1.6	3.2	
	0.78	3.5	3.0			3.0	0.4	0.1	0.6	3.1		6.8	3.5	7.6			
	1.56	1.8				3.4	1.5	1.4	0.1	1.0	1.1		1.8	3.8	1.6	1.1	
B	3.13	5.3		1.1	3.8	1.9	2.2	0.9	0.8		3.3	0.7	5.3	6.3		1.1	0.9
	6.25	1.8	1.5	1.1		1.7	2.2	0.6	0.8		1.1	1.4	1.8	2.5	1.6		
	12.5		1.5	2.3		1.1	1.3	0.7	0.4	1.0	2.2			1.3	1.6		0.9
C	25.0	1.8	1.5	1.1	3.8	1.1	0.6	0.5	0.8		3.3	0.7	1.8		1.6	1.1	0.9
	50.0			2.3		1.4	1.3	1.0	0.4		1.1	1.4		1.3			
	100≦	31.3	19.9	32.4	34.7	14.1	22.8	29.1	33.2	11.5	6.8	10.1	31.3	21.4	25.4	18.2	29.1
	Total (%)	100	100	100	100	100	100	100	100	100	100	100	100	100	100	100	100

A: High-sensitivity group. B: Intermediate-sensitivity group. C: Low-sensitivity group.

sensitivities were very different between sources of isolation, we analyzed the strains from the following four specimens for sensitivity to erythromycin: pus, pharyngeal mucus, sputum and urine. *Staphylococcus aureus* was most frequently isolated in these four specimens, as shown in Table II.

The strains of the low-sensitivity group, as shown in Table IV, were the most frequent in urine, then pus, sputum and pharyngeal mucus in this order.

It is also obvious that the tendency of annual changes of sensitivities was very similar among the four sources of isolation. However, pus showed the most typical patterns and urine had minimal changes.

Multiple-drug resistance

With regard to multiple-drug resistances, a number of studies have already been reported (*1, 5*). Among them, however, few have been investigated by the year and statistically analyzed. Therefore, we reviewed our results to determine the suitability for this type of analysis.

1. The strains tested
From the above-mentioned results, which showed that the degrees of drug sensitivity were very different between the sources of isolation, we used only those strains from the same source of isolation, namely, pus specimens.

2. Differentiation between sensitive and resistant strains
We have divided the strains into sensitive and resistant, according to the following criteria of their M.I.C. values. The strains showing M.I.C. values equal to or higher than those listed on page 13 were regarded as resistant and the others, as sensitive.

3. Results on seven drugs including erythromycin
The frequencies of multiple-drug-resistant strains were studied annually for the four periods. According to the results shown in Table V, single-drug-resistant and two-drug-resistant strains

TABLE V
Annual Frequencies of Single-drug-resistant and Multiple-drug-resistant Strains of S. aureus Isolated from Pus Specimens
(Drugs tested: PC-G, SM, EM, CP, KM, TC and SIM)

	1965		1966		1967		1968		Total	
	No. of strains	%	No. of strains	%	No. of strains	%	No. of strains	%	No. of strains	%
Total	682	100	662	100	797	100	712	100	2853	100
Sensitive to 7 drugs	241	35.3	161	24.3	211	26.5	260	36.5	873	30.6
Total resistant	441	64.7	501	75.7	586	73.5	452	63.5	1980	69.4
Resistant to 1 drug	108	24.5†	152	30.3	172	29.4	107	23.7	539	27.2
Resistant to 2 drugs	51	11.6	59	11.8	61	10.4	31	6.9	202	10.2
Resistant to 3 drugs	90	20.4	59	11.8	79	13.5	57	12.6	285	14.4
Resistant to 4 drugs	97	22.0	71	14.2	110	18.8	98	21.7	376	19.0
Resistant to 5 drugs	65	14.7	103	20.6	100	17.1	112	24.8	380	19.2
Resistant to 6 drugs	26	5.9	42	8.4	43	7.3	34	7.5	145	7.3
Resistant to 7 drugs	4	0.9	15	3.0	21	3.6	13	2.9	53	2.7

† Among total resistant strains which are expressed as 100%.

Drug	M.I.C. (μg/ml)
PC-G	$3.13\leqq$ (u/ml)
CP	$25\ \leqq$
EM	$3.13\leqq$
SM	$25\ \leqq$
TC	$25\ \leqq$
KM	$25\ \leqq$
CET*	$25\ \leqq$
CER*	$25\ \leqq$
AB-PC*	$3.13\leqq$
SIM	$125\ \leqq$

* A description of these three antibiotics is in the latter part of this paper, because none of the strains tested was resistant to CET and CER, and AB-PC was tested only on the strains isolated in 1968.

showed a tendency to decrease, whereas four-drug-resistant and five-drug-resistant strains showed a tendency to increase. Almost no change was observed in the frequencies of six-drug-resistant and seven-drug-resistant strains.

Frequently observed combinations of drug resistances—We compared the theoretically possible combinations of drug resistances with the actual observed combinations in examining those combinations of resistances with the above-listed seven drugs, except for CET, CER and AB-PC. As seen in Table VI, the combinations of three drug resistances and four drug resistances were most abundant. Many different combinations were actually observed. If

TABLE VI
Theoretically Possible Combinations and Actually Observed Combinations of Drug Resistances with Their Frequencies in *S. aureus*

(For total 4-year period from 1965 to 1968)

Type resistant to	No. of theoretically possible combinations	No. of actually observed combinations	Frequency of strains
1 drug	7	7	27.2
2 drugs	21	15	10.2
3 drugs	35	22	14.4
4 drugs	35	22	19.0
5 drugs	21	17	19.2
6 drugs	7	7	7.3
7 drugs	1	1	2.7
Total	127	91	100.0%

TABLE VII
Theoretically Possible Combinations and Actually Observed Combinations of Drug
Resistances Expressed for Each Drug Resistance in *S. aureus*

(For total 4-year period from 1965 to 1968)

Type resistant to	No. of theoretically possible combinations	No. of actually observed combinations including resistance to						
		PC-G	SM	EM	CP	KM	TC	SIM
2 drugs	6	5	5	5	3	2	4	6
3 drugs	15	11	12	10	10	3	10	10
4 drugs	20	13	13	15	11	9	14	13
5 drugs	15	11	13	13	12	11	12	13
6 drugs	6	6	6	6	6	6	6	6
Total	62	46	49	49	42	31	46	48

we examine the data for each drug, however, considerable differences are found in the frequencies of the drug-resistant strains
(Table VII).

In the frequencies of the actual observed drug-resistant strains,
single-drug-resistant strains were the most frequent (27.2%). Four-
drug-resistant and five-drug-resistant strains were 19.0% and
19.2%, respectively. Three-drug-resistant strains were 14.4%;
two-drug-resistant strains, 10.2%; six-drug-resistant strains, 7.3%;
and seven-drug-resistant strains, 2.7%. These frequencies were not
related to the types of combinations of drug resistances (Table VI).

Table VIII shows the data on the frequencies of various types
of drug-resistant strains for the four years. As seen here, annual
changes are not obvious except for some types of drug-resistant
strains. In the two-drug-resistant strains, our attention is drawn
to those strains resistant to PC-G plus SIM-type, which were as
frequent as 42.6%; strains resistant to TC plus SIM-type, 19.8%;
and strains resistant to SM plus PC-G-type, 9.9%. Indeed, these
three types together occupy 73% of the total two-drug-resistant
strains. In the three-drug-resistant strains, PC-G, SIM plus TC-
type was 49.1%; and TC, SM plus SIM-type and PC-G, SM plus
SIM-type were 10.5% and 10.9%, respectively. These three types
together occupy 70% of the total three-drug-resistant strains. In
the four-drug-resistant strains, PC-G, TC, SM plus SIM-type was

41.5%; and PC-G, TC, EM plus SIM-type, 31.1%. These two types together were 73% of the total four-drug-resistant strains. The latter type of the four-drug-resistant strains showed a tendency toward annual increase. In the five-drug-resistant strains, PC-G, SM, TC, EM plus SIM-type was 63.9%; and PC-G, EM, TC, CP plus SIM-type, 13.9%. These two types together occupied about 78% of the total five-drug-resistant strains. The former type of the five-drug-resistant strains showed a tendency to increase annually, as was true with the four-drug-resistant strains. In the six-drug-resistant strains, EM, TC, CP, SM, PC-G plus SIM-type was 53.1%; and KM, EM, TC, SM, PC-G plus SIM-type, 33.1%. These two types together were 86% of the total six-drug-resistant strains. It is interesting to note that KM resistance appeared here for the first time in the main drug-resistance combinations.

Among the total single-drug-, two-drug-, three-drug-, four-drug-, five-drug-, six-drug- and seven-drug-resistant strains, EM, TC, SM, PC-G plus SIM-type was 12.3%; TC, SM, PC-G plus SIM-type, 7.9%; TC, PC-G plus SIM-type, 7.1%; EM, TC, PC-G plus SIM-type, 5.9%; PC-G plus SIM-type, 4.3%; and EM, TC, CP, SM, PC-G plus SIM-type, 3.9%. The total of these six types was 41% among the total resistant strains.

4. Results on erythromycin
The frequency of the total EM-resistant strains showed a remarkable chronological increase, particularly in the four-drug-resistant strains, which had increased considerably (Table IX).

Combinations of EM resistance with other drug resistances—The observed types of combinations of EM resistance with other drug resistances were the most numerous (Table VII). The most frequent combinations with EM resistance were four-drug-resistant strains (22.9%) and five-drug-resistant strains (42.0%). The following combinations were the most frequent types among the observed combinations. The percentage indicates the frequency among the total EM-resistant strains.

Two-drug-resistant : EM plus PC-G-type, 1.2%.
Three-drug-resistant: EM, TC plus SIM-type, 1.9%.
Four-drug-resistant : EM, TC, PC-G plus SIM-type, 13.6%.

TABLE VIII
Main Types of Combinations of Drug Resistances and Their Frequencies in *S. aureus*

Type resistant to	Order	Combination	1965 No.	1965 %	1966 No.	1966 %	1967 No.	1967 %	1968 No.	1968 %	Total No. (B)	Total %	(B)/(A) %
		all	51	100	59	100	61	100	31	100	202	100	10.20
2 drugs	1	SIM, PC-G	14	27.5	35	59.3	26	42.6	11	35.5	86	42.6	4.34
	2	SIM, TC	17	33.3	10	16.9	9	14.8	4	12.9	40	19.8	2.02
	3	SM, PC-G	1	2.0	4	6.8	9	14.8	6	19.4	20	9.9	1.01
		all	90	100	59	100	79	100	57	100	285	100	14.39
3 drugs	1	SIM, TC, PC-G	39	43.3	36	61.0	38	48.1	27	47.4	140	49.1	7.07
	2	SIM, SM, PC-G	12	13.3	6	10.2	7	8.9	6	10.5	31	10.9	1.57
	3	SIM, TC, SM	19	21.1	5	8.5	3	3.8	3	5.3	30	10.5	1.52
		all	97	100	71	100	110	100	98	100	376	100	18.99
4 drugs	1	SIM, TC, SM, PC-G	65	67.0	31	43.7	39	35.5	21	21.4	156	41.5	7.88
	2	SIM, EM, TC, PC-G	13	13.4	18	25.4	44	40.0	42	42.9	117	31.1	5.91
	3	SIM, EM, SM, PC-G	1	1.0	5	7.0	7	6.4	6	6.1	19	5.1	0.96
	3	SIM, EM, TC, SM	5	5.2	2	2.8	5	4.5	7	7.1	19	5.1	0.96
		all	65	100	103	100	100	100	112	100	380	100	19.19
5 drugs	1	SIM, EM, TC, SM, PC-G	32	49.2	69	67.0	62	62.0	80	71.4	243	63.9	12.27
	2	SIM, EM, TC, CP, PC-G	12	18.5	8	7.8	16	16.0	17	15.2	53	13.9	2.68
	3	SIM, EM, TC, CP, SM	11	16.9	9	8.7	2	2.0	5	4.5	27	7.1	1.36
		all	26	100	42	100	43	100	34	100	145	100	7.32
6 drugs	1	SIM, EM, TC, CP, SM, PC-G	21	80.8	21	50.0	23	53.5	12	35.3	77	53.1	3.89
	2	SIM, KM, EM, TC, SM, PC-G	0	0	16	38.1	13	30.2	19	55.9	48	33.1	2.42
	3	SIM, KM, EM, TC, CP, SM	5	19.2	4	9.5	2	4.7	0	0	11	7.6	0.56
7 drugs		SIM, EM, TC, CP, SM, KM, PC-G	4		15		21		13		53		2.68
Total strains resistant to from 1 to 7 drugs											1980	(A) 100	

TABLE IX
Strains of *S. aureus* Resistant to Erythromycin

	1965		1966		1967		1968		Total	
	No. of strains	%	No. of strains	%	No. of strains	%	No. of strains	%	No. of strains	%
Total	682	100	662	100	797	100	712	100	2853	100
Sensitive to EM	542	79.5	460	69.5	537	67.4	454	63.8	1993	69.9
Total EM-resistant	140	20.5	202	30.5	260	32.6	258	36.2	860	30.1
Resistant to EM alone	5	3.6†	4	2.0	8	3.1	6	2.3	23	2.7
Resistant to EM+1 drug	6	4.3	3	1.5	8	3.1	6	2.3	23	2.7
Resistant to EM+2 drugs	14	10.0	9	4.5	19	7.3	18	7.0	60	7.0
Resistant to EM+3 drugs	24	17.1	34	16.8	68	26.2	71	27.5	197	22.9
Resistant to EM+4 drugs	61	43.6	96	47.5	94	36.2	110	42.6	361	42.0
Resistant to EM+5 drugs	26	18.6	41	20.3	42	16.2	34	13.2	143	16.6
Resistant to EM+6 drugs	4	2.9	15	7.4	21	8.1	13	5.0	53	6.2

† Among total EM-resistant strains which are expressed as 100%.

TABLE X
Strains of *S. aureus* Resistant to from 1 to 8 Drugs[a]

(Year of isolation: 1968)

	All eight		PC-G		SM		CP		TC		EM		KM		SIM		AB-PC	
	No.	%	No.	%	No.	%	No.	%	No.	%	No.	%	No.	%	No.	%	No.	%
Total	710	100	710	100	710	100	710	100	710	100	710	100	710	100	710	100	710	100
Total sensitive	226	31.8	359	50.6	485	68.3	628	88.2	416	58.6	452	63.7	656	92.4	387	54.5	337	47.5
Total resistant	484	68.2	351	49.4	225	31.7	82	11.5	294	41.4	258	36.3	54	7.6	323	45.5	373	52.5
Single-drug-resistant	84	17.4[b]	13	3.7	12	5.3	4	4.9	6	2.0	4	1.6	0	0.0	13	4.0	32	8.6
Two-drug-resistant	68	14.1	48	13.7	6	2.7	3	3.7	6	2.0	6	2.3	1	1.9	11	3.4	55	14.7
Three-drug-resistant	35	7.2	20	5.7	14	6.2	4	4.9	13	4.4	12	4.7	2	3.7	22	6.8	18	4.8
Four-drug-resistant	55	11.4	40	11.4	20	8.9	5	6.1	40	13.6	23	8.9	5	9.3	47	14.6	40	10.7
Five-drug-resistant	95	19.6	83	23.6	43	19.1	19	23.2	82	27.9	67	26.0	9	16.7	89	27.6	83	22.3
Six-drug-resistant	101	20.9	101	28.8	84	37.3	20	24.4	101	34.4	100	38.8	2	3.7	98	30.3	100	26.8
Seven-drug-resistant	34	7.0	34	9.7	34	15.1	15	18.3	34	11.6	34	13.2	23	42.6	31	9.6	33	8.8
Eight-drug-resistant	12	2.5	12	3.4	12	5.3	12	14.6	12	4.1	12	4.7	12	22.2	12	3.7	12	3.2

a None of the 710 strains was resistant to CET, CER.   b Among total resistant strains which are expressed as 100%.

TABLE XI

Correlation between Two Individual Drugs in the Incidence of Resistant Strains of *S. aureus*

(Year of isolation: 1968. Total strains tested: 710)

Resistant to	PC-G	SM	CP	TC	EM	KM	SIM	CET	CER	AB-PC
PC-G: (351)[a]	—	(176)[a]	(59)	(248)	(213)	(41)	(268)	0	0	(328)
100[b]		50.1[b]	16.8	70.7	60.7	11.7	76.4			93.4
SM: (225)	(176)	—	(40)	(177)	(168)	(53)	(184)	0	0	(176)
100	78.2		17.8	78.7	74.7	23.6	81.8			78.2
CP: (82)	(59)	(40)	—	(68)	(65)	(20)	(64)	0	0	(60)
100	72.0	48.8		82.9	79.3	24.4	78.0			73.2
TC: (294)	(248)	(177)	(68)	—	(223)	(45)	(269)	0	0	(243)
100	84.4	60.2	23.1		75.9	15.3	91.5			82.7
EM: (258)	(213)	(168)	(65)	(223)	—	(51)	(223)	0	0	(212)
100	82.6	65.1	25.2	86.4		19.8	86.4			82.2
KM: (54)	(41)	(53)	(20)	(45)	(51)	—	(38)	0	0	(40)
100	75.9	98.1	37.0	83.3	94.4		70.4			74.1
SIM: (323)	(268)	(184)	(64)	(269)	(223)	(38)	—	0	0	(266)
100	83.0	57.0	19.8	83.3	69.0	11.8				82.4
CET: (0)	0	0	0	0	0	0	0	—	0	0
0										
CER: (0)	0	0	0	0	0	0	0	0	—	0
0										
AB-PC: (373)	(328)	(176)	(60)	(243)	(212)	(40)	(266)	0	0	—
100	87.9	47.2	16.1	65.1	56.8	10.7	71.3			

[a] No. of resistant strains. [b] Their frequency (%) when the figures in left column are expressed as 100%.

Five-drug-resistant: EM, TC, PC-G, SM plus SIM-type,
                        28.3%.
Six-drug-resistant: EM, TC, CP, SM, PC-G plus
                        SIM-type, 9.0%.
                        EM, TC, KM, SM, PC-G plus
                        SIM-type, 5.6%.
Seven-drug-resistant: EM, TC, CP, SM, PC-G, KM plus
                        SIM-type, 6.2%.

Discussion and conclusions

As described above, we have been able to discover the changes in bacterial sensitivities to each drug by comparing the annual changes of the high-sensitivity group, intermediate-sensitivity group and low-sensitivity group, which had been so classified by their M.I.C. values. Our previous method had been by comparison of the annual averages of the M.I.C. values and was not as accurate as our new method.

In *S. aureus*, the high-sensitivity group and the intermediate-sensitivity group decreased and the low-sensitivity group increased, regarding EM during the test period 1965–1968.

The frequencies of multiple-drug-resistant strains of *S. aureus* were investigated for seven drugs for the same period.

The drug-resistance markers most commonly observed in the strains resistant to four and five drugs were PC-G, SM, TC and SIM. The most common drug-resistance markers in the strains resistant to four, five and six drugs were EM and CP and the one in the strains resistant to six and seven drugs was KM.

The possible processes for the development of the main types of multiple-drug-resistant strains were examined in light of their frequencies. The drug-resistance markers common to the various types of multiple-drug resistances were TC, PC-G and SIM. It was inferred that various types of multiple-drug-resistant strains may be formed by the successive addition of SM, EM, CP and KM markers in this order to the TC, PC-G and SIM markers. This model is shown in Fig. 3.

The frequencies of multiple-drug-resistant strains of *S. aureus*

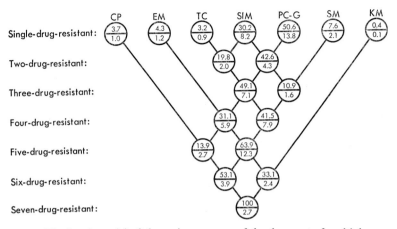

Fig. 3. A model of the main processes of development of multiple-drug-resistant strains of *S. aureus*. Figures above the line in the circles represent the frequency (%) among the strains resistant to each corresponding number of drugs, and the figures below the line represent the frequency (%) among the total resistant strains and the data used for calculation are the same as shown in Table XIII.

isolated in 1968 are summarized in Table X for ten drugs. Table XI shows the relationship of two drugs.

REFERENCES

1 Mitsuhashi, S. 1967. Epidemiological and genetical study of drug resistance in *Staphylococcus aureus*. *Japan. J. Microbiol.*, **11**, 49–68.
2 Otaya, H., and Inoue, E. 1967. Report on the drug resistance of staphylococci and *Escherichia coli* against antibiotics and sulphonamide. I. (in Japanese). *Mod. Med.* **22**, 2545–2568.
3 Otaya, H., Inoue, E., and Machihara, S. 1967. Report on the drug resistance of staphylococci and *Escherichia coli* against antibiotics. II. The statistical analysis of sensitivity (in Japanese). General meeting of the west-Japan branch Society of Chemotherapy. P. 11–12, Dec. 22, Hiroshima.
4 Otaya, H., Okamoto, S., and Inoue, E. 1969. Report on the drug resistance of staphylococci and *Escherichia coli* against antibiotics (in Japanese). General meeting of the Japan Society of Chemotherapy. P. 37, Apr. 24–26, Osaka.
5 Research Committee on Drug Resistance. Drug resistance in *Staphylococcus aureus*. *Chemotherapy*, **14**, 1–8 (1966); **14**, 392–396 (1966); **14**, 633–640 (1966); **15**, 195–197 (1967); **16**, 843–846 (1968).

RESISTANCE TO MACROLIDE ANTIBIOTICS AND LINCOMYCIN IN *STAPHYLOCOCCUS AUREUS*

Susumu Mitsuhashi, Hiroshi Oshima, Matsuhisa Inoue and Yoriko Yamaguchi

Department of Microbiology, School of Medicine, Gunma University, Maebashi, Japan

The introduction and extensive use of antibacterial agents have contributed greatly to improved treatment of infectious diseases and surgical infections. However, the extensive and frequently indiscriminate use of antimicrobial agents set the stage for the emergence of bacterial strains resistant to these agents. It should be noted that most strains of *Staphylococcus aureus*, in addition to gram-negative enteric bacteria, constitute a major group of resistant microorganisms seen in hospitals, and many studies concerning drug-resistance of staphylococci have been reported (*17–19, 38*).

Since 1961 this laboratory has collected strains of *S. aureus* isolated from infected lesions of inpatients, and the resistance patterns and phage types of these organisms have been determined. The present article describes the results of investigations that have been specifically focussed on resistance to macrolide(Mac) antibiotics and lincomycin(LCM).

Materials and methods

1. Bacterial strains

About 6,000 strains of *Staphylococcus aureus* isolated from infected lesions of inpatients in hospitals geographically dispersed throughout Japan were used in this study. In addition, 100 erythromycin resistant strains, isolated in the United States, were kindly provided by Dr. H. D. Isenberg, Long Island Jewish Hospital, N. Y. The strains used in these studies were all stock cultures from this laboratory, and were collected and stocked from the following research projects: "Studies on the infection and immunity of staphylococcal strains" (Chief: K. Ishiwara, School of Medicine, Gunma University), with the cooperation of 10 participating laboratories from 1961 through 1962, and "Studies on the drug-resistance of staphylococci" (Chief: T. Ichikawa, The 1st National Hospital, Tokyo), with the cooperation of 24 participating laboratories from 1961 to the present.

Other strains were collected by this laboratory from the following Institutes: School of Medicine, Gunma University; Kitasato Institute; Gunma Prefectural Institute of Health; and Shizuoka Prefectural Institute of Health.

2. Determination of drug resistance

All bacterial suspensions were prepared in peptone broth and grown in stationary culture for 18 hr at 37° C. Each culture was spotted onto heart infusion agar plates that contained serial two-fold dilutions of each drug, using a small capillary pipette or an apparatus fitted with many stainless steel loops. Drug resistance was expressed as the maximal concentration of each drug which allowed visible growth to the same level as that on the control plate without any drugs.

3. Drugs

Tetracycline (TC), dihydrostreptomycin (SM) and penicillin G (PC) were used. Sulfisomidine was used for the determination of resistance to sulfanilamide (SA). Erythromycin (EM), oleandomycin (OM), josamycin (JM), leucomycin (LM), spiramycin (SP), lincomycin and 7-chlorolincomycin (CL–LCM) were all working standards for the determination of drug resistance.

Epidemiological features of drug resistance

1. Drug resistance
It is known that the isolation frequency of the strains resistant to SA, TC, SM and to PC is very high among the staphylococcal strains isolated from clinical sources. Annual changes in isolation frequency of the strains resistant to TC, PC, SM, and to SA are shown in Fig. 1.

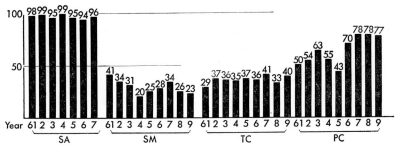

Fig. 1.   Isolation frequency of drug-resistant strains of *S. aureus*. Results based on 4,900 strains of *S. aureus* isolated from 1961 to 1969.

The frequencies with which the strains resistant to either SA, SM, TC or PC were isolated were almost the same during the survey period of 1961 through 1969, and represent the maximum frequency of isolation. These results indicate that, as suggested previously (*38*), there are factors which limit the isolation frequency of strains resistant to a given drug in a particular area such as a country, state or hospital. These limiting factors result in a maximum population of strains resistant to a given drug (M.P.R.). The M.P.R. for SA, SM, TC, and PC among the strains of *S. aureus* isolated in Japan was 94–99%, 20–41%, 29–41%, and 43–78%, respectively. The M.P.R. is governed by the amount of drug used, duration of its use, and also by the genetic characters of the staphylococci themselves. Genetic characters which govern the rate of mutation to resistance and characters which govern pathogenicity, infectivity and parasitic ability, play a large role in the acquisition of resistance; they increase the chance of contact with drug and affect distribution of the resistant strains among the host. Resistance patterns of staphylococcal strains with reference to TC, SA, SM and PC are summarized in Fig. 2.

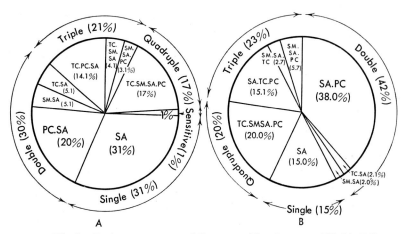

Fig. 2.   Resistance patterns of *S. aureus* with reference to TC, SA, PC and SM. A: Summary of results from 2,099 strains of *S. aureus* isolated from 1961 to 1965; B: Summary of results from 2,801 strains of *S. aureus* isolated from 1966 to 1969.

Ninety-seven to 99% of the staphylococcal strains isolated in Japan were resistant to either one or more of the four drugs. Of the strains, those showing multiple resistance were isolated more frequently and the TC- and SA-resistance markers were found most frequently among multiple resistant strains.

2. Macrolide resistance
Soon after the introduction of macrolide antibiotics into clinical use, Garrod (*9*) described two types of resistance to Mac antibiotics; double (EM. OM) and dissociated type (EM). His observations are now completely explainable by the notion of inducible resistance to Mac antibiotics. In our surveys, we noticed that the values for EM- and OM-resistance in some strains, as determined by the laboratories participating in this survey, varied widely from

the values obtained in this laboratory, where the assays were repeated (Mitsuhashi et al., unpublished data). Later, it was found in this and another laboratory (21-24, 55) that the dissociated resistance of S. aureus to EM possessed the characteristics of an inducible resistance. On the basis of this finding, we surveyed cross-resistance to Mac antibiotics and classified them into three groups (25, 38): group A, resistant to all Mac antibiotics and mostly to LCM; group B, resistant to both EM and OM where these antibiotics act as inducers; group C, resistant to EM where only EM acts as an active inducer. When a strain carrying inducible resistance was inoculated in a broth containing subinhibitory concentrations of inducer, the strain acquired a high resistance to all Mac antibiotics and to LCM. But the resistance of an induced population was lost after growth in the absence of an inducer. These results indicate that there are two types of resistance to Mac antibiotics: constitutive and inducible. The former showed resistance to all Mac antibiotics and mostly resistance to LCM. The resistance was stable and high, but in some strains it was further heightened after prior treatment with EM. The latter is found to be inducible, and the induction of high resistance to both Mac and LCM occurred after prior treatment with inducers such as EM and OM, and the resistance of induced cells was lost when grown in the absence of an inducer. Therefore the Mac-resistant strains consistently carry EM-resistance, even though their resistance is of the constitutive or inducible type.

In 1965, we conducted an examination of cross-resistance to Mac antibiotics in both Japan and the United States; group A was 10 to 15%, and groups B and C were 85 to 90% (25, 26, 38). Since then, the constitutive type of Mac-resistance has been increasing remarkably. Isolation frequency of the resistant strains of S. aureus to Mac antibiotics and LCM is shown in Table I. The isolation frequency of EM-resistance was the highest, and that of resistance to other Mac antibiotics and LCM was almost the same.

As stated before, the isolation frequency of staphylococcal strains carrying either triple- or quadruple-resistance with reference to TC, SA, SM and PC was found to be remarkably high (38). The frequency of the distribution of resistance to Mac,

TABLE I
Isolation Frequency of Resistant Strains of *S. aureus* to Macrolide Antibiotics and Lincomycin

Drug	Percent of resistant strains isolated in							
	1961	62	63	64	65	66	67	68
EM	8	5	9	7	16	19	27	31
OM	3	4	6	4	12	14	20	16
LM	1	2	9	4	19	13	17	15
SP						13	17	15
LCM						13	17	14

Results based on surveys of 4,485 strains of *S. aureus* isolated from 1961 to 1968. Resistance to either SP or LCM was not examined from 1961 to 1965.

chloramphenicol (CM), dimethoxyphenyl penicillin (DMP), novobiocin (NB), and kanamycin (KM) was highest in triple- and quadruple resistant strains with reference to the aforementioned four drugs. The frequency of distribution of either a constitutive or inducible type of Mac-resistance among the resistant strains with special reference to four drugs (TC, SA, SM and PC) is shown in Table II. The isolation frequency of the strains carrying either the constitutive or inducible type was highest in triple- and quadruple-resistant strains followed by double-resistant strains.

TABLE II
Isolation Frequency of Resistance to the Macrolide Antibiotics with Reference to Resistance Patterns to TC, SM, SA and PC.

Resistance patterns to TC, SA, SM and PC	Macrolide antibiotics (%)	
	Constitutive	Inducible
Single		
1961–1965 (31%)	9.9	9.1
1966–1969 (15%)	7.0	7.0
Double		
1961–1965 (30%)	12.0	28.0
1966–1969 (42%)	21.0	25.0
Triple and quadruple		
1961–1965 (38%)	78.1	62.9
1966–1969 (43%)	79.0	68.0

Results based on surveys of 2,099 strains isolated from 1961 to 1965, and 2,801 strains isolated from 1966 to 1969. Figures in parentheses indicate the total isolation frequency for each resistance pattern in two surveys from 1961 to 1965 and from 1966 to 1969, respectively.

TABLE III
Classification of the Macrolide Resistance in Staphylococcal Strains of Clinical Origin

Group	Subgroup	Level of resistance	Resistance pattern	
			Before induction	After induction
Constitutive	stable	stable, high	Mac.LCM (or LCMs)	Mac.LCM (or LCMs)
	variable[a]	variable, high or intermediate	Mac.LCM (or LCMs)	Mac.LCM (or LCMs)
Inducible	EM	variable, low before induction	EM	Mac.LCM
	EM.OM	variable, low before induction	EM.OM	Mac.LCM
	EM.LM[b]	variable, low before induction	EM.LM	Mac.LCM

[a]Resistance is elevated by treatment with EM.   [b]This mutant was isolated by treatment with nitrosoguanidine from S. aureus MS537, in which EM was an active inducer (54).   Mac indicates resistance to EM, OM, LM and SP.

The inducible group is divided into two subgroups: EM and (EM.OM) types, in which EM or both EM and OM are active inducer(s), respectively. We have never isolated the strains from clinical sources in which LM, JM or SP are active inducers in addition to both EM and OM. There are subgroups in constitutive-resistant strains which are classified as stable and variable. The variable group shows resistance to all Mac antibiotics, so far as tested, but its resistance is variable and is heightened by prior treatment with EM. The stable one shows a high resistance to all Mac antibiotics and its resistance is constitutive. The results are summarized in Table III.

The isolation frequency of Mac-resistant strains including those that were both constitutive and inducible was investigated and compared with that of PC-resistant strains. As shown in Table IV, Mac-resistant strains were isolated mostly from among the PC-resistant strains. Genetic analysis indicated that the determinants responsible for both Mac- and PC-resistance in some staphylococcal strains were jointly eliminated or jointly transduced (13, 24, 35, 37). By contrast, the determinant for PC-resistance was not cotransduced with those responsible for resistance to TC,

SA and SM (*36*). Namely, the determinants governing both Mac- and PC-resistance were located in the same genetic element and close to each other, and in some strains both determinants were located on a plasmid.

TABLE IV
Isolation Frequency of the Mac-Resistant Strains among PC-Resistant Staphylococci

PC-Resistance	No. of Mac-resistant strains
PC-Resistant strains	722 (87.8 %)
PC-Sensitive strains	106 (12.2 %)
Total	828

Numbers in parentheses indicate the percent of the isolation frequency of Mac-resistant strains in either PC-resistant or PC-sensitive strains. Mac-resistance includes both the constitutive and inducible type of resistance. The results are based on surveys of 2,801 strains of *S. aureus* isolated from 1966 to 1969.

As reported in previous papers (*14, 54*) we obtained several mutants carrying either a constitutive or inducible type of Mac-resistance from the Mac-inducible strain MS537 (EM) in which EM was the only active inducer. As shown in Fig. 3, most of the mutants were found to be Mac-constitutive and resistant to both Mac antibiotics and LCM. Two types of Mac- inducible strains were isolated from MS537 (EM), *i.e.*, MS537 (EM.OM) and MS537 (EM.LM), in which both OM and LM became active inducers in addition to EM. Recent surveys have indicated a rapid increase in the number of Mac-constitutive strains of staphylococci, and the rate of isolation of Mac-constitutive strains has been increasing among Mac-resistant strains. Based on these results and those of other genetic studies, the process of development of Mac-resistant strains can be accounted for by the following: a) appearance of EM-inducible strains of staphylococci after the introduction of EM for clinical use; b) appearance of the (EM. OM)-inducible or Mac-constitutive strains after the following introduction of OM; and c) appearance of the Mac-constitutive strains from either EM- or (EM.OM)-inducible strains by the wide use of OM, LM, JM, SP *etc.* By contrast, the number of strains carrying an inducible type of Mac-resistance in which both EM and OM were active inducers did not increase remarkably.

It should be noted, however, that we had not yet been able to isolate the mutants of Mac-inducible strains from clinical isolates, in which LM, JM, or SP is an active inducer in addition to both EM and OM.

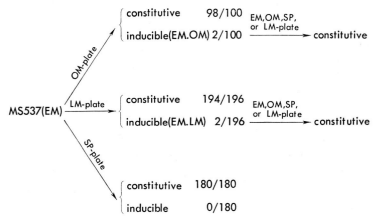

Fig. 3. The mutation process of Mac-resistance in *S. aureus*. The drug in parentheses indicates the inducer for Mac-resistance. Selective plates contained 6.3 μg/ml of each drug. Denominator indicates the number of total colonies examined among the mutants obtained on each selective plate. Numerator indicates the number of colonies carrying the indicated resistance type.

In interpreting these facts, it is relevant to note that a) the repressor of the structural gene(s) for Mac-resistance has an affinity for the chemical structures of EM, OM, and of other macrolide antibiotics in decreasing order, and b) the mutation rate of the loss of repression for the regulator gene(s) is much higher than that of the increase in number of inducers in addition to EM or OM. These results are summarized in Fig. 3.

Most of the staphylococcal strains carrying the constitutive type of Mac-resistance were also resistant to both lincomycin (LCM) and 7-chlorolincomycin (CL–LCM). Few of the strains of the Mac-constitutive type of staphylococci were found to be sensitive to both LCM and CL-LCM. However, the strains carrying the inducible type of Mac-resistance are sensitive to both LCM and CL-LCM, indicating that the drugs are incapable of becoming inducers for Mac-resistance. The strains acquired, however, high resistance to both Mac antibiotics and LCM after induction. In all cases of LCM-resistance, the level of resistance to CL-LCM was found to be much lower than to LCM. This fact can be interpreted by the notion that the resistance mechanisms to either LCM or CL-LCM are the same but the penetration of CL-LCM into bacterial cells is much higher than that of LCM (*24, 39*).

Genetics of resistance to Mac and LCM

Barder reported in 1949 that the PC-sensitive variant colonies appeared from the penicillinase-producing strains of *S. aureus* (*3*). But it was not known at that time that there were two types of genetic determinants in microorganisms located either on plasmid or chromosome. According to whether the elimination of drug-resistance in gram-negative enteric bacteria was spontaneous or artificial (*32–34*), we performed the same experiment with staphylococcal strains carrying Mac-resistance to confirm whether the determinants governing cross-resistance to Mac antibiotics were located on either the plasmid or chromosome. We selected two strains of staphylococci; MS66 and MS258, from our stock cultures that were isolated from patients with staphylococcal infections. Both strains carried multiple resistance to TC, SA, PC, EM, OM, LM and to other Mac antibiotics. In 1963 we found that EM-, OM- and LM-resistance of *S. aureus* MS66 and MS258 was jointly eliminated by treatment with acriflavine. Conversely, EM-, OM- and LM-resistance was jointly transduced to Mac-sensitive strains obtained from either MS66 or 258 even at lower multiplicities of infection of 0.1. These results indicated that the Mac-resistance of *S. aureus* MS66 and MS258 was controlled by a gene(s) governing cross-resistance to Mac antibiotics and the genetic element was located probably on a cytoplasmic element, *i.e.*, plasmid (*35*).

   In 1965, the determinants of penicillinase production (PCase⁺, *i.e.*, PCʳ) and resistance to Mac antibiotics were irreversibly eliminated by treatment with acridine or with ultraviolet irradiation. Among the strains tested, PCase⁺ and Mac-resistance were eliminated from all strains except one, which lost only PCase$^+$ but not Mac-resistance. The characters of PCase$^+$ and Mac-resistance were jointly transduced, with the aid of phage lysates obtained from the resistant donors by ultraviolet irradiation, into staphylococcal strains sensitive to both PC and Mac antibiotics. Segregation of PCase$^+$ and Mac-resistance was rarely observed after transduction. These results indicated that the determinants of both PCase$^+$ and Mac-resistance of staphylococci are located close together on a single genetic element, *i.e.*, a plasmid, which exists extrachromosomally (*37*).

It was known that there are two types of resistance to LCM in the constitutive type of Mac-resistance; resistance to both Mac and LCM, and resistance to Mac but sensitivity to LCM. By contrast, the strains carrying the inducible type of Mac-resistance acquired high resistance to both Mac antibiotics and LCM after induction (*14, 24*). Therefore, it may be predicted that the genes governing the resistance to both Mac antibiotics and LCM are the same in both the inducible and constitutive type of Mac-resistance carrying LCM-resistance. However, the precise analysis of the genes governing LCM-resistance still remained to be carried out. Consequently, a series of plasmids (*52, 53*) were identified in *S. aureus* and they fall into several groups: the penicillinase plasmids (*43–45, 48*), which occur in a homologous series with various marker patterns (*48*) responsible for penicillinase production and

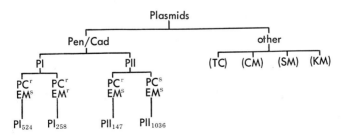

Fig. 4.   Plasmids of *S. aureus*. Pen/Cad indicates a plasmid carrying the genetic determinants for both penicillinase production and resistance to cadmium (*45, 46, 48*). Parentheses indicate uncertainty about extrachromosomal status of plasmids carrying each resistance marker. PI_{258}: See the footnote of Table V.

control (*43*); resistance to EM (*13, 35*); and resistance to a series of inorganic ions, *i.e.*, mercury (*50*), arsenite, arsenate, cadmium and lead (*45*), and bismuth (*48*). In some strains of *S. aureus*, resistance to other drugs, namely resistance to TC, CM, KM (*1, 2, 5, 27, 29, 49*), or SM (*41*), seems to be plasmid-born but more detailed studies will be needed to establish the plasmids which determine resistance to such drugs. The four resistance determinants (TC, SA, SM and CM (*16, 20, 36*)) are linked neither to one another nor to penicillinase production.These relationships are shown in Fig. 4, and the DNA of the episome or plasmid is shown in Table V.

TABLE V
Episome- or Plasmid-specific DNA

Episome or plasmid	Host	Contour lengths[a] (μm)	Monomer mol. wt. (in millions of daltons)	Total[b] DNA (%)	References
Col El	*Proteus*	2.3,4.7,6.9	4.5	0.2–0.3	*11,52*
Col V,B,Cys,Trp	*Proteus*	54.5	107	5	*14a*
F	*E.coli*		45	2	*8*
R222	*Proteus*	7,28,35	69		*42*
R15	*Proteus*	18	35		*42*
PI$_{258}$	*S.aureus*	9.4	18.8		*53*

R indicates the transmissible drug-resistance factor (*40*). *S. aureus* MS258 was isolated in this laboratory and the genes governing resistance to both Mac antibiotics and PC were jointly eliminated and jointly transduced, indicating that the genes are located on a plasmid (*13, 37*). This plasmid was termed by Novick PI$_{258}$ (*46*).
[a] Mostly measurements of open circular forms seen in the electron microscope.
[b] Estimates of total amount of DNA per chromosome.

SUMMARY

According to epidemiologic and genetic studies, it is notable that the staphylococcal strains isolated from clinical specimens were multiple-resistant. Some of their resistances were found to be labile and could be irreversibly eliminated by storing in broth or by artificial treatment (*1–5, 7, 13, 29, 35, 37*). It should be noted, moreover, that multiple-resistant strains of staphylococci were confined to a specific phage group and most of these staphylococcal strains were found to be lysogenic. According to sequential cultures from a single source, such as nasal carriers, or cultures from different colonies from one primary culture plate, differences between members of these sets of cultures indicated some changes in typing patterns that occurred from day to day. It was shown that changes in the phage typing pattern in staphylococci resulted from artificial lysogenization, probably as a result of serologically specific prophage immunity (28, 47, 51).

Transduction of drug resistance in staphylococci has been reported by many investigations (6, 12, 30, 31). According to our studies of transduction of drug resistance by phage lysates obtained from multiple-resistant strains, almost every strain was found to be a competent recipient of TC-resistance in various combinations of donors and recipients (36). Moreover, joint transduction of (TC.SM), (TC.SA.SM), (Mac.PC) and (CM.TC) indicated to us that many determinants responsible for drug resistance in staphylococci are located close together and form a cluster (16, 20, 36, 37). From these results, one of the present authors (SM) has presented the theory that transduction of resistance by phage lysates obtained from lysogenic strains is mainly responsible for the rapid acquisition of drug resistance, widespread occurrence of multiple-resistant strains and for changes in the phage typing patterns occurring in our clinical populations (36, 38).

It is also interesting to note that there are many reports concerning the induction of drug resistance in staphylococci, i.e., PC-resistance (10), Mac-resistance (14, 23–25, 55), CM-resistance (27) and TC-resistance (15), but the mechanisms of induction of Mac-resistance have been the most extensively studied. There are two types of resistance to Mac antibiotics in staphylococci; the inducible and the constitutive. The inducible type of resistance is raised after prior treatment with subinhibitory concentrations of the inducer such as EM or OM, and the induced population acquires a high resistance to both Mac antibiotics and LCM. But the resistance of the induced cells is lost when they are again grown in a drug-free medium. The strains carrying the constitutive type of resistance are also mostly resistant to LCM.

Of the inducible strains, EM is the best inducer, followed by OM. However, we have never isolated strains from clinical speci-

mens in which JM, LM and SP were active inducers and the isolation frequency of the strains, in which both EM and OM were
active inducers, is also rather low. From these results and other
genetic studies, the mutation process of Mac-resistance in staphylococci is predicted as follows: the EM-inducible, (EM.OM)-
inducible and Mac-constitutive type of resistance.

The determinants governing Mac-resistance in some strains of
staphylococci were found to be located on a plasmid, and some
of them were linked to the determinant responsible for penicillinase
production. The strains carrying Mac-resistance were isolated
most frequently from among the strains harboring triple or
quadruple resistance with special reference to TC, SA, SM and
PC, especially from PC-resistant strains of staphylococci.

REFERENCES

1   Asheshov, E. H. 1966. Chromosomal location of the genetic elements
    controlling penicillinase production in a strain of *Staphylococcus aureus*.
    Nature, **210**, 804–806.
2   Asheshov, E. H. 1966. Loss of antibiotic resistance in *Staphylococcus
    aureus* resulting from growth at high temperature. *J. Gen. Microbiol.*,
    42, 403–410.
3   Barber, M. 1949. The incidence of penicillin-sensitive variant colonies
    in penicillinase-producing strains of *Staphylococcus pyogenes*. *J. Gen.
    Microbiol.*, **3**, 274–281.
4   Bondi, A., Kornblum, J., and de Saint Phalle, M. 1953. Isolation of
    penicillin-susceptible mutants from penicillinase-producing strains of
    Micrococcus pyogenes. *Proc. Soc. Exptl. Biol. Med.*, **83**, 527–530.
5   Chabbert, Y. A., Baudens, J. G., and Gerbaud, G. R. 1964. Variations
    sous l'influence de l'acriflavine et transduction de la résistance à la kana-
    mycine et au chloramphénicol chex les staphylocoques. *Inst. Pasteur*,
    107, 678–690.
6   Collins, A. M., and Roy, T. E. 1963. Transduction of chloramphenicol
    and novobiocin resistance in staphylococci. *Canad. J. Microbiol.*, **9**, 541–
    547.
7   Fairbrother, R. W., Parker, L., and Eaton, B. R. 1954. The stability of
    penicillinase-producing strains of *Staphylococcus aureus*. *J. Gen. Micro-
    biol.*, **10**, 309–316.
8   Freifelder, D. R., and Freifelder, D. 1968. Studies on *E. coli* sex factors.
    11. Some physical properties of F'*lac* and F DNA. *J. Mol. Biol.*, **32**,
    25–35.

9   Garrod, L. P. 1957. Erythromycin group of antibiotics. *Brit. Med. J.*, July **13**, 57–62.
10 Geronimus, L. H., and Cohen, S. 1957. Induction of staphylococcal penicillinase. *J. Bacteriol.*, **73**, 28–34.
11 Goebel, W., and Helinski, D. R. 1968. Generation of higher multiple circular DNA forms in bacteria. *Proc. Natl. Acad. Sci. U.S.*, **61**, 1406–1413.
12 Goto, S., Niwa, C., Kuwahara, S., and Mikami. Y. 1964. Transfer of drug-resistance in staphylococci. IV. Transduction of resistance to chloramphenicol by typing phage 80. *Medicine and Biology*, **68**, 38–41 (in Japanese).
13 Hashimoto, H., Kono, M., and Mitsuhashi, S. 1964. Elimination of penicillin resistance of *Staphylococcus aureus* by treatment with acriflavine. *J. Bacteriol.*, **88**, 261–262.
14 Hashimoto, H., Oshima, H., and Mitsuhashi, S. 1968. Drug resistance of staphylococci. IX. Inducible resistance to macrolide antibiotics in *Staphylococcus aureus*. *Japan. J. Microbiol.*, **12**, 321–327.
14a Hickson, F. T., Roth, T. F., and Helinski, D. R. 1967. Circular DNA forms of a bacterial sex factor. *Proc. Natl. Acad. Sci. U.S.*, **58**, 1731–1738.
15 Inoue, M., Hashimoto, H., and Mitsuhashi, S. 1969. Mechanism of tetracycline resistance in strains of *Staphylococcus aureus*. *In* "Progress in Antimicrobial and Anticancer Chemotherapy (Proc. 6th International Congress of Chemotherapy)," University of Tokyo Press, Tokyo, Vol. I, p. 433–439.
16 Inoue, M., Hashimoto, H., Yamagishi, S. and Mitsuhashi, S. 1970. Transduction of the genetic determinants for chloramphenicol resistance in staphylococci. *Japan. J. Microbiol.*, **14**, 261–268.
17 Isenberg, H. D. 1964. A comparison of nationwide microbial susceptibility testing using standardized discs. *Health Lab. Sci.*, **1**, 185–256.
18 Isenberg, H. D. 1965. The consistency of *in vitro* microbial response: a survey of the Americas, Europe and Japan. *Health Lab. Sci*, **2**, 163–178.
19 Ishiwara, K., Tanaka, A., and Tajima, S. 1959. Phage-typing of staphylococci from pyogenic lesions and carriers in and outside the hospital. *Japan. J. Microbiol.*, **3**, 427–442.
20 Kasuga, T., Hashimoto, H., and Mitsuhashi, S. 1968. Drug-resistance of staphylococci. VII. Genetic determinants responsible for the resistance to tetracycline, streptomycin, sulfanilamide and penicillin. *J. Bacteriol.*, **95**, 1764–1766.
21 Kono, M., Hashimoto, H., and Mitsuhashi, S. 1964. Relation between inducible resistance to macrolide antibiotics and lincomycin. Record of the 12th East Branch Meeting of Japan Chemotherapeutic Assoc. Oct., Sendai.
22 Kono, M., Hashimoto, H., and Mitsuhashi, S. 1964. Drug resistance of

staphylococci. Inducible resistance of macrolide antibiotics. Record of the Kanto Branch Meeting of Japan Bacteriol. Assoc., Nov., Tokyo; 1965. *Japan. J. Bacteriol.*, **20**, 122–123.

23   Kono, M., Hashimoto, H., and Mitsuhashi, S. 1965. Inducible resistance of macrolide antibiotics in *Staphylococcus aureus*. *Japan. J. Bacteriol.*, **20**, 122–123.

24   Kono, M., Hashimoto, H., and Mitsuhashi, S. 1965. Antibacterial action of lincomycin on staphylococci. *J. Antibiotics, Ser. B*, **18**, 53–55.

25   Kono, M., Hashimoto, H., and Mitsuhashi, S. 1966. Drug resistance of staphylococci. III. Resistance to some macrolide antibiotics and inducible system. *Japan. J. Microbiol.*, **10**, 59–66.

26   Kono, K., Kasuga, T., and Mitsuhashi, S. 1966. Drug resistance of staphylococci. IV. Resistance pattern to some macrolide antibiotics in *Staphylococcus aureus* isolated in the United States. *Japan. J. Microbiol.*, **10**, 109–113.

27   Kono, M., Ogawa, K., and Mitsuhashi, S. 1968. Drug resistance of staphylococci. VI. Genetic determinant for chloramphenicol resistance. *J. Bacteriol.*, **95**, 886–892.

28   Lowbury, E. J. L., and Hood, A. M. 1953. The acquired resistance of *Staphylococcus aureus* to bacteriophage. *J. Gen. Microbiol.*, **9**, 524–535.

29   May, J. W., Houghton, R. H., and Perret, C. J. 1964. The effect of growth at elevated temperatures on some heritable properties of *Staphylococcus aureus*. *J. Gen. Microbiol.*, **37**, 157–169.

30   Morse, M. L. 1959. Transduction by staphylococcal bacteriophage. *Proc. Natl. Acad. Sci. U.S.*, **45**, 722–727.

31   Morse, M. L., and Labelle, J. W. 1962. Characteristic of a staphylococcal phage capable of transduction. *J. Bacteriol.*, **83**, 775–780.

32   Mitsuhashi, S., Harada, K., and Kameda, M. 1960. Drug resistance of enteric bacteria. Elimination of transmissible drug-resistance by treatment with acriflavine. *Tokyo Iji Shinshi*, **77**, 462 (in Japanese).

33   Mitsuhashi, S., Hashimoto, H., Harada, K., Suzuki, M., Kameda, M., and Matsuyama, T. 1960. Multiple resistance of *S. flexneri* 3a and *E. coli* isolated from the epidemy in Gunma Prefecture. *Japan. J. Bacteriol.*, **15**, 844–848 (in Japanese).

34   Mitsuhashi, S., Harada, K., and Kameda, M. 1961. Elimination of transmissible drug-resistance by treatment with acriflavine. *Nature*, **189**, 947.

35   Mitsuhashi, S., Morimura, M., Kono, M., and Oshima, H. 1963. Elimination of drug resistance of *Staphylococcus aureus* by treatment with acriflavine. *J. Bacteriol.*, **86**, 162–163.

36   Mitsuhashi, S., Oshima, H., Kawaharada, U., and Hashimoto, H. 1965. Drug resistance of staphylococci. I. Transduction of tetracycline resistance with phage lysates obtained from multiply resistant staphylococci. *J. Bacteriol.*, **89**, 967–976.

37   Mitsuhashi, S., Hashimoto, H., Kono, M., and Morimura, M. 1965. Drug resistance of staphylococci. II. Joint elimination and joint transduction of the determinants of penicillinase production and resistance to macrolide antibiotics. *J. Bacteriol.*, **89**, 988–992.

38   Mitsuhashi, S. 1967. Epidemiological and genetical study of drug resistance in *Staphylococcus aureus*. *Japan. J. Microbiol.*, **11**, 49–68.

39   Mitsuhashi, S., Kasuga, T., and Saito, T. 1969. Antibacterial activity of 7-chlorolincomycin. *Chemotherapy*, **17**, 763–765.

40   Mitsuhashi, S. 1971. *In* "Transferable drug resistance factor R," University of Tokyo Press, Tokyo p. 25–32.

41   Morimura, M., Watanabe, K., Mori, H., and Mitsuhashi, S. 1970. Lability of streptomycin resistance in *Staphylococcus aureus*. *Japan. J. Microbiol.*, **14**, 253–256.

42   Nisioka, T., Mitani, M., and Clowes, R. 1969. Composite circular forms of R factor deoxyribonucleic acid molecules. *J. Bacteriol.*, **97**, 376–385.

43   Novick, R. P. 1963. Analysis by transduction of mutations affecting penicillinase formation in *Staphylococcus aureus*. *J. Gen. Microbiol.*, **33**, 121–136.

44   Novick, R. P., and Richmond, M. H. 1965. Nature and interactions of the genetic elements governing penicillinase synthesis in *Staphylococcus aureus*. *J. Bacteriol.*, **90**, 467–480.

45   Novick, R. P. 1967. Penicillinase plasmids of *Staphylococcus aureus*. *Federation Proc.*, **26**, 29–38.

46   Novick, R. P. 1969. Extrachromosomal inheritance in bacteria. *Bacteriol. Rev.*, **33**, 210–235.

47   Oshima, H., Kawaharada, U., Kasuga, T., and Mitsuhashi, S. 1967. Changes in the phage-typing patterns of staphylococci following lysogenization. *Japan. J. Microbiol.*, **11**, in press.

48   Peyru, G., Wexler, L., and Novick, R. P. 1969. Naturally occurring penicillinase plamids in *Staphylococcus aureus*. *J. Bacteriol.*, **98**, 215–221.

49   Poston, S. M. 1966. Cellular location of the genes controlling penicillinase production and resistance to streptomycin and tetracycline in a strain of *Staphylococcus aureus*. *Nature*, **210**, 802–804.

50   Richmond, M. H., and John, M. 1964. Co-transduction by a staphylococcal phage of the genes responsible for penicillinase synthesis and resistance to mercury salts. *Nature*, **202**, 1360–1361.

51   Rountree, P. M. 1959. Changes in the phage-typing patterns in staphylococci following lysogenization. *J. Gen. Microbiol.*, **20**, 620–633.

52   Roth, T. F., and Helinski, D. R. 1967. Evidence for circular DNA forms of a bacterial plasmid. *Proc. Natl. Acad. Sci. U.S.*, **58**, 650–657.

53   Rush, M. G., Gordon, C., Novick, R. P., and Warner, R. 1969. Circular DNA from *Staphylococcus aureus* and *Shigella dysentheriae* Y6R. *Federation Proc.*, **28**, 532.

54   Saito, T., Hashimoto, H., and Mitsuhashi, S. 1970. Macrolide resistance in *Staphylococcus aureus*. Isolation of a mutant in which leucomycin is an active inducer. *Japan. J. Microbiol.*, **14,** 473–478.

55   Weaber, J. R. and Pattee, P. A. 1964. Inducible resistance to erythromycin in *Staphylococcus aureus*. *J. Bacteriol.*, **88,** 574–580.

JOSAMYCIN, A NEW MACROLIDE ANTIBIOTIC OF RESISTANCE NON-INDUCING TYPE

Takashi Osono and Hamao Umezawa

Central Research Laboratories, Yamanouchi Pharmaceutical Co., Ltd., Tokyo, Japan and Institute of Microbial Chemistry, Tokyo, Japan

For the past ten years, we have been endeavoring to isolate a new macrolide antibiotic for treatment of diseases caused by drug-resistant staphylococci. During that time, many physicians began to feel that penicillin and tetracyclines were becoming less and less effective in the treatment of staphylococcal infections in patients. Later it was found that multiple drug-resistant staphylococci—most of which are resistant to tetracycline, penicillin, streptomycin and sulfa drugs, or to 2 or 3 of these—were becoming dominant in Japan. In fact, they now amount to about 70 percent of staphylococci isolated from clinical sources. There was clearly an urgent need for antibiotics effective against these multiple drug-resistant staphylococci. As a result, two laboratories cooperated in carrying out screening studies for new macrolides.

Many thousands of streptomycetes strains were isolated from soil samples at H. Umezawa's laboratory at the Institute of Microbial Chemistry, and all the strains which appeared to produce macrolides in the preliminary screening were sent to T. Osono's laboratory at the Yamanouchi Pharmaceutical Co. for further screening. In 1964, a new macrolide antibiotic was discovered from culture broth of a *Streptomyces* strain, A 204-P 2, collected at a mountain recess far up the Yoshino River of Shikoku Island, Japan. The antibiotic was named Josamycin after Tosa province, the ancient name of the region where the strain originated. The strain, A 204-P 2, was classified as a new variety of *Streptomyces narbonensis* from a taxonomical study by Y. Okami, and was given name *S. narbonensis* var. *josamyceticus* nov. var. (*1, 3*).

Josamycin was obtained as white needle crystals melting at 130 to 133°C, which had a slightly bitter taste and an ultraviolet absorption maximum at 232 mμ. It showed strong antimicrobial activity against gram-positive bacteria and mycoplasmas, and excellent *in vivo* activity superior or equal to erythromycin in subcutaneous staphylococcal infection in mice which we had selected as the most reliable criterion for clinical usefulness (*1, 2, 4*).

In 1967, clinical studies on josamycin began at 33 university clinics and hospitals which included all the institutions engaged in significant antibiotic research in Japan. At the 16th Annual Meeting held in May 1968 at Tokyo, the Japan Society of Chemotherapy devoted a symposium to a clinical evaluation of josamycin under the chairmanship of K. Fukushima, professor of Internal Medicine, Yokohama City University. The clinical results collected at the 33 institutions were summarized and presented at this symposium. Josamycin was confirmed to be as effective as erythromycin in the treatment of staphylococcal and gram-positive infections in patients. Impressively, it showed only minimal side effects consisting mainly of mild anorexia, and it was thus determined to be a safe remedy suitable for prolonged or outpatient use (*11*).

Further, unlike erythromycin, the study of S. Mitsuhashi, professor of Microbiology, Gunma University, showed that josamycin did not induce macrolide resistance in staphylococci. As stated elsewhere in this book, most erythromycin-resistant staphylococci belong to Group C or Group B of Mitsuhashi's classification in which erythromycin, or in the case of Group B, erythromycin and oleandomycin, induces macrolide-resistance. Josamycin, however, is effective for these erythromycin-resistant staphylococci which have become prevalent in Japan and the United States in recent years (*12*).

1. Screening criteria (*67*)

It is obvious that the discovery of an antibiotic depends on the methods and criteria of evaluation. We adopted the following criteria at the start of the present screening studies.

1) Ability to be isolated easily as crystals from culture products
Macrolide antibiotics are a compound whose structure consists of a macrocyclic lactone with between one and three sugar moieties attached. More than 70 macrolides and their components have been reported in the literature as having streptomycetes origin.

Many new antibiotics have been differentiated by biological characteristics, even when they were isolated as a mixture of components. However, this does not apply to macrolides as the large number of reported substances in the same group makes differentiation very difficult. Complete differentiation is possible only when the macrolide can be obtained as a crystal of a single substance. With a crystal in hand, we can use the melting point, one of the most important means of identification in chemistry. Elementary analysis and other physical measurements such as IR and NMR are useful only when the unity of the substance is guaranteed. For these reasons we selected only those substances which may be crystallized.

However it is not easy to get macrolides as crystals, as most have rather large molecular weights and they are often accompanied by several components resembling one another in the structure. It was important to find an efficient means to recognize and distinguish minute amounts of substances which showed only minor differences in their structures. Early adoption of the thin layer chromatography of Stahl (*46*), which has now become routine in antibiotic research, proved to be an effective method.

Selection of easily crystallizable substances offered some unexpected advantages. We selected organisms which predominantly produced a single substance for ease of crystallization. This resulted in easy industrial production of a good yield of crystals. Commercial macrolide products, except for oleandomycin and erythromycin, are sold as a mixture of several components. In such cases, it is unavoidable to find some inter-lot fluctuation of component ratios, which have been known to be altered by the improvement of producing strains or fermentation conditions. Thus, it has been our experience that some lots of a commercial macrolide differed in their *in vivo* activity from other lots in spite of the same *in vitro* antibacterial potency. In purified crystal form, josamycin could be produced as a commercial product of the same *in vivo* and *in vitro* activities. Further, contaminations responsible for clinical side effects were easily eliminated as josamycin could be crystallized free from other by-products of fermentation.

2) Ability to show strong protective effect against subcutaneous staphylococcal infection in mice

Whereas the first criterion was for identification or differentiation, we considered the second criterion as the most important to predict clinical usefulness.

New antibiotics have been determined useful from their *in vivo* activity. Today's routine procedure for that purpose is the use of the mouse infection of a septic type such as intraperitoneal infection with *Staphylococcus aureus* Smith strain. When evaluated by

TABLE I

Protection in Septic Staphylococcal Infection in Mice (4)†

Dosage (mg/kg)	Survival after 7 days				
	JM	LM	EM	SPM	Control
200 × 5	10	10	10	10	
100 × 5	10	6	10	7	
50 × 5	2	1	10	4	
25 × 5	1	1	5	1	
12.5 × 5	0	0	2	0	
6.25 × 5	0	0	0	0	
0					0
ED_{50} (mg/kg)	287	405	111	308	

† Infected intraperitoneally with 100 MLD of *S. aureus* Smith strain (with mucin); treated orally at 1, 4, 8, 12 and 16 hr after infection; 10 male ddN mice in each group; 15 mice in control group.

this method, erythromycin shows unusually good results among commercial macrolides. As seen from Table I, the ED_{50} of erythromycin is 1/3 that of spiramycin and 1/4 that of leucomycin (4). Further, not shown in the table, the findings for oleandomycin suggest that erythromycin should be twice as strong in its activity. However, when used in the treatment of clinical infections, erythromycin never shows such conspicuously good results when compared with the other macrolides. The required dosage of erythromycin is not half that of oleandomycin or leucomycin, but the same. This suggested that the septic type infection is not an adequate criterion for evaluation.

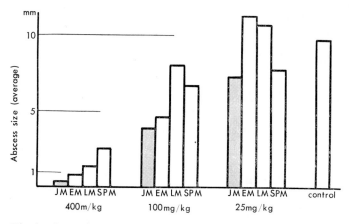

Fig. 1.   Protection in subcutaneous staphylococcal infection in mice (4). They were infected subcutaneously with 10^8 cells of *S. aureus* No. 226 strain; treated orally immediately after infection; 10 male ddN mice in each group; 15 mice in control group.

For this reason, we sought an alternative method for evaluation which would reflect clinical effectiveness with greater fidelity. Most of the staphylococcal infections frequently seen at clinics are local ones such as respiratory or suppurative infections, but not severe life threatening sepsis conditions. We paid attention to a subcutaneous infection in mice which had been developed for the purpose of immunological study by I. Tadokoro, professor of Bacteriology, Yokohama City University (10, 47). In this method, mice were infected with *S. aureus* strain No. 226 isolated by I. Tadokoro from a dead case of infantile pneumonia which produced coagulase, deoxyribonuclease and α-hemolysin. Drugs were given immediately after the infection. Forty-eight hours later, the animals were sacrificed, the skin of the back cut open, and the size of abscess formed were measured (*cf.* Photo 3). A representative result is given in Fig. 1, which coincided with the tendency seen among clinical effectiveness of commercial macrolides. Among many antibiotics we screened, josamycin equalled or surpassed the effectiveness of erythromycin. Thus we selected this substance at the beginning of 1964. Later, it was found that it was as effective as erythromycin in clinical trials also, and the reliability of this method was confirmed.

3) Ability to be stable in acidic solution

It has been shown that erythromycin is very labile in acidic pH, being destroyed by gastric juice. Figure 2 shows a crossover experiment on blood levels after oral administration using 4 dogs (7). The peak of blood levels was highest in josamycin and lowest in erythromycin. This tendency runs parallel with acid-stability of

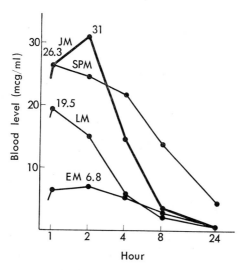

Fig. 2. Blood levels of macrolides after oral administration (7) (average in 4 dogs given 100 mg/kg).

these macrolides. Erythromycin was converted to a more acid-stable and blood level-elevating derivative, propionyl erythromycin estolate. However, this chemical change of erythromycin molecule resulted in an incidence of liver toxicity. Thus, we stressed this criterion. As seen from Table II, josamycin was found stable in acidic solution (4), and was judged able to meet our new criteria.

TABLE II
Stability of Josamycin in Aqueous Solution[†]

Drug	pH	0.5	1	2	3	4	5	6	7 (hr)
	2	93	97		71	55	59.5	55	40
	3	100	100	100	100	97	80	80	80
	4	100	100	100	100	100	100	100	100
JM	5	100	100	100	100	100	100	100	100
	6	100	100	100	100	100	100	100	100
	7	100	100	100	100	100	100	100	100
	8	100	100	100	100	100	100	100	100
	9	100	100	100	100	100	100	100	100
	2	2	1.2	trace					
	3	6	1.6	trace					
	4	19.5	17.5	trace	trace	trace	trace	trace	
EM	5	100	85	72.5	42.5	55	41	52.5	
	6	100	100	100	100	100	100	100	100
	7	100	100	100	100	100	100	100	100
	8	100	100	100	100	100	100	100	100
	9	100	100	100	100	100	100	100	100

† Residual potency given as % of initial when kept at 37°C (*B. subtilis* assay).

4) Ability not to be irritating to conjunctiva of rabbit eyes
Some commercial macrolides were known to be so irritating that they could not be used as ophthalmic instillations. We adopted this as an auxiliary criterion. Josamycin was found to show no irritation when applied to rabbit eyes for 7 days as a 1.0 percent solution.

2. Isolation and physicochemical properties

Josamycin is produced by streptomycetes strains belonging to *S. narbonensis* var. *josamyceticus* represented by strain A 204-P 2.

The strain was isolated from a soil sample collected at Motoyama, Nagaoka-gun, Kochi Prefecture, located in a lonely mountain recess far up the Yoshino River of Shikoku Island. On solid synthetic media, the strain A 204-P 2 formed yellowish brown growth carrying aerial mycelia of brown grey color. Neither spirals nor whorls were formed on the aerial mycelium. No soluble pigment was produced on synthetic and organic media (*cf.* Photo 2). When cultured aerobically, the strain produced josamycin in the fermentation fluid which could be isolated as crystals in good yield by solvent extraction followed by benzene crystallization (*1*).

Photograph 1 shows a polarized microphotograph of josamycin crystals thus obtained. Josamycin produced white needle crystals melting at 130 to 133° C. It showed a specific rotation of $-70°$, a pKa' value of 7.1 and an absorption maximum at 232 mμ in the ultraviolet region. The molecular formula of josamycin will be ultimately determined after completion of its structure elucidation just as in the cases of many rather high molecular weight antibiotics, but it was tentatively assigned $C_{40}H_{69}NO_{14}$. Josamycin was soluble in most organic solvents such as alcohols, acetic esters, chloroform or benzene and also in acidic water, but practically insoluble in neutral water or petroleum solvents. It gave red violet color in the erythromycin test using sulfuric acid, which changed to dark violet on heating. It developed a red color in the carbomycin test by the addition of hydrochloric acid. Its ultraviolet and infrared absorption spectra are given in Figs. 3 and 4, and its nuclear magnetic resonance spectrum is shown in Fig. 5 (*1*).

The structural study of josamycin is now in progress. It is known that josamycin has one molecule each of isovaleric acid, mycarose, mycaminose and macrocyclic lactone containing $-CHO$, $-OCH_3$, $-OCOCH_3$ and $-C=C-C=C-C-OH$ groups. However, the entire structure of the macrocyclic lactone is not yet determined.*

Some mention should be made of the relationship between josamycin and leucomycin A_3. On the isolation of josamycin as a crystal in 1964, we compared it with all the known macrolides which had been reported, and differentiated it from all of them in-

---

* Paper on the structure of josamycin is now in preparation.

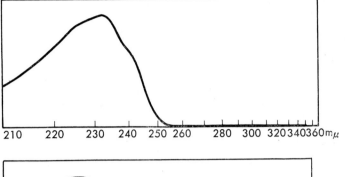

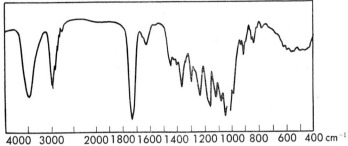

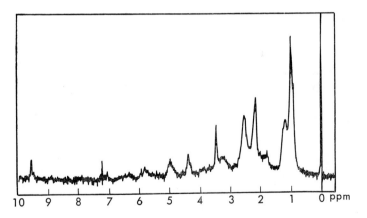

Fig. 3 (top).   UV spectrum of josamycin.
Fig. 4 (middle).   IR spectrum of josamycin.
Fig. 5 (bottom).   NMR spectrum of josamycin.

cluding reported components of leucomycins. Thus it was concluded to be a new substance (*1, 3*). Two years later, Omura
et al., Kitasato Institute, isolated from crude material of leucomycins a new minor component, leucomycin A_3, as a crystal, and
presented its structure (*48*). It was found that leucomycin A_3 was
the one most resembling josamycin among all the macrolides, including those reported after our discovery of josamycin (*68*). However some discrepancies are seen between them, as in the melting
point of some of its derivatives. The differentiation will be conclusive on the structure elucidation now in progress. Leucomycin
A_3 was shown by Omura *et al.* to be less toxic and to give higher
blood levels than leucomycin A_1, the main component of leucomycins (*49*). However, no results of detailed animal experiments
or clinical studies have as yet been reported.

3. Biological activities

1) In vitro activities (2, 4, 11)

Josamycin shows strong antimicrobial activities against gram-
positive bacteria, some gram-negative organisms and mycoplasmas, but weak action against enteric organisms. The antimicrobial
spectrum measured by the standard agar dilution method of the
Japan Society of Chemotherapy (*50*) using nutrient agar is shown
in Table III and that using heart infusion agar in Table IV. Josamycin was active against *S. aureus* at 0.39 to 0.78 mcg/ml, against
Streptococcus pyogenes at 0.19 mcg/ml, against *Diplococcus pneumoniae* at 0.78 mcg/ml, against *Corynebacterium diphtheriae* at
0.04 mcg/ml, against *Neisseria meningitidis* at 0.04 mcg/ml, against
Neisseria gonorrhoeae at 0.09 mcg/ml, against *Bordetella pertussis*
at 0.09 mcg/ml and against *Escherichia coli, Salmonella* and
Shigella at 100 to 500 mcg/ml. Josamycin did not show cross-
resistance to penicillin, streptomycin, tetracycline or chloramphenicol, but did exhibit cross-resistance to other macrolides.
When a more nutrient-rich medium was used, the minimum inhibitory concentrations of josamycin were expressed one to two
dilutions lower. The influence of the pH of the medium, the addition of serum, and the effect of inoculum size are given in Table V.

TABLE III
Antibacterial Spectrum of Josamycin (4)[a]

Organism	MIC (mcg/ml)	Organism	MIC (mcg/ml)
Bacillus megaterium 10778	0.19	*Mycobacterium* 607	3.1
" APF	0.39	*Mycobacterium phlei*	3.1
Bacillus cereus	0.39	*Corynebacterium diphtheriae* A-7[b]	0.04
Bacillus subtilis ATCC 6633	0.19	*Neisseria meningitidis* 13077[b]	0.04
Sarcina lutea PCI 1001	0.005	" *gonorrhoeae*[b]	0.09
Staphylococcus citreus	0.39	*Bordetella pertussis*[b]	0.09
Staphylococcus aureus Terajima	0.39	*Escherichia coli* O-1	125
" Smith	0.78	" O-12	100
" 209 P	0.39	" O-25	25
" 226	0.78	" O-124	500
" resistant to		" NIHJ	100
Streptothricin	0.39	*Aerobacter aerogenes* C-12	25
Penicillin	0.39	*Klebsiella pneumoniae* PCI 602	25
Amphomycin	0.39	*Salmonella paratyphi* A 1015	200
Telomycin	0.19	" *typhimurium* 1406	100
Actinomycin	0.19	" *typhi* H 901 W	125
Carbomycin	> 50	*Shigella dysenteriae* Hanabusa	125
Erythromycin	20	" *flexneri* 2a 1675	50
TC, EM	6.25	" " 3a 102349	100
CP, TC, PC	0.78	" *sonnei* II 37148	250
Streptococcus pyogenes SS 458[b]	0.19		
Diplococcus pneumoniae I			
(Neufeld)[b]	0.78		

[a] Standard agar dilution method of Japan Society of Chemotherapy using nutrient agar. [b] Using heart infusion agar with 10% serum.

Josamycin was more active at alkaline pHs, as many of basic antibiotics are, but serum addition or inoculum size had no influence differing from the results found with lincomycin or clindamycin (51). The action of josamycin was mainly bacteriostatic, but bactericidal effect was observed at more than 100 mcg/ml. On serial transfers of *S. aureus*, resistance to josamycin developed rather slowly as shown in Fig. 6 (4).

It is very important for the prediction of clinical usefulness to make a study on the pathogenic strains isolated from clinical sources. Results from 29 university clinics and hospitals were summarized and presented at the "Josamycin Symposium" of the Japan Society of Chemotherapy, 1968 (11–14, 18–44). The distribu-

TABLE IV
Antimicrobial Spectrum of Josamycin (4)[a]

Organism	MIC (mcg/ml)			
	JM	LM	SPM	EM
Bacillus megaterium 10778	0.39	0.39	1.56	0.19
" APF	0.39	0.39	1.56	0.19
Bacillus cereus	0.39	0.78	3.13	0.19
Bacillus subtilis ATCC 6633	0.19	0.39	0.78	0.09
Sarcina lutea PCI 1001	0.04	0.04	0.09	0.04
Micrococcus flavus	0.09	0.19	0.19	0.39
Staphylococcus citreus	1.56	1.56	6.25	0.78
Staphylococcus aureus Terajima	1.56	1.56	6.25	0.78
" Smith	0.78	0.78	6.25	0.78
" 209P	1.56	1.56	6.25	0.78
" Streptothricin-resistant	1.56	1.56	6.25	0.39
" Amphomycin "	0.78	1.56	6.25	0.78
" Penicillin "	1.56	1.56	6.52	0.78
" Carbomycin "	>100	>100	>100	0.78
" Telomycin "	0.78	1.56	6.25	0.78
" Onuma (EM, OL, LM, SM, KM, PC, CL, SA-resistant)	>100	>100	>100	>100
" Shimanishi (EM, OL, LM, SM, PC, CL, SA-resistant)	>100	>100	>100	>100
" Sugioka (EM, OL, LM, SM, CL, SA-resistant)	>100	>100	>100	>100
" Tanaka (SM, CP, TC, SA-resistant)	1.56	1.56	6.25	0.78
Torula utilis	50	100	>100	50
Mycobacterium 607	1.56	1.56	3.13	3.13
" *phlei*	1.56	3.13	3.13	0.78
Haemophilus influenzae 9327 type a[d]	12.5		100	3.13
" 9332 type d[d]	12.5		100	3.13
" 9833 type f[d]	12.5		100	3.13
Mycoplasma pneumoniae Mac.[b]	0.03			
" Campo[b]	0.1	0.3		10
" *gallisepticum* C30 as[c]	0.03	0.03	0.03	>0.01
" " S6[c]	0.03			>0.001
" " KP-13[c]	0.03			>0.001
" " 396S[c]	0.03			>0.001
" " TTC[c]	0.03			>0.001
Vibrio coli 34E[e]	6.25		6.25	
" Tohgen[e]	0.78		1.56	
Escherichia coli O-1	>100	>100	>100	>100
" O-12	>100	>100	>100	>100
" O-111	25	50	>100	25
" O-124	>100	>100	>100	>100
" NIHJ	>100	>100	>100	>100

Escherichia coli SM-resistant		>100	>100	>100	>100
"	CP-resistant	>100	>100	>100	>100
"	NM-resistant	>100	>100	>100	>100
"	K12 • R5 (SM, KM,	>100	>100	>100	>100
CP, TC, SA-resistant)					
Aerobacter aerogenes C-12		>100	>100	>100	>100
Klebsiella pneumoniae PCI 602		12.5	25	>100	12.5
Salmonella paratyphi A 1015		>100	>100	>100	>100
"	*typhimurium* 1406	>100	>100	>100	>100
"	*cholerae-suis* 1348	>100	>100	>100	>100
"	*typhi* H 901 W	>100	>100	>100	>100
"	*enteritidis* 1891	12.5	25	100	6.25
Shigella dysenteriae Hanabusa		>100	>100	>100	>100
"	*flexneri* 2a 1675	100	100	>100	100
"	" 3a 102349	>100	>100	>100	>100
"	*sonnei* II 37148	>100	>100	>100	>100
Shigella flexneri 2a 59 (CP, TC, SA-		>100	>100	>100	>100
	resistant)				
"	2a 133 (TC, SA-	>100	>100	>100	>100
	resistant)				
"	2a 311 (SA-resistant)	>100	>100	>100	>100
"	2a 511 (SM, CP, SA-	>100	>100	>100	>100
	-resistant)				

[a] Standard agar dilution method of Japan Society of Chemotherapy using heart infusion agar. [b] Using PPLO agar Difco with 15% serum incubated for 5 days. [c] *M. gallisepticum* agar Eiken with 15% serum incubated for 4 days. [d] Using chocolate agar. [e] Using brain heart infusion agar with 10% blood.

tion of the minimum inhibitory concentrations (MICs) measured by the standard agar dilution method of the Society is given in Table VI and Figs. 7 and 8. Among 1316 strains of *S. aureus*, 75 percent showed the MIC to be below 3.2 mcg/ml, and the peak of distribution was at 1.6 mcg/ml. The peaks in *Streptococcus* and *D. pneumoniae* were at 0.2 mcg/ml and less than 0.1 mcg/ml respectively, and most of the strains were inhibited at less than 0.4 mcg/ml. Against anaerobes, josamycin also showed strong activity, and most strains were inhibited at less than 1.6 mcg/ml as seen from Table VII. As mentioned above, josamycin was shown not cross-resistant to commercial antibiotics, except for macrolides, from studies on laboratory strains. This was also confirmed on clinical isolates as seen from Table VIII. The table and Fig. 9 show the distribution of MICs of those strains in which the measurement against five antibiotics had been made on the same strain among

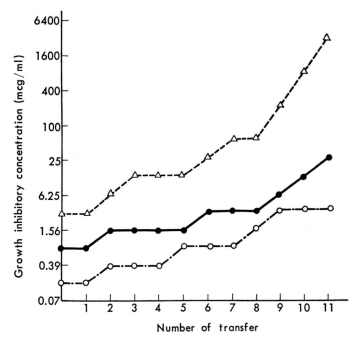

Fig. 6. Development of resistance in *S. aureus* 209P Strain (4) by tube dilution method using nutrient agar. △, SPM; ●, JM; ○, EM.

1316 staphyloccal isolates referred to in Table VI. Recently, multiple drug-resistant staphylococci have increased year by year, and about 70 percent of the clinical isolates show multiple resistance to tetracycline, streptomycin, penicillin and sulfa drugs, or to a combination of 2 or 3 of them. This tendency is seen also from the table. Josamycin was shown to be effective against tetracycline- and/or penicillin-resistant staphylococci, and was expected to be useful in the treatment of multiple drug-resistant staphylococcal infections.

2) In vivo activities

Effect of josamycin against staphylococcal infections has already been explained in Chapter 1. Here are given some data on its effect in subcutaneous infections in mice as seen in Tables IX and X. The activity of josamycin slightly surpassed or equalled that of erythromycin (4).

JOSAMYCIN, A NEW MACROLIDE ANTIBIOTIC 55

TABLE V
Effect of Medium pH, Serum Addition and Inoculum Size against Antibacterial Activity of Josamycin (4)[†]

		JM (mcg/ml)									
		12.5	6.25	3.12	1.56	0.78	0.39	0.19	0.09	0.04	0.02
pH	5	−	−	−	+	+	+	+	+	+	+
	6	−	−	−	+	+	+	+	+	+	+
	7	−	−	−	−	−	+	+	+	+	+
	8	−	−	−	−	−	−	+	+	+	+
	9	−	−	−	−	−	−	−	+	+	+
Serum	0%	−	−	−	−	−	−	+	+	+	+
	10	−	−	−	−	−	−	+	+	+	+
	25	−	−	−	−	−	−	+	+	+	+
	50	−	−	−	−	−	−	+	+	+	+
Inoculum	Broth	−	−	−	−	−	−	+	+	+	+
	10^{-1}	−	−	−	−	−	−	+	+	+	+
	10^{-2}	−	−	−	−	−	−	+	+	+	+
	10^{-3}	−	−	−	−	−	−	+	+	+	+

[†] Agar dilution method using heart infusion agar; inoculated with a loopful of 18-hr broth culture of S. aureus 209P; incubated for 20 hr.

TABLE VI
MIC Distribution of Josamycin in Clinical Isolates[a]

Organism[b]	No. of strains	MIC (mcg/ml)										
		≤0.1	0.2	0.4	0.8	1.6	3.2	6.3	12.5	25	50	100≤
Staphylococcus	1316	3	13	103	228	457	183	21	4	10	10	284
Streptococcus	176	14	92	50	3	6	2	2		5	2	
Diplococcus	21	12	9									
Anaerobes	51	13	3	4	7	7	6	2	3		2	4
Enterococcus	45				1	10	6				17	11
Klebsiella	50											50
Pseudomonas aeruginosa	63											63
Proteus	12							1		1		10
Escherichia coli	105										3	102

[a] Standard agar dilution method of Japan Society of Chemotherapy. [b] As described by clinicians.

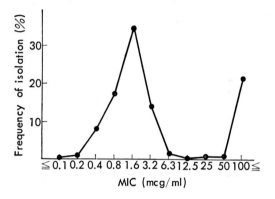

Fig. 7.   MIC distribution of josamycin in *S. aureus*.

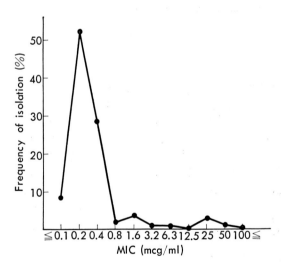

Fig. 8.   MIC distribution of josamycin in *Streptococcus*.

TABLE VII
MIC Distribution of Josamycin in Anaerobic Clinical Isolates (Kosakai *et al.* (13))

Organism	No. of strains	MIC (mcg/ml)								
		≤0.1	0.2	0.4	0.8	1.6	3.1	6.3	12.5	12.5<
Peptococcus	4				1	2	1			
Peptostreptococcus	4		2	2						
Clostridium welchii	2						1	1		
Anaerobic *Corynebacterium* and non-sporulating gram-positive bacilli	4		2				1		1	
Veillonella	4							1	1	2
Bacteroides	9			2	2	4				1

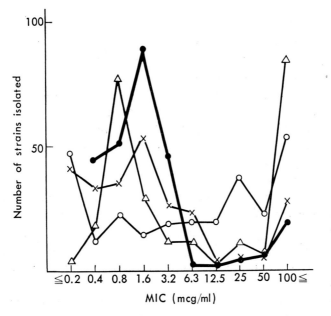

Fig. 9. MIC distribution of antibiotics in *S. aureus.* ○, PC-G; ×, KM; △, TC; ●, JM.

TABLE VIII
MIC Distribution of Antibiotics in *S. aureus*

Drug	MIC (mcg/ml)									
	<0.2	0.4	0.8	1.6	3.2	6.3	12.5	25	50	100≦
JM	......	45	51	89	46	2	2	5	6	20
PC-G	47	12	23	13	19	20	19	38[a]	22	53
KM	41	33	45	54	26	24	4	5	5	28
TC	4	18	77	29	11	12	3	11[b]	7	84
CP	....	3	4	101	93	24	9	9	24	

[a] Includes 16 strains of >25 mcg/ml.   [b] Includes 10 strains of >25 mcg/ml.

Further, results in septic type infections are found in Table XI. Josamycin was not effective in *E. coli* infections just as other macrolides were not. The conspicuous effect of spiramycin against pneumococcal infections is a characteristic of this antibiotic (*4*).

Josamycin is effective also against some other nonbacterial infections. It shows a strong antimycoplasma activity as stated in the previous section. As seen from Table IV, josamycin was active against *Mycoplasma pneumoniae* causing human respiratory infections, at 0.03 mcg/ml, and against *M. gallisepticum*, the causative organism of chronic respiratory disease of chicks (CRD), at 0.03 mcg/ml. In accord with these *in vitro* activities, josamycin was shown to be effective for CRD in veterinary field trials, and also for lung mycoplasmosis of children in clinical trials as will be mentioned later (*31*).

M. Goto at the Dermatology Department of Kyushu University showed that it was effective in experimental syphilis in rabbits. Table XII presents results of josamycin treatment of a syphiloma formed by the intracutaneous inoculation of *Treponema pallidum* Nicols strain (*34*). These results were later confirmed by other workers.

M. Murata, A. Kawamura and others at the Institute of Medical Science of the University of Tokyo showed josamycin to be effective in rickettsial infections in mice. As seen from Table XIII, it completely inhibited *in vivo* multiplication of *Rickettsia orientalis* Ozeki strain, and was found to be twice as effective as erythromycin (*5*).

TABLE IX
Protection in Subcutaneous Staphylococcal Infection in Mice (4)†

Drug	Dosage (mg/kg)	Abscess size (mm)										Average (mm)
JM	400	0	0	0	2×2	1×1	0	1×1	0	1×1	0	0.5
	100	4×5	4×5	4×6	3×6	1×1	3×3	5×6	3×4	3×4	4×4	3.9
	25	7×8	8×9	8×8	5×5	8×9	5×5	5×6	7×8	8×8	7×8	7.1
LM	400	4×5	0	2×2	2×2	1×1	0	0	1×1	1×1	0	1.2
	100	6×7	7×7	5×5	10×10	10×10	12×12	6×6	7×8	6×9	8×8	8.0
	25	12×13	11×11	9×10	9×13	10×12	13×13	11×11	9×10	8×10	8×11	10.7
EM	400	0	2×2	1×1	0	2×2	0	0	2×2	1×1	0	0.8
	100	7×7	3×4	7×7	4×4	4×7	3×4	3×3	3×4	4×5	4×5	4.7
	25	11×13	12×13	9×9	13×15	13×11	8×14	11×12	12×12	8×9	8×10	11.2
SPM	400	4×5	2×4	0	0	3×3	1×1	5×5	2×2	3×4	2×3	2.5
	100	4×8	5×8	5×8	6×7	7×7	8×8	4×5	8×9	7×8	5×7	6.7
	25	8×10	10×10	5×6	8×8	8×8	7×8	7×7	4×6	8×9	7×8	7.6
Control		12×12 8×9	10×10 8×11	10×10 7×8	7×7 8×12	9×9 12×12	10×12	10×12	11×11	9×9	7×8	9.7

† Infected subcutaneously with 10^8 cells of *S. aureus* No. 226 strain; treated orally immediately after infection; 10 male ddN mice in each group; 15 mice in control group.

TABLE X
Protection in Subcutaneous Staphylococcal Infection in Mice (4)†

Drug	Dosage (mg/kg)	Abscess size (mm)										Average (mm)
JM	400	0	3×3	3×3	3×3	2×2	3×3	0	2×4	0	2×2	1.8
	200	3×3	4×5	3×3	3×5	4×4	3×3	1×1	3×3	1×1	3×5	3.1
	100	5×6	5×5	5×8	5×6	5×6	4×4	4×4	7×7	5×5	5×6	5.4
	50	12×11	13×13	12×12	9×9	9×9	8×9	12×12	8×8	8×8	8×10	10.2
	25	10×10	12×13	15×16	12×13	10×10	11×11	14×15	13×13	15×15	12×14	12.6
LM	400	3×3	2×2	3×4	3×5	5×5	5×6	3×3	0	4×4	5×5	3.5
	200	5×5	4×4	4×5	3×3	6×6	5×6	6×6	7×5	6×6	6×6	5.2
	100	7×7	7×7	8×8	6×7	6×7	7×8	9×11	8×8	6×10	8×8	7.3
	50	15×15	10×12	8×8	10×12	9×10	9×9	10×12	10×12	10×14	11×15	11.0
	25	15×15	15×15	15×15	15×13	12×15	10×10	10×12	11×11	14×14	13×13	13.2
EM	400	4×5	3×3	3×3	1×1	2×2	2×2	2×2	0	3×3	0	2.3
	200	3×3	5×5	5×4	3×4	1×1	4×4	4×5	8×8	2×2	4×4	3.3
	100	4×4	5×5	5×7	5×5	7×8	4×5	3×3	5×6	7×7	7×7	5.5
	50	8×8	6×8	11×12	8×10	9×10	7×7	5×10	6×6	6×6	6×9	7.9
	25	11×10	8×9	15×15	15×15	15×14	15×16	9×10	10×10	12×12	12×12	12.3
SPM	400	4×5	4×5	2×2	3×5	0	1×1	2×2	0	3×3	3×3	2.4
	200	5×6	4×4	5×7	4×5	4×5	8×8	5×5	2×2	3×3	2×4	4.6
	100	4×4	3×5	5×5	8×8	6×7	8×10	8×8	9×9	5×5	8×9	6.7
	50	8×9	11×10	10×10	8×11	10×11	8×9	9×11	12×15	8×12	7×10	10.0
	25	12×12	12×13	10×10	8×10	10×12	10×10	10×10	14×15	14×16	8×8	11.2

Drug	Inoculum (×10⁸ cells)	Abscess size (mm)										Average (mm)
Control	2	15×10	12×16	12×10	13×10	16×12	16×9	16×10	14×8	10×10	13×10	12.1
	1	10×12	13×6	9×9	8×8	15×11	12×10	15×9	11×13	12×10	13×7	11.2
	0.5	6×4	5×5	10×13	8×11	7×9	13×6	9×11	12×11	9×11	8×12	9.0
	0.25	8×8	4×5	4×4.5	3×3	4×3	5×1	4×6	5×3	5×3	4×2	4.2
	0.13	1×5	1×1	1×1	4×1	3×1	6×3	3×1	1×1	1×1	2.5×2.5	2.0
	0.06	2×1	0	0	4×2	0			1×1	0	0	0.6
	0.03	0	0	0.5×0.5	0	1×1			2×3	0	0	0.4

† Infected subcutaneously with 10⁸ cells of *S. aureus* No. 226 strain; treated orally immediately after infection; 10 male ddN mice in each group.

TABLE XI
Protection in Septic Type Infections in Mice (4)[†]
Staphylococcus aureus Smith strain (infected with 100 MLD with mucin)

Dosage (mg/kg)	Survival after 7 days				
	JM	LM	EM	SPM	Control
200 × 5	10	10	10	10	
100 × 5	10	6	10	7	
50 × 5	2	1	10	4	
25 × 5	1	1	5	1	
12.5 × 5	0	0	2	0	
6.25 × 5	0	0	0	0	
0					0
ED_{50} (mg/kg)	287	405	111	308	

Streptococcus pyogenes S-23 strain (infected with 100 MLD with mucin)

Dosage (mg/kg)	Survival after 7 days				
	JM	LM	EM	SPM	Control
200 × 5	10	10	10	10	
100 × 5	10	9	10	10	
50 × 5	9	2	10	10	
25 × 5	5	1	8	7	
12.5 × 5	1	0	1	4	
6.25 × 5	0	0	0	0	
0					0
ED_{50} (mg/kg)	125	306	95	83	

Diplococcus pneumoniae Type I Neufeld strain (infected with 100 MLD)

Dosage (mg/kg)	Survival after 7 days				
	JM	LM	EM	SPM	Control
400 × 5	10	10	10	10	
200 × 5	10	7	10	10	
100 × 5	8	4	10	10	
50 × 5	3	2	6	10	
25 × 5	2	1	1	10	
12.5 × 5	0	0	0	7	
6.25 × 5	0	0	0	5	
3.13 × 5	0	0	0	0	
0					0
ED_{50} (mg/kg)	288	534	217	40	

Escherichia coli NIHJ strain (infected with 10 MLD)   (cont'd)

Dosage (mg/kg)	Survival after 7 days					
	JM	LM	EM	SPM	CP	Control
400 × 5	1	0	2	1	10	
200 × 5	0	1	0	0	10	
100 × 5					10	
25 × 5					5	
12.5 × 5					0	
0						0
ED_{50} (mg/kg)					125	

† Infected intraperitoneally with each organism as shown in the table; treated orally at 1, 4, 8, 12 and 16 hr after infection; 10 male ddN mice in each group; 15 mice in control group.

TABLE XII
Treatment of *T. pallidum* Infection in Rabbits (Goto and Muramoto (*34*))†

Drug	Rabbit No.	Before treatment	Days after treatment					Result	Local finding
			1	2	3	4	5		
Control	63	+ + +	+ + +	+ + +	+ + +	+ + +	+ + +		worsened
EM	64	+ + +	+ + +	+ +	+	−	−	good	improved
JM	68	+ + +	+ + +	+ +	+ +	+	+	poor	improved
	69	+ + +	+ + +	+ + +	+ +	+	−	good	improved

† Infected intracutaneously with 7.6×10^5 cells of *T. pallidum* Nichols strain; after syphiloma formation, treated intramuscularly with 50 mg/kg per day for 5 days, + + +, more than 5 cells; + +, 1 to 5 cells; +, less than 1 cell; 0, no cell per microscopic field.

The same authors also studied its action against *Miyagawanella psittaci* infections in mice, and some life span prolongation was observed in mice infected intracranially with *M. psittaci* California 10 strain by 3 oral doses of 10 mg per mouse. However, other routes of infection or treatment were considered necessary to get conclusive results (*5*).

4. Absorption, distribution, excretion and metabolism

1) General aspects (4, 7)
Josamycin is absorbed well from intestine. Table XIV shows the distribution of radioactivity after oral administration of ³H-labeled josamycin in mice. Three hours after administration, radioactivity remaining in contents of alimentary canal and feces were

TABLE XIII

Treatment of *R. orientalis* Infection in Mice (Murata *et al.* (5))†

Drug	Dosage (mg/mouse)	Days after infection											Dead/Total
		11	12	13	14	15	16	17	18	19	20	21	
JM	5 mg×9											O O O O O — — — — — O O O O — — — —	0/10
	10 mg×9	◉◉ — —										O O O O O — — — — O O O — —	0/8
EM	5 mg×9									● ● ● + +	●● +	O O O O + + + + ● + O +	5/10
	10 mg×9	◉ —										O O O O + + + + O O O + + +	0/9
Control	not treated			●●●● + + + +	●●● + + +		● +					10/10
	Saline			●●● + + + +	●●● + + + +			●●● + + + +	● +				10/10

† Male ddN mice were infected intraperitoneally with 10 MLD of *R. orientalis* Ozeki strain; treated orally at 6, 12 and 18 hr after infection, and once daily for 6 days thereafter: O, alive; ●, dead; ◉, dead from accident. +, *Rickettsia* positive; −, *Rickettsia* negative.

TABLE XIV

Distribution of ³H-Josamycin Given Orally to Mice (7)[a]

Organ	1 hr after medication		3 hr after medication	
	dpm/mg or dpm/μl	Recovery (%)	dpm/mg or dpm/μl	Recovery (%)
Brain	36.0	0.03	68.6	0.05
Heart	119.0	0.03	6435.0	1.34
Liver	1812.0	3.23	1648.0	3.28
Lung	347.5	0.10	26910.0	8.47
Kidney	593.1	0.37	534.5	0.34
Submaxillary gland	221.5	0.04	241.7	0.04
Spleen	255.3	0.04	263.3	0.04
Muscle	104.8	1.57	108.2	3.23
Blood	247.8	0.42	424.0	0.72
Bile	6760.0	2.44	4962.0	0.71
Thymus	144.2	<0.01	4170.0	0.91
Adrenal	259.4	<0.01	259.1	<0.01
Testicle	49.0	0.01	258.2	0.08
Stomach	2111.0	0.66	468.6	0.16
Small intestine	4312.0	10.46	1085.0	2.94
Large intestine	3131.0	1.96	1802.0	1.44
Contents of stomach		1.14		1.50
Contents of small intestine		29.20		15.77
Contents of large intestine		4.23		20.50
Feces	2998.0	0.38	3808.0	1.44
Urine		16.93		25.90
Total recovery		73.23		88.14[b]

(3 hr contents rows bracketed: 39.21)

[a] Male ICR-JCL mice were given orally 200 mg/kg ³H-Josamycin of 5.07 mCi/g specific radioactivity.   [b] Remaining 12% is assumed to be distributed in skin and bone not examined in this experiment.

about 40 percent of total activity originally administered. When high excretion into the bile was taken into consideration, more than 60 percent of the josamycin given orally was considered to be absorbed from intestine in the lapse of 3 hr.

One hour after administration, radioactivity was distributed at high concentrations in the liver (1,812 dpm/mg) and at 3 times as high a level in the bile (6,760 dpm/μl), but the levels of activity were low in the peripheral blood and tissues with the exception of high retention in the walls of stomach and intestines. Three

TABLE XV

Distribution of ^{3}H-Josamycin Given Orally to Mice (7)†

Organ	1 hr after			3 hr after		
	JM from bioassay	JM from radioactivity	Activity ratio	JM from bioassay	JM from radioactivity	Activity ratio
Liver	11.6 mcg/g	161.1 mcg/g	7.2%	1.5 mcg/g	146.5 mcg/g	1.0%
Lung	2.4 "	30.9 "	7.8	16.6 "	2392 "	0.7
Kidney	6.1 "	57.7 "	10.6	12.2 "	47.5 "	25.7
Blood	2.6 mcg/ml	22.9 mcg/ml	11.3	0.6 mcg/ml	53.4 mcg/ml	1.1
Urine	133 mcg/total	1032 mcg/total	12.9	400 mcg/total	1607 mcg/total	25.0

† Same experiment as Table XIV; activity ratio=JM from bioassay/JM from radioactivity.

hours after, concentrations in alimentary walls decreased and those in the liver and bile also declined. But radioactivity appeared in the lungs at a very high concentration amounting to 5 times as high a level as in the bile (26,910 dpm/mg). Higher levels were also observed in the heart and thymus.

These results show the distribution characteristics: a) Excretion into the bile encounters few difficulties; b) after biliary excretion slows down, it goes through from the liver into the blood stream; and c) possibly from a high affinity for tissues, it is trapped in the lungs, the first tissue it reaches, at a very high concentration and in a very large quantities (as much as 8.47 percent of the originally administered drug). It is also suggested from the table that it is excreted fairly well into urine (as much as 25.9 percent in 3 hr).

Table XV presents a ratio of the biologically active form among the josamycin distributed as shown in Table XIV. From the

TABLE XVI
Distribution of ^{3}H-Bleomycin in Mice (54)†

Organ	BLM from radioactivity		BLM from bioassay	Activity ratio
	(mcg)	(mcg/g)	(mcg)	(%)
Liver	20.3	7.4	<0.50	<2.4
Spleen	3.6	5.6	<0.11	<3.0
Kidney	35.5	62.2	1.10	3.1
Testicle	1.9	14.6	0.10	5.2
Urinary bladder	2.6	162.5	0.07	2.7
Stomach	2.3	7.8	<0.08	<3.4
Large intestine	7.8	6.9	<0.20	<2.5
Small intestine	41.3	12.8	1.06	2.6
Heart	1.6	10.6	0.01	0.6
Lung	3.5	9.5	0.38	10.9
Brain	1.6	2.2	<0.13	<8.1
Tongue	1.8	16.5	0.05	2.8
Skin	154.8	22.6	43.80	28.3
Bone	10.1	8.0	0.44	4.4
Muscle	44.5	6.0	8.80	19.8
Peritoneum	18.9	21.2	1.68	8.9
Diaphragm	1.1	11.5	<0.03	<2.7
Urine	791.3		273.00	34.5
Feces	13.3		<1.90	<14.3
Blood	11.6		25.5	219.8

† ddY mice were given subcutaneously 0.9 mg/mouse ^{3}H-bleomycin of 4.75×10^6 dpm/mg specific activity; 1 hr after the administration assays were made.

TABLE XVII
Inactivation of Josamycin by Tissue Homogenates (4)[†]

Organ	Mouse			Rat		
	1	2	4 (hr)	1	2	4 (hr)
Liver	5	4	3.5	5	4.5	4
Spleen	90		80	85		80
Small intestine	75	70	68	80	73	70
Muscle				95		90
Serum	85	87	83			

[†] Residual potency given as % of initial when incubated at 37°C with homogenates from male ddN mice or Donryu rats for period given in the table (*B. subtilis* assay).

TABLE XVIII
Binding of Josamycin to Red Blood Cells and Serum Protein (4)
Adsorption of josamycin to red blood cells[a]

Incubation	Residual potency (mcg/ml) after incubation with red blood cell suspension at			
	0	12.5	25	50 (%)
30 min	100	96	103	103
60	100	99	102	105

Dialysis of josamycin through cellophane bag[b]

	Against buffer	Against serum
Outer layer mcg/ml	70	49
Inner layer mcg/ml	55	48

[a] Rabbit red blood cell suspension at a concentration given in the table was kept with 100 mcg/ml josamycin at room temperature for a period indicated in the table.
[b] 100 mcg/ml josamycin in phosphate buffer at pH 7.8 and in bovine serum were placed in cellophane bags and dialyzed against the same vehicles for 48 hr in refrigerator; assayed with *B. subtilis*.

columns of activity ratio, it is observed that inactivation of the josamycin proceeded with time and that the liver played the most important role in inactivation as the ratios were almost equal to that in the liver except for higher ratios in the kidneys and urine at the 3rd hour. The latter fact suggested that inactivated josamycin was more easily adsorbed in the peripheral tissues. At first sight, as the results found in the table indicate, josamycin may be considered too easily inactivated to maintain significant blood levels. However, it should be noted that easy inactivation is rather a requisite for minimizing side effects. This ability was later recognized to be a significant characteristic. A harmless and effective drug should be easily destroyed in the body, while maintaining adequate activity in the remaining portion or intermediates. Table XVI shows a similar study on bleomycin (54). Bleomycin is known as a less toxic anticancer antibiotic, and also shows very low activity ratios, as shown in the table.

Turning to inactivation of josamycin in various tissues, Table XVII presents inactivation by tissue homogenates. Josamycin is seen to be inactivated mainly in the liver. Serum and other tissues including the muscle, small intestine and spleen did not contribute much to the inactivation process. Further, the lungs and kidneys were shown to be insignificant in the inactivation of josamycin (18).

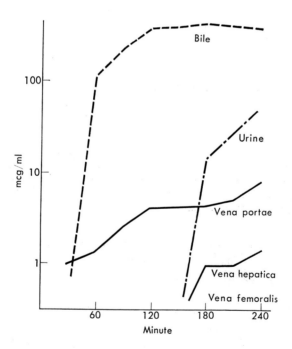

Fig. 10.   Josamycin levels after gastric administration in dogs (Mashimo et al. (18)). Dogs under thiopental anesthesia were given 200 mg/kg josamycin into stomach; blood and bile were collected from cannulae inserted operatively.

Table XVIII presents the binding to red blood cells and serum proteins. Adsorption of josamycin to these blood constituents is not significant. However, adsorption to the liver, lung and kidney tissues seems substantial (*18*).

K. Mashimo, professor of Internal Medicine at Hokkaido University, performed a smart and clear experiment showing the distribution characteristics of josamycin (*18*). Dogs were operated upon using thiopental anesthesia, and had cannulae inserted for collection of the bile, urine, and blood from portal, hepatic and femoral veins. Two hundred mg/kg of josamycin was administered into the stomach, and the levels were watched closely. The results

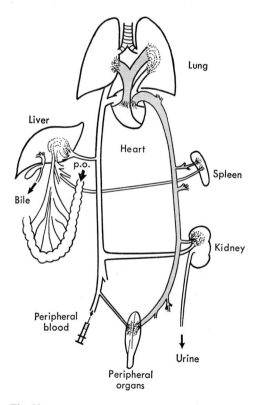

Fig. 11.

are presented as Fig. 10. Josamycin appeared in the portal vein after its absorption from the intestine, and at the same time, excretion into the bile began at a very high concentration. When biliary excretion approached a high threshold value, it flooded over to the hepatic veins, resulting in a simultaneous excretion into the urine. It was not detected in the femoral vein in this experiment, but that phenomena are often seen in anesthetized dogs.

Figure 11 illustrates anatomic features related to distribution. Orally-given josamycin is absorbed from the intestine, and reaches the liver through the portal vein. Here, a part is inactivated. However, it is excreted predominantly into the bile, then it may be reabsorbed from intestine, entering into enterohepatic circulation. As Fig. 10 indicates, only after the biliary excretion is saturated, will it flood into the hepatic veins and join the main flow of inferior vena cava. The whole amount of josamycin, having flooded from the liver, is carried to the lungs through the right heart and pulmonary arteries and is trapped within the huge capillary beds of the lungs, resulting in a very high tissue level there. That which escapes lung adsorption now goes to the greater circulation through the left heart and aortic arch, and is distributed to various parts of the body in proportion to the sizes of the arteries feeding them. Only a fraction is carried to the kidneys through renal vessels which constitute only a smaller bypass in the greater circulation. Thus carried to peripheral tissues, it is again adsorbed there, and escaping josamycin appears for the first time in the peripheral veins.

Josamycin shows a relatively high tissue affinity and a high biliary excretion rate. In the case of aminoglycosidic antibiotics such as kanamycin or gentamicin, the tissue affinity and the rate of biliary excretion are low. Injected antibiotics are kept in the blood stream without being trapped within tissues, and they are excreted only from the kidneys. Higher blood levels, lower tissue levels and high urinary excretion rates are characteristic of these antibiotics. On the other hand, enduracidin, a bacitracin-like polypeptide antibiotic, provides an example of the opposite extreme. Enduracidin shows such a very high tissue affinity that it scarcely penetrates into blood stream from the injection site. The tissue binding value of enduracidin was shown to be 95 percent in various tissues (*55*). Josamycin is located between these two extremes. Because of relatively high tissue affinity, it can pass through the liver and is then adsorbed and distributed in the lungs at a high level and in other peripheral tissues at moderate levels, but at levels adequate to manifest infection-suppressing activity. It is a matter of course that the peripheral blood level is rather low and fluctuating, but high tissue levels are maintained even after the blood level has declined, as shown in the next section.

2) Results in man and animals (4)
In the following, the results of tests in man and animals are given as figures and tables. Blood and tissue levels after oral administration in rats and rabbits are shown in Figs. 12 and 13. In accord with biologically assayed tissue levels in Table XV, high concentrations

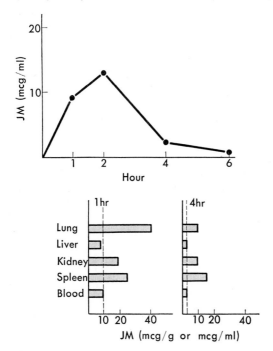

Fig. 12.   Blood and tissue levels of josamycin in rats (*4*) (average in 3 male Donryu rats given 400 mg/kg josamycin orally).

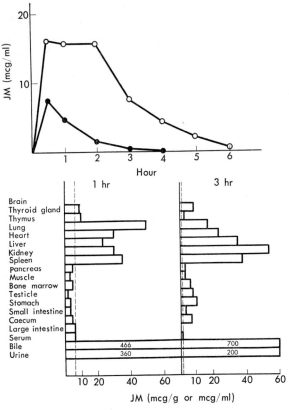

Fig. 13.   Blood and tissue levels of josamycin in rabbits (4) (average in 2 male rabbits given 200 and 400 mg/kg josamycin orally). Bloos levels with O, 400 mg/kg; ●, 200 mg/kg (upper). Tissue levels with 200 mg/kg (lower).

were detected in the bile, lungs, kidneys, spleen and liver. In Fig. 13 as well as 12, it is shown that tissue levels were maintained conspicuously higher than blood levels even after the latter had decreased with time. This result seems to indicate relatively high tissue affinity and suggests a clinical usefulness for josamycin.

Blood levels in orally medicated dogs have been already given as Fig. 2. As stated in the previous section, high levels in the lungs and high excretion into bile are characteristic of josamycin. Figure 14 presents biliary excretion of josamycin after oral administration in dogs and rabbits (*18, 36*). As can be seen from the figure, bile levels reached 100 times concentrations of those in the blood. Pharmacodynamic data calculated on intravenously medicated dogs are given as Table XIX (*18*). The halflife in blood (T/2) was 1.13 hr, distribution volume was 26.8 liters, rate of removal from serum was 0.63, and clearances from urine and bile were 61.5 and 8.6 ml/min, respectively.

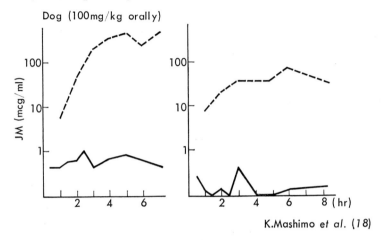

K.Mashimo *et al.* (*18*)

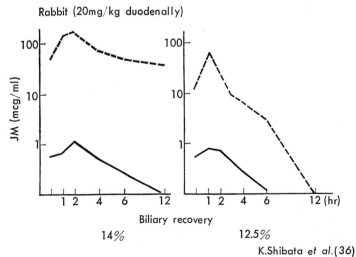

K.Shibata *et al.*(*36*)

Fig. 14.   Blood and bile levels of josamycin. ------, bile; ——, blood.

TABLE XIX
Halflife (T/2), Distribution Volume (DV), Clearances and Rates of Removal of Josamycin in Dogs (Mashimo *et al.* (*18*))†

Drug		T/2 (hr)	DV (*l*)	Clearance (ml/min) from			Rate of removal from		
				Serum	Urine	Bile	Serum	Urine	Bile
JM	Dog C	1.05	35.6	397.2	106.7	10.8	0.67	0.18	0.018
	Dog D	1.2	18.0	174.0	16.9	6.3	0.58	0.05	0.021
	Average	1.13	26.8	258.6	61.5	8.6	0.63	0.12	0.02
EM	Average	1.18	66.1	682.2	36.7	12.2	0.6	0.04	0.01

† Thiopental-anesthetized dogs were given intravenously 20 mg/kg josamycin.

TABLE XX
Blood Levels and Urinary Excretion of Josamycin in Healthy Male Human Adults Given Orally 1.0 g Josamycin (*4*)
Blood levels (mcg/ml)

Dosage (mg/kg)	Hours after administration			
	1	2	4	6
17	3.8	1.65	0.89	0.59
17	4.2	1.7	0.92	0.55
18	2.9	3.1	0.64	0.25
15	1.9	4.9	2.11	0.98
18	1.5	2.5	4.1	1.5
Average	2.86	2.77	1.73	0.77

Urinary excretion

Dosage (mg/kg)	Urinary concentration (mcg/ml) 2-4 4-6 6-8 8-10 10-12 12-24 (hr)	Urinary excretion (mg) 2-4 4-6 6-8 8-10 10-12 12-24 total (hr)	Urinary recovery (%)
17	90 21 ..... 12	15.7 5.6 ..... 3.3 .... 24.6	2.46
17	145 .... 100 ...... 34	31.9 .... 27.0 ...... 5.6 .... 64.5	6.45
18	210 ..... 30 6.3 trace	26.2 ..... 3.3 0.69 .... 30.2	3.02
15	130 380 .... 160 37 28	11.7 28.1 24.5 6.63 0.97 71.9	7.19
18	50 28 ..... 15 7 2	11.0 6.6 ..... 3.0 1.2 0.9 22.7	2.27

Table XX gives the blood levels and urinary recoveries after a single oral administration of 1.0 g in healthy human adults. Blood levels showed peaks in 1 to 2 hr. The peak level was 2.86 mcg/ml on the average of 5 persons. Urinary recoveries ranged from 2.27 to 7.19 percent in the first 24 hr.

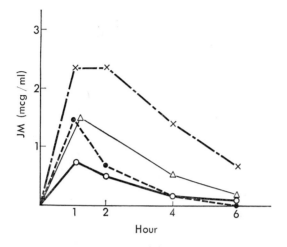

Fig. 15.   Blood levels of josamycin given orally to human adults.
○, 400 mg; ●, 600 mg; △, 800 mg; ×, 1,000 mg.

An extensive study on administration in humans was carried out at 22 university clinics and leading hospitals in cooperation, and the result was summarized and presented at the "Josamycin Symposium" of the Japan Society of Chemotherapy, 1968 (*11, 18, 19, 21, 23–29, 31, 33, 35–44*). Figure 15 illustrates the summarized average blood levels in human adults. After a single oral administration, the peaks of blood levels appeared in 1 hr except in the case of 1,000 mg medication, when josamycin was still detectable after 6 hr. By a single oral dose of 600 mg, there were obtained peak levels enough to inhibit most of clinical isolates of staphylococci. However, when the much higher tissue levels characteristic of josamycin were taken into consideration, 400 mg was sufficient as a single dose to obtain clinical effects. Figure 16 shows the blood levels in children. A single oral dose of 10 to 20 mg/kg gave comparable blood levels to those with 800 to 1,000 mg in adults (*29, 31*). Urinary recoveries in this study were also summarized and are given as Table XXI. On the average, orally given josamycin was recovered as much as 7.2 percent in 24 hr.

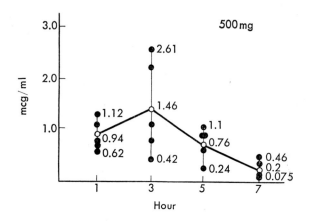

Blood levels (mcg/ml)

Age	Sex	Body weight (kg)	Dosage (mg)	Hours after administration			
				1	3	5	7
7 yr.	female	25.5	500	0.75	1.12	0.92	0.12
8 yr.	female	26.0	"	1.35	0.84	0.64	0.075
8 yr.	male	28.4	"	0.62	2.32	0.92	0.46
10 yr.	male	35.5	"	1.12	2.61	1.1	0.31
11 yr.	male	46.0	"	0.86	0.42	0.24	0.02
		Average		0.94	1.46	0.76	0.2

Fig. 16.   Blood levels of josamycin given orally to children (Naka-zawa *et al.* (*31*)).

Josamycin penetrated well into human milk. Levels in milk were almost equal to the mother's blood levels after a single oral dose of 500 mg. However, levels in the umbilical blood were 1/2 to 1/5 as high as in the mother's blood, those in amniotic fluid were still lower, and no josamycin was detected in the peripheral blood of newborns (*40, 41*). Good penetration into ocular tissues and the aqueous humor was also demonstrated, as shown in Fig. 17. Oral administration resulted in good penetration into the aqueous humor, but subconjunctival application and eye drop instillation gave much higher humor levels. After oral administration of 500 mg to rabbits, high concentrations were obtained in the extraocular muscles, retina and choroid, lids, conjunctiva, cornea, and iris

TABLE XXI
Urinary Recovery of Josamycin Given Orally to Human Adults

Dosage (mg)	0–2	0–4	0–6	0–8	0–12	0–24	(hr)
1000	3.4	4.6	3.6		4.4	5.5	%
800			2.5	3.5			
600	1.7	2.2	2.5	2.9			
500	1.9	3.5	4.0				
400	4.9	13.4	6.9		8.8	8.8	
200			5.0		5.6		
Average	3.0	5.8	4.0	3.2	6.3	7.2	

and ciliary body (*43, 44*). Josamycin was demonstrated also to appear in the sputum. After intravenous medication of 200 mg to a bronchiectasia patient, as much as 17.4 mcg/ml of josamycin was found in sputum collected 3 hr later, as shown in Table XXII (*25*).

TABLE XXII
Sputum and Urinary Recoveries of Josamycin after Intravenous Administration of 200 mg to 47–Year-old Male Patient with Bronchiectasia (Ito *et al.* (*25*)).

	Hours after administration							Recovery for 24 hr (mg)
	1	2	3	4	6	12	24	
Blood level (mcg/ml)	0.69	0.34	0.30	0.17	trace	trace	—	
Urinary level (mcg/ml)	240.0	38.0	37.0	23.0	17.5	6.0	3.8	
Urinary excretion (mg)	28.8	2.7	2.6	2.4	4.4	3.9	2.9	47.7 (23.9)[†]
Sputum level (mcg/ml)	6.0	7.8	17.4	6.7	6.5	3.7	3.3	
Sputum excretion (mg)	0.12	0.16	0.09	0.05	0.07	0.19	0.10	0.76(0.38)[†]

† Numbers in parentheses show percentage.

3) Some aspects of metabolism (62)

As discussed above, easy inactivation is considered a characteristic of josamycin which guarantees minimum side effects. Studies on the metabolism of josamycin will be taken up next.

Many thin-layer and paper chromatographic studies have been reported on the metabolism of macrolide antibiotics. However, only a few papers have been presented on the identification of the

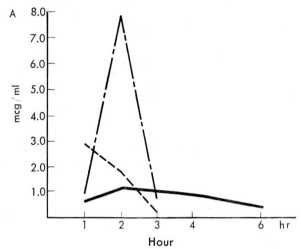

Administration	Hours after administration				
	1	2	3	4	6
Orally, 500 mg	0.58	1.07		0.96	0.29
By instillation 1% solution	2.9	1.76	0.15		
Subconjunctivally 1%, 0.5 ml	0.8	7.8	0.95		

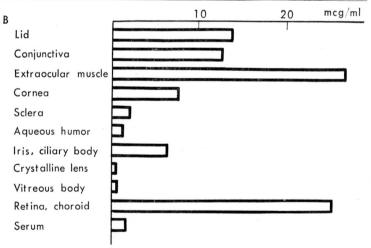

Fig. 17.   Josamycin levels in ophthalmic tissues of rabbits (Mikuni et al. (44)). A: Levels in aqueous humor (mcg/ml). —, orally; ---, by eye drop instillation; ———, subconjunctivally. B: Levels in ophthalmic tissues (mcg/g or mcg/ml), orally 500 mg, 2 hr after.

isolated metabolites (see Table XXIV). J. S. Welles of the Lilly Research Laboratories isolated a colorless crystalline metabolite from the bile collected from duodenal fistula in dogs given erythromycin intravenously. He identified it as des-N-methyl erythromycin by comparing X-ray diffraction patterns and IR spectra with a synthesized authentic sample (56). Similar des-N-methylation was also confirmed in a lincomycin derivative, clindamycin, which is not a true macrolide (57). H. Takahira of the Kyowa Hakko Kogyo Co., isolated a des-acetylated metabolite from acetyl spiramycin treated with rabbit liver homogenate and identified it as spiramycin itself by UV and IR spectra (58). However in this study, no precaution was taken to exclude the occurrence of nonenzymatic hydrolysis which often takes place in esters. Further, it is suspected that most of the acetyl spiramycin is absorbed after its hydrolysis to spiramycin by the action of esterases in the intestinal canal. Strictly speaking, this should be considered "outside body" metabolsim. Another such instance is glycoside hydrolysis of spiramycin to neospiramycin which takes place in the stomach, nonenzymatically, by the action of acid (58). However, these reactions may also be included in the "metabolism in the body," as orally given antibiotics are forced to undergo these enzymatic or nonenzymatic reactions as a natural metabolic fate. The same situation is encountered in the case of propionyl erythromycin. When blood from individuals having taken propionyl erythromycin was examined, erythromycin and propionyl erythromycin were found at a ratio of about 1 : 3. However, propionyl erythromycin was easily hydrolyzed in phosphate buffer at pH 7.4, while hydrolysis in the blood was much slower than in the buffer (60).

From complexity of chemical structures of macrolides, identification of metabolites is not conclusive except in the few cases referred to above. Many metabolites have been detected only chromatographically and their structures could only be assumed. In such cases, it will be instructive to consult studies on drug-metabolizing enzymes which will suggest possible chemical changes macrolides may undergo. Table XXIII presents a list of such enzyme fractions and their types of reactions. Drugs are metabolized through these surprisingly limited reactions and change to

TABLE XXIII
Drug-metabolizing Enzymes (Kato, 1968 (61))

Type of reaction	Fraction showing enzyme activity
Oxidation	
oxidation of alcohols	supernatant
oxidation of aldehydes	supernatant
oxidation of alkyl side chains	microsome
hydroxylation of aromatic rings	microsome
N-dealkylation	microsome
O-dealkylation	microsome
N-oxidation	microsome
S-oxidation	microsome
dehalogenation	microsome
aromatization	mitochondria
Reduction	
azo-reduction	microsome
nitro-reduction	microsome
Conjugation	
glucuronidation	microsome
sulfate conjugation	supernatant
glycine conjugation	mitochondria
acetylation	supernatant
methylation	microsome
Hydrolysis	
esterase	microsome
	serum
lactonase	microsome
	serum
glucuronidase	lysosome
arylsulfatase	lysosome
	microsome
amidase	
glucosidase	

more polar or more water-soluble forms which are then more easily excreted into the urine. Among these enzymes, those in liver microsomes are the most important, and striking progress has been made recently on them (61). Liver microsomal drug-metabolizing enzymes are those enzyme systems bound firmly to lipoid-rich smooth microsomes in liver cells, oxidizing various drugs with NADPH and molecular oxygen and reducing various drugs with

NADPH. These show rather wide substrate specificity and are induced by pretreatment with several drugs such as phenobarbital. Many central acting drugs are lipid-soluble and can hardly be excreted into urine as they are reabsorbed from the renal tubules. Thus they are necessarily oxidized by the microsomal enzymes to give hydroxylated compounds. Also concerning macrolides,

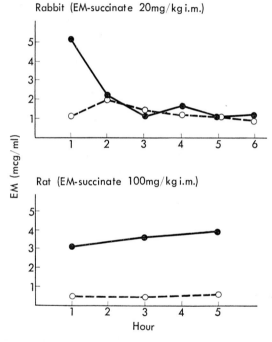

Fig. 18. Blood levels of erythromycin after phenobarbital pretreatment (Furukawa (*59*)). Rats and rabbits were pretreated with 80 mg/kg phenobarbital (i.p. and i.m. respectively); 48 hr after were given intramuscularly erythromycin succinate; each value shows average of 3 rats or 2 rabbits. ●, EM only; ○, with phenobarbital (80 mg/kg, 48 hr before EM).

H. Furukawa at the Department of Internal Medicine, Hokkaido University, demonstrated participation of liver microsomal enzymes (*59*). As shown in Fig. 18, blood levels of erythromycin were lower on pretreatment with phenobarbital. This suggested that more erythromycin was metabolized by the action of induced microsomal enzymes. Actually, marked increase in aminopyrine N-demethylase activity was confirmed in the liver of these animals, suggesting that erythromycin was metabolized to des-N-methyl erythromycin having activity 1/10 that of the parent erythromycin. However, antibiotics are less lipid-soluble than central acting drugs and are not as suited to metabolization at lipoid-rich smooth microsomes. It may be possible that more roles are played by extramicrosomal enzymes than were previously realized. In Table XXIV, enzyme reactions which may participate or are assumed to participate in macrolide metabolism are arranged from the list in Table XXIII, and the above-mentioned instances are supplemented in them.

As mentioned previously, the metabolism of josamycin occurs mainly in the liver. Thus, we studied it using enzyme fractions of liver cells, and compared it with the metabolism of its 3 acetyl derivatives shown in Fig. 19 (62). After 24-hr fasting, male ddN mice had their livers excised and homogenated. The homogenate was centrifuged at 10,000 $\times g$ for 30 min to separate the mitochondrial fraction. The supernatant was further centrifuged at 105,000 $\times g$ for 60 min, and the microsome fraction and its supernatant were obtained. The microsome fraction thus obtained was contaminated with less than 5 percent of total mitochondrias when cytochrome c oxidation was measured as a representative mitochondrial enzyme activity. Homogenates or fractions corresponding to liver from a mouse were incubated with josamycins in phosphate buffer at pH 7.2 for a definite time at 37°C. After reactions were stopped by heating, the reaction mixture was extracted with equal volume of ethyl acetate. In control runs, homogenates or fractions thereof were used after heating at 100°C for 10 min. A definite amount of the ethyl acetate extract was spotted on alumina thin-layer plates and developed with a solvent system consisting of butyl acetate, methylethylketone and water (80 : 18 : 2 v/v). Detection of spots was performed by a spraying of 10 percent sulfuric acid followed by heating at 110°C for 15 min, a spraying of Dragendorff reagent or bioautography using *Bacillus subtilis*.

TABLE XXIV

Drug-metabolizing Enzymes Possibly Participating in Macrolide Metabolism

1. Oxidation
      1a oxidation of alcohols
      1b oxidation of aldehydes
      1c oxidation of alkyl side chains
      1d hydroxylation of homocyclic rings
      1e O-dealkylation

      1f N-Dealkylation

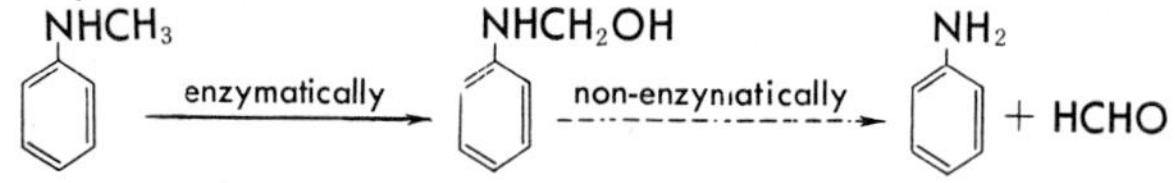

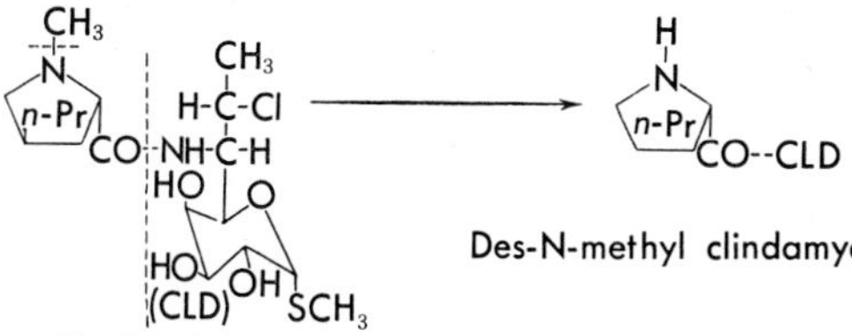

Des-N-methyl clindamycin (57)

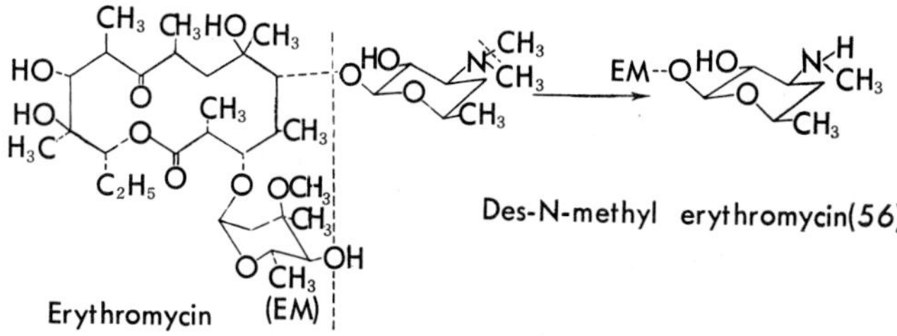

Clindamycin

Des-N-methyl erythromycin(56)

Erythromycin (EM)

2. Hydrolysis
      2a Esterase

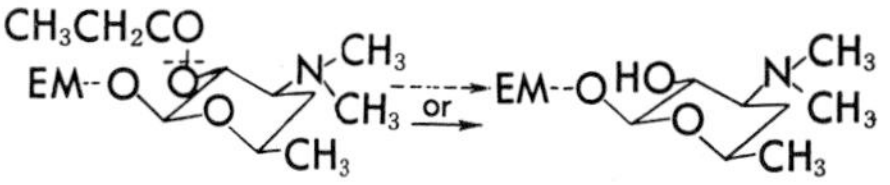

Propionyl erythromycin   Erythromycin (60)

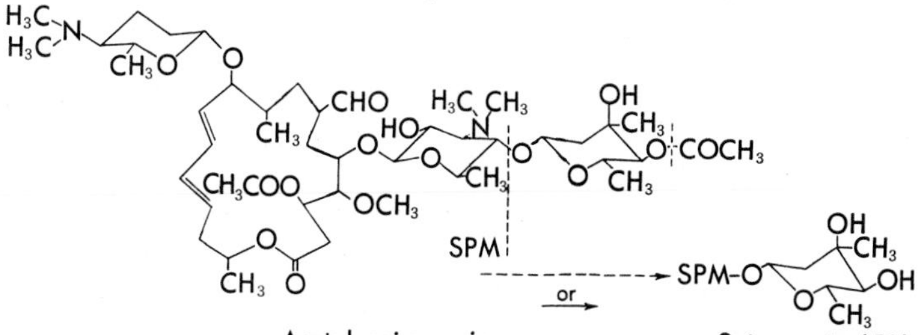

Acetyl spiramycin   Spiramycin (58)

      2b Lactonase
      2c Glucosidase

When diacetyl josamycin was incubated with the liver homogenate, a metabolite (*Rf* 0.30) appeared in 1 hr which showed deeper coloration with sulfuric acid at the 3rd hour, and two more polar metabolites (*Rf* 0.19 and 0.15) were detected 5 hr after.

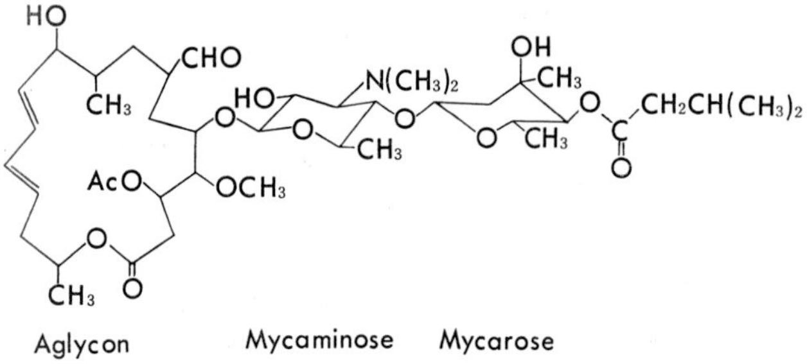

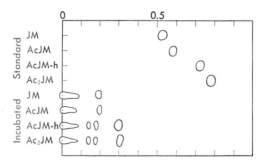

Aglycon   Mycaminose   Mycarose

	Acetyl at	mp
JM : Josamycin	—	130 to 133°C
AcJM : Acetyl josamycin	mycaminose-OH	182 to 183°C
AcJM-h : Acetyl josamycin-h	aglycon-OH	128 to 131°C
Ac₂JM : Diacetyl josamycin	mycaminose-OH aglycon-OH	152 to 153°C

Fig. 19.   Acetyl derivatives of josamycin.

Fig. 20.   Thin-layer chromatogram of metabolites of josamycins incubated with mouse liver homogenate (*62*). They were incubated at 37°C for 5 hr; detected by spraying of 10% sulfuric acid followed by heating at 110°C for 15 min.

Figures 20 and 21 show thin-layer chromatogram of metabolites and their densitogram. Under the same conditions, josamycin gave a spot at Rf 0.20. These spots were biologically active and showed positive Dragendorff color reactions. Josamycin and acetyl josamycin showed the same chromatographic pattern, while diacetyl josamycin and acetyl josamycin-h also showed another same pattern. A similar experiment using 10,000 $\times g$ supernatant is shown in Fig. 22. Clearer separation of spots was observed from a less lipid content extracted into ethyl acetate samples. However, the same metabolic patterns were confirmed as in the homogenate. From these results, des-N-methylation seen in erythromycin does not seem to participate in the metabolism of josamycins, as all the spots of metabolites including those at the origin were Dragendorff-positive, indicating a remaining tertiary amine, that is, the dimethylamino group. Acetyl group at mycaminose-OH is considered to be easily hydrolyzed enzymatically while that at aglycon-OH not so, as josamycin and acetyl josamycin, and diacetyl josamycin and acetyl josamycin-h, in each case gave the same metabolites. The isovaleryl group attached to mycarose is seemingly difficult to hydrolyze from the violet sulfuric acid-coloration of metabolite spots which should have changed to green. The spot corresponding to josambose which lacks an isovaleryl mycarose was not detected, while the reference substance showed an Rf of 0.12 and pale brown color with sulfuric acid.

Josamycins were next incubated with the microsome fraction and its supernatant (105,000 $\times g$ supernatant). No metabolite was detected with the microsome fraction. On the other hand, the 105,000 $\times g$ supernatant gave the same metabolites as the homogenate or 10,000 $\times g$ supernatant as shown in Fig. 23. Thus josamycins were shown to be metabolized mainly by enzymes in the microsome supernatant.

Among drug-metabolizing enzymes in the liver, a number of esterases have been demonstrated in microsomes (61). However, deacetylation of josamycins seemed to occur in the microsome supernatant. Possibly some esterases differing in their substrate specificity may exist in the supernatant. We prepared josamycins attached with ^{14}C-acetyl: acetyl josamycin-^{14}C containing labeled acetyl at mycaminose-OH and diacetyl josamycin-^{14}C containing it at aglycon-OH. These labeled josamycins were treated with the 10,000 $\times g$ supernatant as in the above experiments.

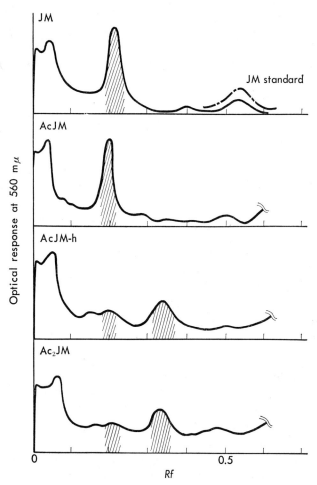

Fig. 21.   Densitogram of metabolites of josamycins incubated with mouse liver homogenate (62). They were incubated at 37°C for 5 hr; detected by spraying of 10% sulfuric acid followed by heating at 110°C for 15 min and by bioautography using *B. subtilis*. ▨: Biologically active.

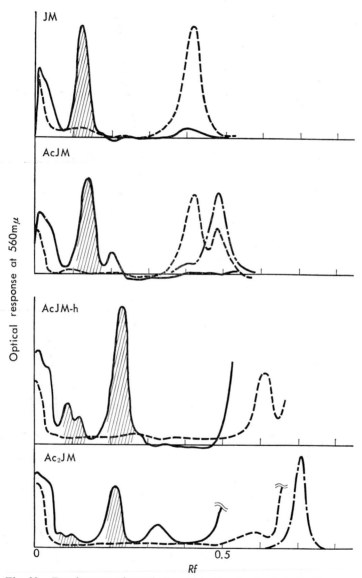

Fig. 22.   Densitogram of metabolites of josamycins incubated with
mouse liver 10,000×g supernatant (62). They were incubated at 37°C
for 2.5 hr; detected by spraying of 10% sulfuric acid followed by
heating at 110°C for 15 min and bioautography using *B. subtilis*;
⧄: Biologically active; control was incubated with heated supernatant.
—, incubated; ···, control; ---, standard.

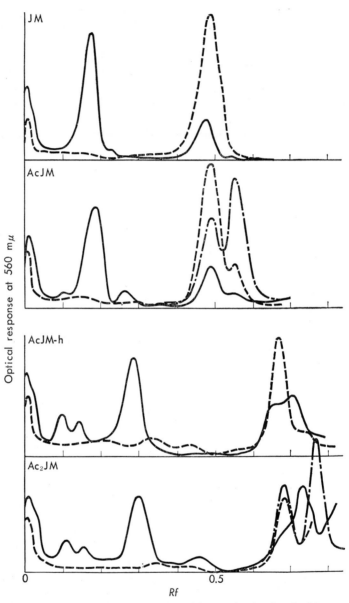

Fig. 23.   Densitogram of metabolites of josamycins incubated with mouse liver 105,000 × g supernatant (62). They were incubated at 37°C for 2 hr; detected by spraying of 10% sulfuric acid followed by heating at 110°C for 15 min; control was incubated with heated supernatant. —, incubated; ···, control; ---, standard.

Figure 24 shows the results. Differing from propionyl erythromycin, hydrolysis of josamycins was shown to be much less rapid in phosphate buffer at pH 7.2 from a preliminary study. It was demonstrated that acetyl josamycin-^{14}C was deacetylated and changed to nonlabeled more polar metabolites losing labeled mycaminose acetyl. Diacetyl josamycin-^{14}C was deacetylated also at mycaminose as shown by the disappearance of the original compound after incubation. However, only a part of the labeled acetyl at the aglycon was recovered in the spot at *Rf* 0.30. Seemingly, the acetyl at aglycon-OH may further be hydrolyzed. These results confirm that josamycins are deacetylated more or less with liver supernatant.

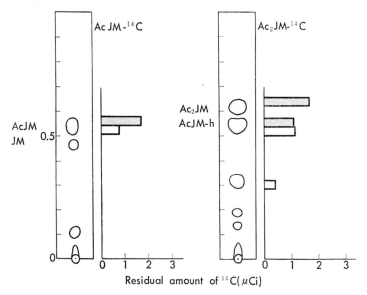

Fig. 24.   Metabolites of (1-^{14}C)-acetyl josamycins incubated with mouse liver 10,000×*g* supernatant (*62*). 5.4 *μ*Ci of AcJM-^{14}C (Ac* at mycaminose, 4.32 *μ*Ci/mg) and 2.325 *μ*Ci of Ac$_2$ JM-^{14}C (Ac* at aglycon, 0.472 *μ*Ci/mg) were incubated at 30°C for 2 hr (AcJM-^{14}C contained *ca.* 50% of JM, Ac$_2$JM contained *ca.* 30% of AcJM-h-^{14}C from hydrolysis during storage at −20°C); scanned with thin-layer radioscanner and detected with sulfuric acid; control was incubated with heated supernatant. ☐, incubated; ▨, control.

For prediction of the josamycin metabolism in man, it is interesting to know the species differences of metabolic patterns among animals. Figure 25 shows thin-layer chromatogram of josamycins metabolized with rat liver 10,000×g supernatant. Figure 26 gives that of josamycin treated with 10,000×g supernatants from mice, rats and guinea pigs, and Fig. 27 that of josamycin incubated with rabbit liver 10,000×g supernatant and that of urine collected from rabbits given oral josamycin. Liver 10,000×g supernatants

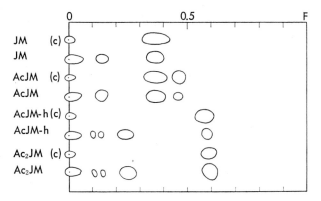

Fig. 25.   Thin-layer chromatogram of metabolites of josamycins incubated with rat liver 10,000×g supernatant (*62*). They were incubated at 37°C for 2 hr; detected by spraying of 10% sulfuric acid followed by heating at 110°C for 15 min; (c): control incubated with heated supernatant.

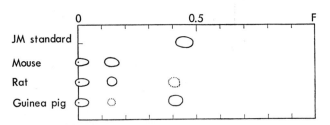

Fig. 26.   Thin-layer chromatogram of metabolites of josamycin incubated with mouse, rat and guinea pig liver 10,000×g supernatant (*62*). They were incubated at 37°C for 2 hr; detected by spraying of 10% sulfuric acid followed by heating at 110°C for 15 min.

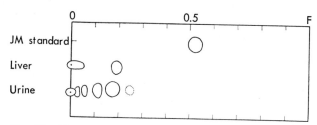

Fig. 27. Thin-layer chromatogram of metabolites of josamycin in rabbits (62). Liver: Josamycin was incubated with liver 10,000×*g* supernatant at 37°C for 2 hr; Urine: Josamycin 1.0 g×4 was given orally to rabbits from which urine was collected for 36 hr; metabolites were detected by spraying of 10% sulfuric acid followed by heating at 110°C for 15 min.

gave the same metabolites in all animals, among which guinea pigs showed the lowest activity. The metabolites found in rabbit urine had undergone a more advanced metabolism than in the liver. In an experiment using the mouse liver 10,000 ×*g* supernatant, the metabolites of josamycin were incubated with fresh 10,000 ×*g* supernatant, but no further change was observed.

These results confirmed that josamycins were metabolized mainly by enzymes in the microsome supernatant of liver cells. The metabolites of josamycins were shown to be more polar, less active substances which possibly lacked acetyl groups but kept a dimethylamino group. The main event in erythromycin metabolism, however, was des-N-methylation at the dimethylamino group, which, it was realized, was catalyzed by microsomal enzymes. Other changes occurring in the josamycin metabolites will become manifest after isolation of a main metabolite which is now in progress.

As explained above, characteristics of josamycin were its relatively high tissue affinity and its easy metabolism in the body. The relatively high tissue affinity resulted in high josamycin levels in the lungs and peripheral tissues, which were the cause of excellent effects in respiratory and suppurative infections. Josamycin's easy metabolism in the body made it a medicament with just few side effects as shown later.

5. Toxicity and general pharmacology (67)

Josamycin was found to be relatively nontoxic, and to be neither antigenic nor teratogenic. No significant pharmacological action was recognized even with amounts exceeding the therapeutic doses and could, thus, be considered safe for use in treatment.

1) Acute toxicity

Table XXV shows LD_{50} in mice and rats. The intravenous LD_{50} was 350 to 400 mg/kg. When given intraperitoneally or subcutaneously, josamycin showed LD_{50} of more than 3,000 mg/kg and more than 5,000 mg/kg, respectively. The oral LD_{50} was found to be more than 7,000 mg/kg. The acute toxicity of josamycin was judged to be very low.

TABLE XXV
Acute Toxicity of Josamycin in ICR-JCL Mice and Wistar Rats Given Josamycin
Base (p.o. and i.p.) or Its Tartrate (s.c. and i.v.)

| | LD_{50} (mg/kg) | | | |
| | Mouse | | Rat | |
Route	Male	Female	Male	Female
p.o.	>7000	>7000	>7000	>7000
i.p.	>3000	>3000	>3000	>3000
s.c.	>5000	>5000	>5000	>5000
i.v.	355	372	390	395
	(335–376)	(346–400)	(366–421)	(367–423)

2) Subacute and chronic toxicity

Subacute and chronic toxicity of josamycin was examined after oral administration to rats dosed daily for 5 weeks and for 6 months (6, 9). Rats were given josamycin up to 3,000 mg/kg per day which was the maximum dosage technically possible. No significant changes attributable to drug action were observed on behavior, food intake, growth curves, organ weights, hematological findings, autoptic and histological findings, or in biochemical examination of sera. Figure 28 shows the growth curves in 6-month tests, and Table XXVI gives the biochemical findings of sera

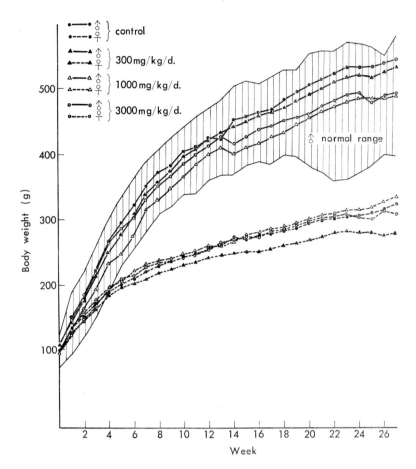

Fig. 28. Growth curves of rats in six-month oral administration of josamycin (9). Wistar rats were given josamycin daily for 189 days by oral syringe.

collected at the end of 6 months of administration. As seen from values of S-GOT, S-GPT and urea N, no toxic changes were detected in liver and kidney functions even with the highest doses of 3,000 mg/kg per day.

Similar examination was performed in dogs given intravenously a more severe daily dosage of up to 240 mg/kg for 4 weeks. Significant toxic changes were not observed. It is worth notice that

TABLE XXVI
Biochemical Findings of Blood after Six-Month Administration of Josamycin (9)

Item Method		Blood sugar (mg/dl) Oxidase method†	S-GOT (Karmen unit/ml) Colorim- etry†	S-GPT (Karmen unit/ml) Colorim- etry†	Alk. Pase (mM unit) Colorim- etry†	Chole- sterol (mg/dl) Colorim- etry†	Urea N (mg/dl) Urease method†	LDH (m unit/ml) Colorim- etry†	Na⁺ (mEq/l) Flame photom- etry	K⁺ (mEq/l) Flame photom- etry	Cl⁻ (mEq/l) Schales- Schales titration	A/G ratio Electro- phoresis	Total protein (g/dl) Refractom- etry
Control	♂	168	112	38	84	150	24	2230	150	6.3	103	0.56	7.6
	♀	150	117	83	54	182	26	1330	146	5.2	99	0.68	7.7
3000 mg/kg/d.	♂	136	90	32	73	114	25	1600	149	5.9	102	0.66	7.4
	♀	116	109	60	60	160	26	1660	150	5.4	104	0.73	7.7
1000 mg/kg/d.	♂	116	105	44	88	97	26	2030	148	5.9	105	0.70	7.5
	♀	122	142	75	88	169	30	1860	149	5.5	103	0.87	8.2
300 mg/kg/d.	♂	171	87	38	103	133	25	1500	146	5.6	102	0.66	7.3
	♀	141	96	54	76	124	26	1630	148	5.2	105	0.79	7.3

† "Test Combination" kits (C. F. Boehringer) were used.

josamycin did not show any sign of hepatic toxicity in prolonged administration.

3) Teratogenic action

The teratogenic action of josamycin was investigated by its administration to pregnant mice and rats (6). With oral josamycin of 300 mg/kg and 3,000 mg/kg per day for 7 days starting from the 7th day of gestation, no significant difference from the control group was observed in litter size, fetal mortality, fetal growth, surviving rate and growth of the young in both mice and rats except for slightly higher fetal mortality and some retardation of fetal growth in mice given 3,000 mg/kg per day. No significant malformation was observed in the animals of both species even with the highest dosage.

4) Antigenicity

Antigenicity of josamycin was studied by testing for anaphylactic shock after intravenous shocking injection in guinea pigs actively sensitized with oral or intraperitoneal josamycin and with intramuscular josamycin with adjuvants, Schultz-Dale phenomenon with excised intestine of guinea pigs sensitized with josamycin with or without adjuvants, and passive cutaneous anaphylaxis in guinea pigs receiving intradermal sensitization with antijosamycin guinea pig serum. Josamycin showed no antigenicity in any of these procedures.

5) General pharmacology (8, 15–17, 53)

In order to examine untoward reactions after josamycin administration, the following pharmacological studies were performed: observations of behavior in mice, cats and rabbits, and of respiration and blood pressure in anesthetized cats, rabbits and dogs, electrocardiography in anesthetized cats and rabbits, electroencephalography in unanesthetized rabbits, observations of spontaneous movement of excised guinea pig and toard hearts, of coronary blood flow in excised guinea pig hearts, of peripheral circulation through ear mussel vessels of rabbits and hind leg vessels of toads, of peripheral vascular permeability affected by intradermal medication in rabbits, of motility of excised intestines of rabbits and guinea pigs, of motility of excised uteri of rats, of effects on neuromuscular preparations of rat diaphragms, and of changes in urine volume in rats and body temperature in rabbits. At the highest doses, josamycin showed sedative action and several sympathomimetic or parasympathomimetic profiles such as fall in blood pressure due to peripheral vasodilation. However, no significant change was observed at 10 mcg/ml which far exceeded the blood levels obtained with oral josamycin.

6. Clinical evaluation (67)

1) Clinical effects (11, 18–45, 69)
Clinical evaluation of josamycin was performed at 33 university clinics and leading hospitals carrying out antibiotic research in Japan. Josamycin was given orally to 785 patients with various infections, and was found to be effective in 643 of them, thus showing an effectivity rate of 81.9 percent. At the 16th Annual Meeting of the Japan Society of Chemotherapy held in May 1968 at Tokyo, a symposium for the clinical evaluation of josamycin was held under the chairmanship of K. Fukushima, professor of Internal Medicine, Yokohama City University. Results submitted by the above 33 institutions were summarized and presented at that time.

TABLE XXVII
Clinical Results with Oral Josamycin

	No. of cases	Clinical result				Effectivity rate (%)
		Excellent	Good	Nil	Unknown	
Internal medicine	127	45	51	30	1	75.6
Surgery	143	111		28	4	77.6
Pediatrics	122	62	45	15		87.6
Gyneco-obstetrics	28	6	18	4		85.7
Dermatology	52	33(+8)		11		78.8
Ophthalmology	44	8	32	2	2	90.9
Urology	23	10	5	8		65.2
Otorhinology	46	29	12	5		89.0
Total	585	475		110		81.2

Table XXVII gives the clinical results on 585 cases collected by that date, the effectivity rate being 81.2 percent. Table XXIX shows the results of the above-mentioned 785 cases classified by disease. Josamycin was thus confirmed to be as effective as erythromycin.

Table XXVIII shows the relationship between dosage of oral josamycin and the clinical results in human adults. Daily dosage was divided into 3 or 4 portions, which were given at an interval of 8 to 6 hr. Dosage of 400 mg per day was not sufficient for good results. Effective doses of 600 mg per day were mostly those given to outpatients with mild cases. Daily doses of 800 to 1,200 mg were enough to obtain good therapeutic results in most infections in internal medicine. When considered not sufficient, dosage was increased to 1,600 mg per day. As explained below, it was found that josamycin seldom caused gastrointestinal disturbances, allowing it to be given at extremely high dosages in severe infection cases. Thus, a case of acute tenonitis was successfully treated with a daily dosage of 2,400 mg. In children, oral 20 to 40 mg/kg per day gave satisfactory results.

Josamycin was effective for superficial and deep suppurative infections, respiratory infections, bacillary dysentery, scarlet fever and ophthalmic infections, as shown in Table XXIX. Among the 785 cases indicated in Table XXIX, causative pathogens were isolated and described in 438, as shown in Table XXX. It was

TABLE XXVIII
Dosage and Clinical Results with Oral Josamycin in Adults

Dosage (mg/day)	No. of cases	Clinical result					Effectivity rate (%)
		Excellent	Good	Slight	Nil	Unknown	
400	8	1	2	1	3	1	50.0
600	26	7	12	4	3	0	88.5
800	97	29	45	6	17	0	82.5
1000	10	3	3	3	1	0	90.0
1200	260	50	139	32	37	2	85.0
1500	3	1	2	0	0	0	100.0
1600	97	11	58	3	24	1	74.2
1800	8	4	2	0	1	1	75.0
2400	3	0	1	0	2	0	33.3

TABLE XXIX
Diseases and Clinical Results with Oral Josamycin

	No. of cases	Clinical result					Effectivity rate (%)	Effective /Total
		Excellent	Good	Slight	Nil	Unknown		
Sepsis	2		2					2/2
Pericarditis	1		1					1/1
Subtotal	3	0	3	0	0	0	100.0	3/3
Folliculitis	7		3	3	1			6/7
Pyoderma	2		2					2/2
Acne vulgaris	6		2	2	2			4/6
Abscess	29	3	19	2	1	4	82.8	24/29
Impetigo	5				5			0/5
Furuncle	65	11	46	4	4		93.8	61/65
Carbuncle	4		3		1			3/4
Phlegmon	14		11		3		78.6	11/14
Pharyngolaryngitis	20	3	13		4		80.0	16/20
Tonsillitis	97	62	24	2	6	3	90.7	88/97
Dacryocystitis	4	1	2	1				4/4
Hordeolum	29	3	17	6	2	1	89.7	26/29
Panaritium	25		21		2	2	84.0	21/25
Furunculosis	14	2	9	1	2		85.7	12/14
Infected atheroma	5	4			1			4/5
Chalazion	6		6					6/6
Postoperative infection	12	1	8		3		75.0	9/12
Infection after burns	8		5		3			5/8
Secondary infection	9		6		3			6/9
Blepharitis	3		2	1				3/3
Subtotal	364	90	199	22	43	10	85.4	311/364
Mastitis	14	2	10		2		85.7	12/14
Lymphangitis -adenitis	13	1	10		2		84.6	11/13
Osteomyelitis	4		2		1	1		2/4
Epididymitis	2	1	1					2/2
Sialoadenitis	1		1					1/1
Spermatocystitis	1	1						1/1
Subtotal	35	5	24	0	5	1	82.9	29/35
Acute, chronic bronchitis	88	3	62	5	18		79.5	70/88
Bronchiectasia	8	2	3	1	2			6/8
Pneumonia bronchopneumonia	62	16	33	6	7		88.7	55/62
Lung mycoplasmosis	3		2		1			2/3
Subtotal	161	21	100	12	28	0	82.6	133/161

Lung abscess	8	1	4	1	2	0	75.0	6/8
Dysentery	25		14	8	3		88.0	22/25
Enteritis	1		1					1/1
Cholecystitis	3	1		1	1			2/3
Subtotal	29	1	15	9	4	0	89.7	25/29
Pyelonephritis	4	2	1		1			3/4
Cystitis	27	10	8		9		66.7	18/27
Urethritis	6	2	1		3			3/6
Adnexitis	8	1	5		2			6/8
Endometritis	6	1	5					6/6
Pelvioperitonitis	1				1			0/1
Gonorrhoea	5	2	1		2			3/5
Subtotal	57	18	21	0	18	0	68.4	39/57
Scarlet fever	34	27	6	1	0	0	100.0	34/34
Turbid cornea	6		6					6/6
Corneal ulcer	2			2				2/2
Acute tenonitis	1			1				1/1
Subtotal	9	0	6	3	0	0	100.0	9/9
Otitis media	43	11	17	2	11	2	69.8	30/43
Sinusitis	7	1	2	2	1	1		5/7
Parotitis	2					2		0/2
Subtotal	52	12	19	4	12	5	67.3	35/52
Miscellaneous	33	4	14	1	8	6	60.6	20/33
Total	785	179	411	53	120	22	81.9	643/785

found to be effective in 81.3 percent of staphylococcal infection cases, in 97.7 percent of streptococcal infection cases and in 92.3 percent of pneumococcal infection cases, the results agreeing with *in vitro* antibacterial activities. Good response in the treatment of dysentery was presumably due to a high local concentration of josamycin in the intestine. MIC levels were measured on some of the isolates. The isolates of streptococci and pneumococci showed MIC levels not higher than 0.8 mcg/ml, which agreed with the high effectivity rates in these infections. In staphylococcal infections, josamycin was effective in about 90 percent of those infected with cocci showing MIC of 3.2 mcg/ml or less, but not in those with resistant cocci showing MIC of 100 mcg/ml or more.

In internal medicine, the response was excellent in 45 and good in 51 cases out of 127 infections. Among them, josamycin was 91

TABLE XXX

Causative Pathogens and Clinical Results with Oral Josamycin

Pathogenic organism†	No. of cases	Clinical result					Effectivity rate (%)
		Excellent	Good	Slight	Nil	Unknown	
Staphylococcus aureus	251	45	143	16	44	3	81.3
Streptococcus pyogenes	86	63	20	1	2	0	97.7
Diplococcus pneumoniae	13	3	8	1	1	0	92.3
Proteus	2	0	0	0	2	0	
Corynebacterium	1	1	0	0	0	0	
Hemophilus	7	1	3	0	3	0	
Morganella	1	0	1	0	0	0	
Enterobacter	1	0	1	0	0	0	
Escherichia coli	4	1	1	0	2	0	
Gram–negatives	1	1	0	0	0	0	
Peptococcus	1	0	1	0	0	0	
Shigella	25	0	14	8	3	0	88.0
Neisseria gonorrhoeae	5	2	1	0	2	0	
Micrococcus	1	0	0	1	0	0	
Anaerobes	1	0	1	0	0	0	
Pseudomonas aeruginosa	2	0	0	0	2	0	
Mixed infection	36	11	14	1	7	3	72.2
Total	438	128	208	28	68	6	83.1

† As described by clinicians.

percent effective in acute pharyngitis, tonsillitis and bronchitis, and the rate of excellent response was 65.6 percent. In rather severe infections, josamycin was effective in 85.2 percent of 27 bacillary pneumonia cases, among which 16 cases showed excellent response and 7 cases good response. However, results were not satisfactory in mixed infections with gram-negative bacteria. As expected from high excretion into the bile, josamycin gave excellent to good relief in 2 cases of biliary infections. Generally speaking, excellent responses were observed in more than 50 percent of infections with staphylococci, hemolytic streptococci and pneumococci. Respiratory infections with *Haemophilus* responded excellently to josamycin in 2, and favorably in 4 out of 10 cases. Three cases infected with enteric gram-negatives failed to respond. Doses of 800 mg per day or less gave excellent results in mild acute infections with gram-positives. Daily doses of 1,200 to 1,600 mg gave excellent therapeutic results in pneumonia, lung abscess and bronchiectasia. In 25 cases of dysentery carriers, 1,200 mg per day for 5 days yielded 88 percent effectiveness.

In surgery, 111 of 143 surgical infections had excellent or good responses to oral josamycin, the effectivity rate being 77.6 percent. Results were excellent in superficial infections. Dosage was 800 to 1,200 mg per day for 4 to 6 days. Josamycin was effective in all cases with staphylococci showing MIC of 1.6 mcg/ml or less.

In pediatrics, josamycin was effective in 87.6 percent of 122 infections, among which 62 showed excellent and 45 showed good responses. Excellent responses were observed in acute respiratory infections, streptococcal infections including scarlet fever, and purulent infections with staphylococci. Dosage of oral josamycin was 20 to 40 mg/kg per day for 2 to 15 days. Two cases with lung mycoplasmosis were cured successfully by josamycin medication. A 10-year-old girl whose case was diagnosed as lung mycoplasmosis from radiograms, CF antibody and cold hemagglutinin titers was treated orally with 1,200 mg per day for 7 days, resulting in disappearance of radiographic shadows accompanied by marked improvement in clinical findings.

In other fields, a high effective rate of 80 to 90 percent effectivity was observed except for urological infections. In ophthalmic infections, it should be remembered that josamycin showed high penetration into the retina, choroid and cornea after oral medication, and into the aqueous humor after eye drop instillation, as mentioned on page 76.

2) Side effects (11, 18–45, 69)
As explained in Chapter 5, josamycin was shown from laboratory studies to be a safe remedy. From clinical trials, josamycin was also confirmed to be a unusually safe remedy showing only rare incidence of side effects. Table XXXI presents side effects observed in a total of 785 cases medicated with oral josamycin. Thirty-one out of 785 cases showed side effects consisting mainly of rather mild gastrointestinal disturbances such as anorexia, epigastric distress or nausea. However, withdrawal of josamycin was not necessary in most of them. High toleration in patients was found

TABLE XXXI
Side Effects with Oral Josamycin

Symptoms as side effects	No. of cases
Epigastric distress, nausea.	6
Anorexia	10
Heartburn	2
Vomiting	3
Borborygmus, abdominal distention	2
Abdominal pain	1
Diarrhea	3
Itching	1
Eruption	3
Total	31

Total cases medicated: 785. Incidence of side effects: 3.9%.

to be an important aspect of josamycin treatment. Josamycin could be given to a patient who could not tolerate the gastrointestinal disturbances from chloramphenicol medication. High tolerability indicated that josamycin could be administered in dosages high enough for complete healing. As mentioned in the previous section, dosage as high as 2,400 mg per day was used in the treatment of acute tenonitis without gastrointestinal disturbance.

Erythromycin estolate and triacetyl oleandomycin have been known to cause hepatic disturbances. Thus, josamycin was examined carefully for hepatic toxicity. As stated previously, josamycin was confirmed to show no sign of hepatic toxicity in animals after prolonged oral administration at a high dosage of 3,000 mg/kg per day for 6 months. Results of the clinical examinations are given in Table XXXII which shows biochemical and hematological findings before and after josamycin treatment. As seen from values of S-GOT, S-GPT and alkaline phosphatase, no hepatotoxic change due to josamycin medication was observed with 1,600 mg per day for 47 days, 38 days, 33 days, 25 days and for 24 days, or with 1,200 mg per day for 31, 31, 30, and for 30 days. Thus, it seemed likely that josamycin would not show hepatic toxicity in clinical trials as well.

TABLE XXXII
Blood and Serum Findings before and after Oral Josamycin (Adults)

Hospital	Name	Age	Sex	Diagnosis	Dosage mg/d.×d.	W.B.C. B[a]	W.B.C. A[b]	Neutrophil (%) B	Neutrophil (%) A	"Links-verschiebung" B	"Links-verschiebung" A	BUN B	BUN A	TTT B	TTT A	GOT B	GOT A	GPT B	GPT A	ALK-P B	ALK-P A
Osaka City Univ. (26)	T.M.	68	♂	Lung cancer + Mixed infection	1600×22	7810	6720	58	51	−	+			1.8	2.9	18	16	7	7	8	8
Hokkaido Univ. (18)	K.O.	35	♂	Acute pneumonia	1200×30	19900	10600	40	70	+	−	20	17								
"	T.N.	26	♀	Bronchopneumonia	1200×7			48	72												
"	S.S.	34	♀	Acute tonsillitis	1000×4	10000	6500							2.1	2.1	12	12	10	10		
"	C.O.	67	♀	Chron. bronchitis	1000×8									3.7	3.2	22	15	7	7		
"	H.T.	32	♂	Acute bronchopneumonia	1000×10	9800	6000							2.0	2.1	10	15	8	8		
"	T.S.	31	♀	Bronchopneumonia	1800×16	15200	9800	72	58												
Univ. Tokyo	Y.T.	56	♂	Pneumonia	1600×5	14500	10700					46	47.5	1	1	16	25	7	11	3	3.6
"	T.Y.	47	♀	Chron. bronchitis	1600×25									3	3	5	7	6	5	1.9	2.2
Keio Univ. (21)	I.F.	57	♀	Acute bronchitis	1200×6	8200	5100	58	48	+	−							5	10	3	3
"	S.H.	62	♂	Bronchiectasia	1200×6	6200	5100											10	5	3	3
"	Y.M.	72	♂	Chron. bronchitis	1200×6	7000	6000	62	58	+	−							21	9	3	4
Tokyo Kyosai Hosp. (23)	R.S.	22	♂	Acute pneumonia	1600×19											15	13	7	7	12.2	8
"	S.K.	71	♂	Lung abscess	1600×16							22.1	24.4			22	16	6	4	6.5	9.3
"	C.S.	64	♂	Acute bronchitis + Chron. nephritis	1200×7							33.1	33.6			21	21	10	17	31.2	32.6
"	H.Y.	60	♂	Pleuritis+Lues	1200×30											56	21	23	10	11.0	13.4
"	A.S.	32	♂	Duodenal ulcer + Lues	1200×31											21	18	7	10	4	4.6
"	T.G.	72	♂	Chron. bronchitis + Lues	1200×25	8000	7500	59	59							14	16	4	6	6.5	11.6
"	S.A.	62	♂	Lung tuberculosis + Lues	1200×30											37	21	17	8	5.3	6.8
"	Y.I.	53	♀	Lung tuberculosis + Lues	1200×31											19	24	9	11	4	4
1st National Hosp. Tokyo (20)	M.Y.	53	♂	Bronchial asthma + Bronchopneumonia	1200×7 2400×7	10800	10100	50	54	+	+			5.2	5.4					11.4	9.8
"	T.M.	24	♀	Bronchitis purulenta +Bronchiectasia	1200×7	9400	7700	64	54												
"	K.K.		♂	Bronchitis + Bronchial asthma	1200×14	5500	4700	48	43	+	+	12.5	13.5			25	18	40	24		
"	S.M.	58	♂	Bronchitis + Bronchial asthma	1200×7	18300	10200	76	61	+	+										
Kawasaki City Hosp. (24)	N.T.	69	♂	Chron. bronchitis	1200×13	4600	5700	43	59	−	−					21	32	45	17	6.0	3.4
Yokohama City Univ. (25)	M.I.	54	♀	Pericarditis	1600×9							16	11			34	44				
"	H.Y.	60	♀	Bronchopneumonia	1600×3	14800	4300	90	66			40	57	5	7						
"	G.H.	45	♂	Bronchopneumonia	1600×21	22300	5000	83	49												
"	H.S.	53	♂	Sepsis	1600×14	4100	6000	52	49					9	6	32	22	22	16	6.4	8.3
"	K.K.	66	♂	Chron. lymph. leukemia	1600×47							27.4	32.4	5	2.5	28	15	11	14	13.4	18.4
"	T.M.	42	♀	Lung abscess	1600×14	10900	6400							1.5	2.5	33	18	12	34	10.2	6.5
"	K.A.	32	♀	Acute bronchitis	1600×10							15	12	5.5	4	13	26			5.0	3.9
"	S.S.	67	♀	Cholangitis	1600×33	17400	10200	84	79	+	−	10	16			144	150	48	55	48	45
"	Y.Y.	27	♂	Lung cancer + Mixed infection	1600×8	6900	9700														
"	M.O.	64	♂	Lung cancer + Mixed infection	1600×38	11800	21500	72	88	−	−	19	28			42	16	15	12		
Kumamoto Univ. (28)	Y.S.	55	♀	Pneumonia	1200×32	10450	6900					17	18								
"	T.I.	59	♂	Lung abscess	1600×24									2.8	3.0	78	34	114	33	6.9	7.2
"	M.G.	71	♂	Lung abscess	1200×26									0.7	0.7	18	28	9	18	8.5	10.2

[a] Before.   [b] After.

7. Josamycin as resistance non-inducing macrolide

We have explained thus far the characteristics and properties of josamycin. Josamycin was shown to be as effective as erythromycin in clinical trials. Further, clinical studies showed it to be suited for out-patient or prolonged medication. Relatively high tissue affinity resulted in high josamycin levels in the lungs and peripheral tissues, which contributed to excellent effects in respiratory and other suppurative infections. Its easy metabolism in the body has led josamycin to be regarded as a remedy showing minimum incidence of mild side effects.

However, the most conspicuous characteristic of josamycin is that it does not induce macrolide resistance in staphylococci. This is the point in which josamycin surpasses erythromycin. Josamycin can be regarded as a "first choice macrolide" as illustrated below.

In antibiotic therapy starting from penicillin, many formerly threatening pathogens are being eradicated, but staphylococci and some gram-negative bacteria have appeared as the "élite of the evil." Nowadays, tuberculosis, pneumonia or typhoid are no longer regarded as terrible diseases. Taking their place, gram-negative and staphylococcal infections appear to annoy us from the most frequent incidence and refractoriness. S. Mitsuhashi, professor of Microbiology, Gunma University, pointed out that "The leading role has been usurped."

Under circumstances of severe attack with antibiotics, only those mutants which have got genetic factors permitting them to develop resistance to antibiotics will be selected and survive. When such genetic factors can infect other individuals of the same species, the tribe of bacteria will spread and hold sway as the fittest after natural selection. Such a condition obtains with the staphylococci and the gram-negative bacteria. In the latter, the R factor transmits resistance to several drugs simultaneously among *Enterobacteriaceae*, not only among cells of the same species, but also from one species to another, from *E. coli* to *Shigella flexneri*, for example. In *S. aureus*, phages play the same role in transduction of multiple-resistant genes. By this infection-like spread of multiple resistance among staphylococci, bacterial populations resistant to tetracycline, penicillin, streptomycin and sulfa drugs, or to 2 or 3 of these, prevail nowadays, and gain increasing clinical importance. Thus, macrolide antibiotics have been in wide use for suppression of these cocci.

TABLE XXXIII
Classification of Macrolide-Resistant *S. aureus* (Mitsuhashi *et al.* (52))

		Pattern of resistance	
Group	Inducer	Before induction	After induction
Group A (constitutive)	—	EM,OL,LM,SPM,JM,(LCM)	EM,OL,LM,SPM,JM,(LCM)
Group B (inducible)	EM,OL	EM,OL	EM,OL,LM,SPM,JM,(LCM)
Group C (inducible)	EM	EM	EM,OL,LM,SPM,JM,(LCM)

With the beginning of mass production and mass use of erythromycin, many staphylococci resistant to that drug were isolated and they now amount to 30 or 40 percent of all strains of staphylococci isolated from clinical sources. As stated elsewhere in this monograph, S. Mitsuhashi classified these erythromycin-resistant *S. aureus* into 3 groups. Table XXXIII shows the classification. Among them, Group A cocci are those constitutive mutants showing high resistance of more than 800 mcg/ml to all the macrolides including erythromycin, oleandomycin, leucomycin, spiramycin and josamycin and in most cases to lincomycin also. Against these cocci, all the macrolides including erythromycin and josamycin have proven ineffective. On the other hand, Groups B and C cocci show inducible macrolide resistance. They are isolated as erythromycin-resistant strains, but they are sensitive to josamycin, leucomycin, spiramycin and carbomycin. Macrolide resistance can be induced, however, when they come in contact with subinhibotory concentrations of erythromycin in as small an amount as 0.1 mcg/ml for a short time (with erythromycin or oleandomycin in the case of Group B). Erythromycin or oleandomycin combines to inactivate repressors which suppress the action of genes controlling macrolide resistance. Thus the resistance gene is brought into operation and there appears the same all-macrolide resistance as seen in Group A. Josamycin does not manifest such an action and therefore is effective in Groups B and C infections except when erythromycin is used concomitantly.

According to studies by S. Mitsuhashi and by others, macrolide antibiotics were shown to be separated into 2 groups, the resistance inducing and resistance non-inducing types, as seen in Figs. 29 and 30. Erythromycin is an effective inducer and oleandomycin is

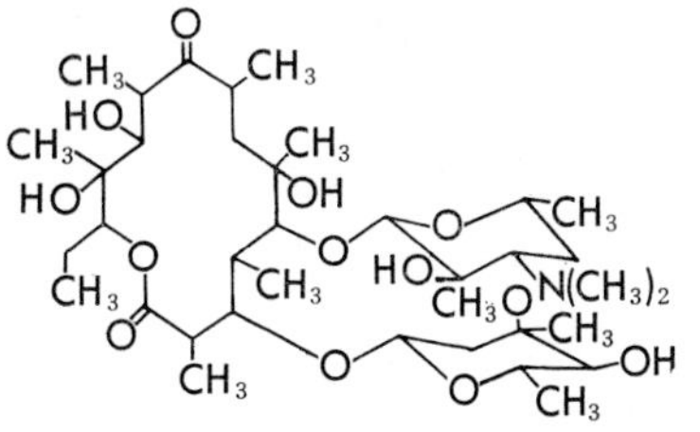

Erythromycin A (52,63)

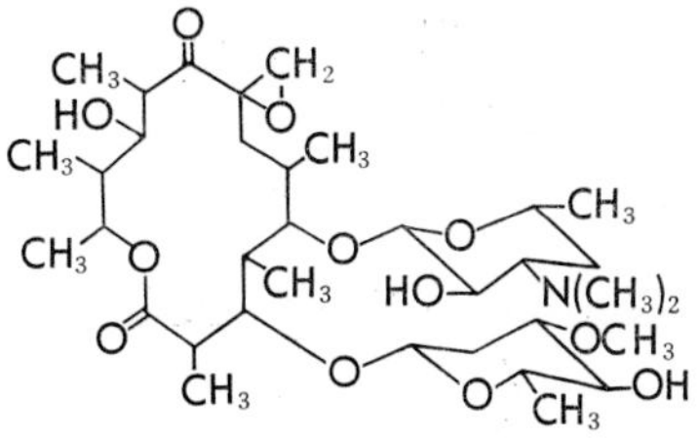

Oleandomycin (52,63)

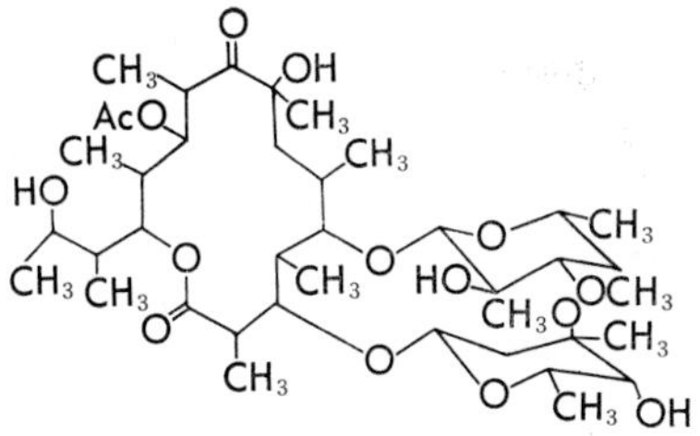

Kujimycin A (64)

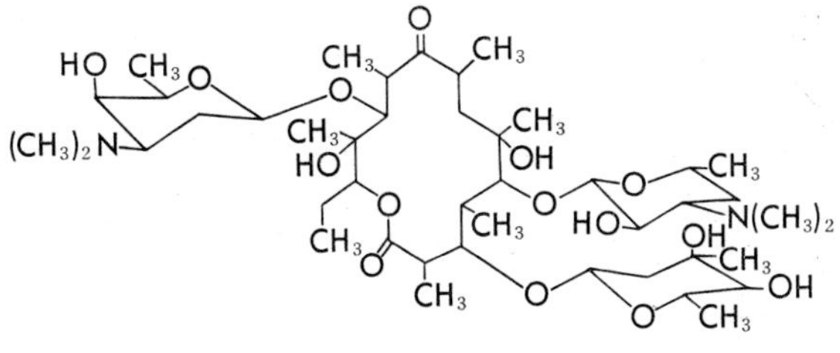

Megalomicin A (65)

Fig. 29. Macrolides of resistance inducing type.

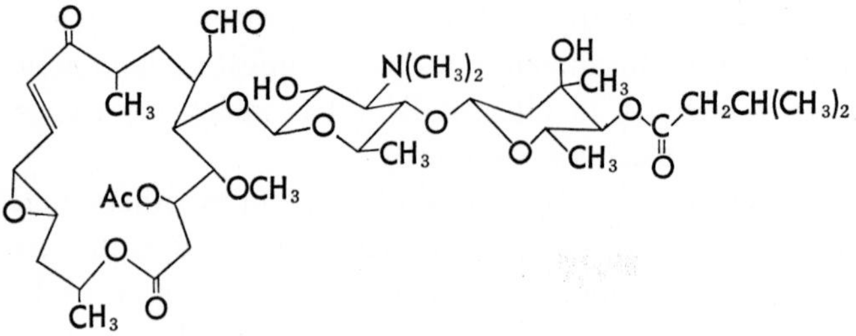

Carbomycin A (Magnamycin A) (63)

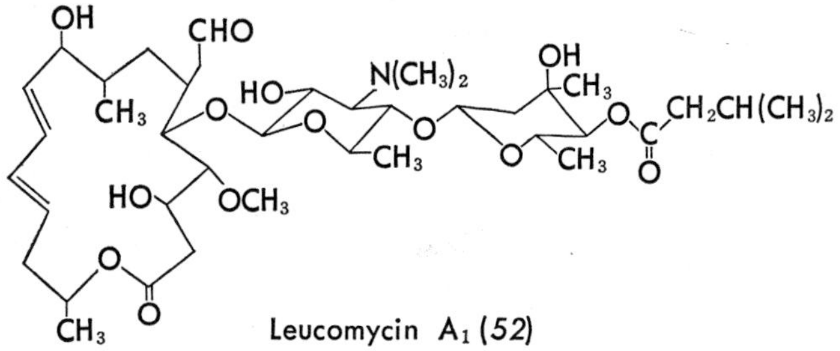

Leucomycin A₁ (52)

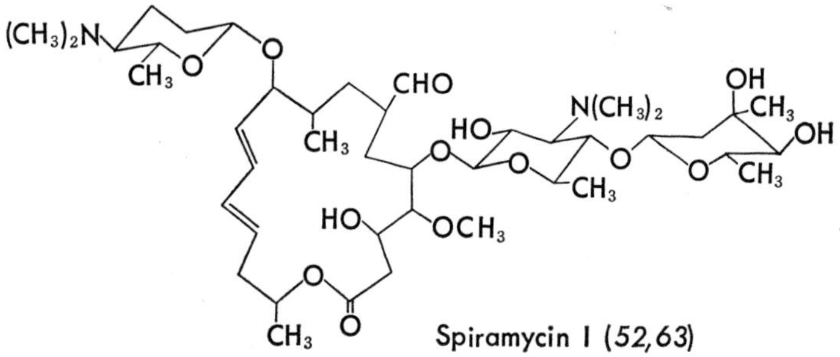

Spiramycin I (52,63)

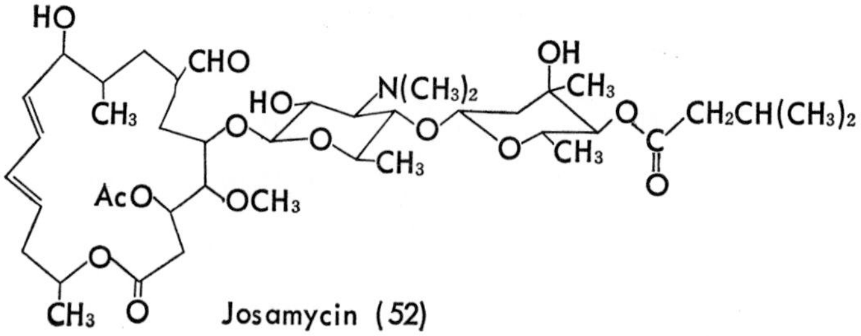

Josamycin (52)

Fig. 30.   Macrolides of resistance non-inducing type.

a less effective one (*52, 63*). Recently kujimycin has been shown to be a potent inducer (*64*), which has a des-acetyl lankamycin structure. Further, megalomicin was confirmed by S. Mitsuhashi to be a more potent inducer than erythromycin (*65*). On the other hand, josamycin (*52*), leucomycin (*52*), spiramycin (*25, 63*) and carbomycin (*63*) are all among those that do not induce macrolide resistance. As seen from Figs. 29 and 30, these two groups have definite structural differences. The most prominent characteristic of non-resistance induction seems to be chain formation of 2 sugars, dimethylamino sugar and neutral sugar, which may provide some steric hindrance on attachment to the enzyme surface. Existence of an aldehyde group may also play some role.

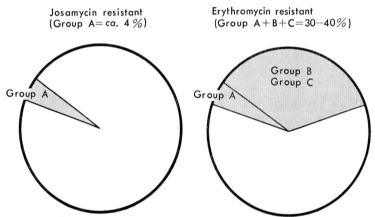

Fig. 31.   Frequency distribution of macrolide-resistant staphylococci.

The next important problem is the frequency at which these mutants occur. From an epidemiological survey of clinical isolates collected by the "Resistant Staphylococci Research Group" of the Japan Society of Chemotherapy, S. Mitsuhashi showed that Group A cocci amounted from 5 to 10 percent of all erythromycin-resistant strains. The remainder consisted of Groups C and B, the latter being few in number. Figure 31 illustrates this. Similar conditions in the United States were confirmed by S. Mitsuhashi on erythromycin-resistant staphylococci supplied by H. D. Isenberg, Long Island Jewish Hospital, New York. Among randomly selected erythromycin-resistant clinical isolates, 13.4 percent belonged to Group A and 86.6 percent to Group C as presented in Table XXXIV.

As a result of the mass use of erythromycin, incidence of many erythromycin-resistant cocci has brought about clinically troublesome problems. However, most of them belong to Groups B and C, as shown in Fig. 31. Group A cocci are less than 10 percent of erythromycin-resistant strains, that is, only less than 4 percent of total staphylococcal isolates from clinical sources. Thus josamycin is effective in all staphylococcal infections except those less than 4 percent caused by Group A.

TABLE XXXIV
Resistance to Macrolide Antibiotics in *S. aureus* Isolated in the United States (52)

Group	No. of strains	Drug resistance (mcg/ml)		
		EM	OL	LM
A	10	12.5<	12.5<	12.5<
C	65	6.25	0.8	0.4–1.6

Thus far josamycin has been shown effective against Group C cocci which constitute the majority of erythromycin-resistant *S. aureus*. In these cocci, erythromycin induces macrolide resistance, but josamycin does not. We should like to examine this fact through laboratory and clinical results.

Table XXXV shows MIC distribution of macrolides in 120 *S. aureus* strains, in which sensitivity to 5 macrolides had been assayed simultaneously on the same strain among 1,316 isolates surveyed at the "Josamycin Symposium" of the Japan Society of Chemotherapy, 1968 (*cf.* Table VI and Fig. 7). As seen from the column of not less than 100 mcg/ml, josamycin was found effec-

TABLE XXXV
MIC Distribution of Macrolides in Clinical Isolates of *S. aureus* (120 strains)

	MIC (mcg/ml)									
	≤0.2	0.4	0.8	1.6	3.2	6.3	12.5	25	50	100≤
JM	......	2	29	49	8	....		6	6	20
EM	28	34	4	....	1	2	1	....	5	45
OM	......	3	17	17	22	18	2	2	1	38
LM	1	3	22	53	8	....				33
SPM	......	1	3	32	22	17	4	2	1	38

tive against half of the strains showing erythromycin or oleandomycin resistance. However, some discrepancy is observed between
this result and the above-mentioned finding of S. Mitsuhashi.
Such a discrepancy has been found between the work of S. Mitsuhashi and of hospital laboratories. Group C cocci used to show
variable results under varying cultural conditions such as inoculum
size or incubation time. In Table XXXVI, such an example is given
for a Group C S. aureus, the B 294 strain. To avoid this variation,
S. Mitsuhashi used plates containing subinhibitory concentrations
of erythromycin as inducer. Only by such methods may reliable
results be obtained on the Group C strains.

TABLE XXXVI
Growth of S. aureus Strain B 294 on Plate Containing Josamycin or Erythromycin[†]

Drug	Medium	Incubation (hr)	Growth on plate containing (mcg/ml)									
			100	50	25	12.5	6.25	3.13	1.57	0.78	0.39	0.19
JM	Nutrient agar	18	—	—	—	—	—	—	—	+	+	+
		24	—	—	—	—	—	—	—	+	+	+
	Tellurite glycine agar	18	—	—	—	—	—	—	—	—	—	+
		24	—	—	—	—	—	—	—	—	+	+
EM	Nutrient agar	18	—	—	—	—	+	+	+	+	+	+
		24	+	+	+	+	+	+	+	+	+	+
	Tellurite glycine agar	18	—	—	—	—	—	—	—	—	+	+
		24	+	+	+	+	+	+	+	+	+	+

† Nutrient agar (pH 7.2) and Tellurite-Glycine Agar "Eiken" for selective isolation
of coagulase-positive staphylococci (0.02% K_2TeO_3, 1% glycine, pH 7.2) containing each antibiotic were inoculated with a loopful of overnight nutrient broth
culture; incubated at 37°C.

Photograph 4 illustrates resistance induction in the same Group
C coccus, B 294 strain. In the course of ordinary antibiotic disc
method practice, a josamycin disc was placed between oleandomycin and erythromycin discs as shown in the photograph. After
overnight incubation, the inhibitory zone of josamycin was not
affected by an oleandomycin disc placed on the left side. But on
the right side, the josamycin zone waned markedly as a result of
resistance induction caused by an erythromycin disc. Thus the
Group C cocci are detected easily without the use of extra materials.

This method is recommended to clinical laboratories as convenient routine practice.

Induction of macrolide resistance was also confirmed in animals. Mice were infected intraperitoneally with the Group C

TABLE XXXVII

Treatment of Murine Infection with *S. aureus* Strain B 294 Belonging to Group C Inducible for Macrolide Resistance[†]

Drug	Dosis (mg/kg)	Observation after 72 hr	Bacterial growth on plate with		
			none	JM 6.25	EM 100 (mcg/ml)
EM	200×3	● ● ● ● ○	+	+	+
	100×3	● ● ● ○ ○	+	+	+
JM	200×3	○ ○ ○ ○ ○	+	−	−
	100×3	● ○ ○ ○ ○	+	−	−
Control		● ● ● ● ●	+	−	±
		● ● ● ● ○			

† Male ddN mice were infected intraperitoneally with 5 MLD (with mucin); treated orally at 2 hr before, 1 and 4 hr after infection; heart blood collected at 72nd hour was streaked on the plate containing josamycin or erythromycin. ○, alive; ●, dead mouse.

staphylococcus, B 294 strain, and 3 medications with an interval of 3 hr were started from 2 hr before instead of immediately after the infection. The results obtained are shown in Table XXXVII. Two hours after the first medication, the erythromycin level in the peritoneal cavity seemed ready for maximum induction of macrolide resistance. Thus, inoculated staphylococci became resistant to erythromycin at more than 100 mcg/ml and also to josamycin as indicated in the columns of isolation study from heart blood. As a result, the resistant cocci killed the animals. However, in the case of josamycin, no resistance was induced and isolated cocci were sensitive to both josamycin and erythromycin. As a matter of course, josamycin cured the animals.

These results clearly show that erythromycin should not be used in Group C infections. In some part of the body or at some time after medication, erythromycin will come down to levels suitable for resistance induction, and refractory relapse will be brought about by resistance-induced populations.

The next instance is a case with a Group C coccus infection and treatment with josamycin (45). The patient was a 40-year-old woman suffering from refractory empyema with a chest sinus complication after tuberculous pneumonectomy. Right pneumonectomy and thoracoplasty had been performed in the preceding year. In spite of massive use of kanamycin, tetracycline and penicillin, the operation was unsuccessful and without primary healing. The operation wound ruptured, resulting in a chest sinus and empyema.

TABLE XXXVIII
MIC and Effect in Subcutaneous Infection in Mice (10)[†]
A. Minimum inhibitory concentration (mcg/ml)

Drug	S. aureus				
	226	Kogure	Smith	209P	Terajima
PC	>400	12.5			
SM	100	>100	0.39	0.39	0.39
KM	0.78	> 50	0.39	0.39	0.39
CP	12.5	50	12.5	6.25	12.5
TC	100	>200			
EM	0.39	100	0.19	0.09	0.19
JM	0.78	0.78	0.39	0.39	0.78

B. Treatment of subcutaneous infection with S. aureus Kogure strain (Group C inducible for macrolide resistance)

Drug	Dose (mg/kg)	Abscess formation		
CP	500	+	+	+
	250	+	+	+
	100	+	+	+
EM	200	+	−	−
	100	+	+	+
	50	+	+	+
JM	200	−	−	−
	100	−	−	−
	50	−	−	−
Control		++	++	++ −

† *Staphylococcus aureus* Kogure strain was isolated from an empyema patient at Tokyo National Chest Hospital; coagulase (+), protease (−), α-hemolysin (+), inducible resistant; B: male ddN mice were infected subcutaneously with 10^9 cells; treated orally immediately after infection.

Thus, the present operation was conducted by K. Yoshimura at Tokyo National Chest Hospital.

Staphylococcus aureus Kogure strain was isolated from the pus of the patient, and was found to belong to the Group C, showing MIC levels as indicated in Table XXXVIII. Kogure strain was resistant to penicillin, streptomycin, kanamycin, chloramphenicol, tetracycline and also to erythromycin, but was sensitive to josamycin. An animal experiment with this strain is also given in the same table. In accord with the *in vitro* results, abscesses formed with chloramphenicol or erythromycin. But no abscesses formed with the use of josamycin.

In thoracic operations, a requisite for healing is the use of at least one antibiotic effective against suppurative pathogens. Other-

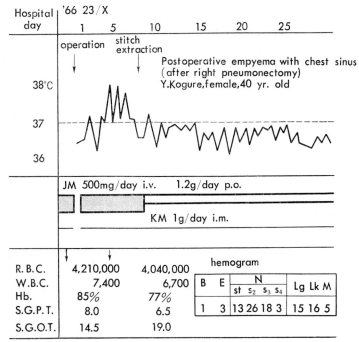

Fig. 32. Treatment of Gronp C staphylococcal refractory empyema with chest sinus (Yoshimura (45)). Pathogen isolated: *S. aureus* Kogure strain Group C inducible for macrolide resistance, coagulase (+), protease (−), α-hemolysin (+), sensitive to JM; resistant to PC, SM, KM, CP, TC, EM.

wise, the operation wounds undergo no primary healing. Remittent fever continues and the wounds rupture again resulting in chest sinus and refractory empyema.

Five hundred mg per day of josamycin was given the patient intravenously for 8 days starting from the day before operation, and oral administration of 1.2 g per day followed for 30 days. As seen from the protocol in Fig. 32, remittent fever disappeared in a few days and no wound rupture occurred after stitch extraction. The wounds underwent primary healing without any side effects or change in liver functions (Fig. 33). The patient suffered from no more relapses after five years and now works at home.

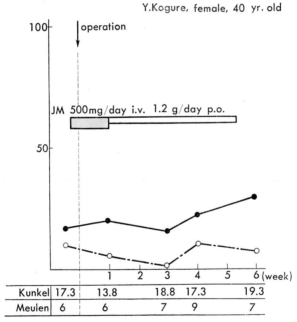

Fig. 33.   Josamycin treatment and liver functions (Yoshimura (45)).
●, GOT; ○, GPT.

Besides the above-mentioned, other results in confirmed Group C infections are being accumulated. At the otological clinic of Nagoya University, A. Ito cured 4 cases of acute and chronic otitis media caused by Group C cocci with josamycin. Dosage was 600 to 1,200 mg per day for 7 days by oral administration (66).

These results indicate that josamycin does not induce macrolide resistance in the Group C staphylococci which constitute the majority of erythromycin-resistant strains. This was confirmed by *in vitro* tests as well as *in vivo* and clinical studies. Thus josamycin was shown useful for the treatment of most erythromycin-resistant staphylococcal infections.

8. Conclusions

A new macrolide antibiotic, josamycin was found from culture fluids of *S. narbonensis* var. *josamyceticus* nov. var. collected in Shikoku, Japan.

Josamycin showed strong antimicrobial activity against gram-positive bacteria and mycoplasmas. It equalled or slightly surpassed *in vivo* activity of erythromycin in protection of subcutaneous staphylococcal infections in mice.

In clinical studies, josamycin was confirmed to be as effective as erythromycin, giving excellent results in the treatment of respiratory and suppurative infections.

Josamycin has been judged through clinical studies to be a safe remedy for outpatient treatment or prolonged medication. Causing few gastrointestinal disturbances, it could be administered to patients showing low chloramphenicol tolerability. No sign of hepatic toxicity was detected even after prolonged administration of 6 months in rats or of more than 1 month in human patients.

Josamycin shows relatively high tissue affinity and easy metabolism in the body.

The relatively high tissue affinity results in high josamycin levels in the lungs and peripheral tissues contributing to high effectiveness in respiratory and suppurative infections.

Josamycin is readily metabolized and inactivated in the body, especially in the liver. This easy inactivation produces few side effects.

One of josamycin's characteristics is its ability not to induce macrolide resistance in staphylococci. In this way josamycin surpasses erythromycin in effectiveness.

After wide scale use of erythromycin, more than 30 percent of staphylococci became resistant to erythromycin. Josamycin is effective against most of them. It does not induce macrolide resistance in Mitsuhashi's Group C staphylococci which constitute the majority of erythromycin-resistant clinical isolates. This fact was confirmed by *in vitro* as well as *in vivo* and clinical studies.

REFERENCES

1 Osono, T., Oka, Y., Watanabe, S., Numazaki, Y., Moriyama, K., Ishida, H., Suzaki, K., Okami, Y., and Umezawa, H. 1967. A new antibiotic, josamycin. I. Isolation and physico-chemical characteristics. *J. Antibiotics, Ser. A*, **20** (3), 174–180.

2 Nitta, K., Yano, K., Miyamoto, F., Hasegawa, Y., Sato, T., Kamoto, N., and Matsumoto, S. 1967. A new antibiotic, josamycin. II. Biological studies. *J. Antibiotics, Ser. A*, **20** (3), 181–187.

3 Umezawa, H., and Osono, T. 1964. Processes for the production of josamycin, a new antibiotic. Japan Patent No. 525, 633 (Jap. Pat. Pub. 21759/66, published on Dec. 19, 1966; filed on June 9, 1964)

4 Osono, T., Yano, K., Miyamoto, F., Watanabe, S., Ishida, H., Hasegawa, Y., Sonezaki, I., Sato, T., and Takahashi, I. 1969. A new antibiotic, josamycin. III. Bacteriological studies, protection against bacterial infections, and absorption, distribution, excretion and metabolism. *Japan. J. Antibiotics*, **22** (2), 159–172.

5 Murata, M., Goto, A., Hamashima, K., and Kawamura, A., Jr. 1969. A new antibiotic, josamycin. IV. Effect on *Rickettsia orientalis* and *Miyagawanella psittaci. Japan. J. Antibiotics*, **22** (2), 173–177.

6 Kuriaki, K., Miki, H., Sejima, Y., Shibata, M., Ida, H., Okazaki, M., and Hashimoto, K. 1969. A new antibiotic, josamycin. V. Studies on toxicity of josamycin. *Japan. J. Antibiotics*, **22** (3), 219–225.

7 Kuriaki, K., Sado, T., Sano, K., Sasaki, H., and Shiobara, Y. 1969. A new antibiotic, josamycin. VI. Absorption and distribution of josamycin. *Japan. J. Antibiotics*, **22** (3), 226–231.

8 Kuriaki, K., Nozaki, Y., Ida, H., Kagami, S., and Odani, Y. 1969. A new antibiotic, josamycin. VII. Studies on pharmacology. *Japan. J. Antibiotics.*, **22** (3), 232–241.

9 Hazato, H., Yamamoto, T., Tadokoro, I., Kawamura, A. Jr., Suzuki, K., Nishioka, K., Okugi, M., Sakamoto, M., Hashimoto, K., Saiki, S., and Sakai, Y. 1969. A new antibiotic, josamycin. VIII. Six month chronic toxicity test on josamycin in rats. *Japan. J. Antibiotics*, **22** (3), 242–253.

10   Osono, T., and Yano, K. 1967. Antibiotics screening using subcutaneous infection in mice. *Modern Media*, **13** (4), 121–126.
11   Fukushima, K., Mitsuhashi, S., Saito, A., Miki, F., Sakai, K., Aratani, H., Nakazawa, S., Takada, M., Goto, M., Hatano, H., Hara, S., and Iwasawa, T. 1969. Proceedings of "Josamycin symposium" at the 16th Annual Meeting of Japan Society of Chemotherapy, Tokyo, May 1968. *Chemotherapy*, **17** (1), 21–28.
12   Mitsuhashi, S. 1969. Laboratory evaluation of josamycin. *Chemotherapy*, **17** (4), 567–571.
13   Kosakai, N., Igari, J., and Oguri, T. 1969. Susceptibility of recently isolated pathogens to josamycin, erythromycin and lincomycin. *Chemotherapy*, **17** (4), 572–575.
14   Nakazawa, S., Ishiyama, M., Otsuki, M., Kakita, K., and Kimura, K. 1969. Bacteriological study on josamycin. *Chemotherapy*, **17** (4), 576–579.
15   Egashira, T., Seki, M., Takashima, H., Arahara, T., Toyoshima, Y., Kawahara, Y., Tokuchi, Y., and Nakano, M. 1969. Pharmacological studies on josamycin, a new antibiotic. I. Comparative studies on the cardiovascular actions of josamycin and macrolide antibiotics. *Chemotherapy*, **17** (4), 580–589.
16   Egashira, T., Seki, M., Yamada, M., Tokuchi, Y., and Nakano, M. 1969. Pharmacological studies on josamycin, a new antibiotic II. Comparative studies on the effect of josamycin and macrolide antibiotics on the smooth muscle, peripheral motor nerve. MAO and ChE activities. *Chemotherapy*, **17** (4), 590–596.
17   Aratani, H., Yamanaka, Y., Ohnishi, R., and Kohno, S. 1969. Pharmacological studies on josamycin, a new antibiotic. *Chemotherapy*, **17** (4), 597–603.
18   Mashimo, K., Kato, Y., Saito, A., Tomisawa, M., Sakuraba, T., Matsumoto, Y., Matsui, K., Chiba, A., Nakayama, I., and Kojima, A. 1969. Laboratory and clinical studies on josamycin. *Chemotherapy*, **17** (4), 604–609.
19   Ueda, Y., Matsumoto, F., Nakamura, N., Saito, A., Noda, K., Omori, M., Furuya, C., and Nakamura, Y. 1969. Study on josamycin. *Chemotherapy*, **17** (4), 610–613.
20   Koya, G., and Misawa, H. 1969. Clinical studies on josamycin in the field of internal medicine. *Chemotherapy*, **17** (4), 614–617.
21   Gomi, J., Aoyagi, T., Tomioka, H., Oana, M., Yoshimura, Y., Mitsuno, Y., Kawai, K., Yamada, Y., Yamada, Y., and Takeshita, T. 1969. Laboratory and clinical studies on josamycin. *Chemotherapy*, **17** (4), 618–620.
22   Kitamoto, O., Fukaya, K., and Tomori, G. 1969. Studies on pharmacokinetics of antimicrobial agents: studies on josamycin. *Chemotherapy*, **17**, (4), 621–625.

23   Nakagawa, K., Shoji, F., Kabe, J., and Yokozawa, M. 1969. Clinical studies on josamycin, a new macrolide antibiotic. *Chemotherapy*, **17** (4), 626–629.
24   Katsu, M., Fujimori, I., Ogawa, J., Osako, R., Ito, S., and Shimada, S. 1969. Fundamental and clinical studies of josamycin. *Chemotherapy*, **17** (4), 630–635.
25   Ito, A., Hasegawa, H., Kurihara, M., and Tarao, K. 1969. Fundamental and clinical studies on josamycin. *Chemotherapy*, **17** (4), 636–641.
26   Miki, F., Higashi, T., Iwasaki, T., Akao, M., Ozaki, T., Sugiyama, H., and Hada, M. 1969. Laboratory and clinical studies on josamycin. *Chemotherapy*, **17** (4), 642–644.
27   Ohkubo, H., Fujimoto, Y., Okamoto, Y., Tsukada, J., and Makino, J. 1969. Basic and clinical studies on josamycin. *Chemotherapy*, **17** (4), 645–649.
28   Soejima, R., Tanaka, S., Notsute, H., Fukuda, Y., Seki, Y., and Hayashi, S. 1969. Laboratory and clinical studies on josamycin. *Chemotherapy*, **17** (4), 650–653.
29   Fujii, R., Ichihashi, H., Konno, M., Uno, S., Takeshita, N., Okada, K., Hachimori, K, and Ubukata, K. 1969. Fundamental and clinical studies of josamycin in pediatrics field. *Chemotherapy*, **17** (4), 654–658.
30   Ichihashi, Y., Oikawa, T., Sakai, M., and Kikuchi, T. 1969. Clinico-laboratory experience with josamycin. *Chemotherapy*, **17** (4), 659–663.
31   Nakazawa, S., Oka, S., Ishihara, K., Sato, H., and Hirasawa, Y. 1969. Laboratory and clinical evaluation of josamycin in pediatrics field. *Chemotherapy*, **17** (4), 664–672.
32   Kawamura, T., Tomizawa, T., Kobayashi, A., and Takahashi, H. 1969. Clinical studies on josamycin in dermatological field. *Chemotherapy*, **17** (4), 673–675.
33   Tanioku, K., Arata, J., Tokumaru, S., Miyoshi, K., and Kodama, H. 1969. Use of josamycin in the field of dermatology. *Chemotherapy*, **17** (4), 676–678.
34   Goto, M., and Muramoto, S. 1969. Josamycin in the treatment of skin infectious diseases and experimental rabbit syphiloma. *Chemetherapy*, **17** (4), 679–684.
35   Ishiyama, S., Sakabe, T., Takahashi, U., Kasagi, T., Nagasaki, Y., Yamagishi, M., Kawakami, I., Nakayama, I., Iwai, S., Iwamoto, H., Oshima, T., and Takatori, M. 1969. Josamycin in surgical infections. *Chemotherapy*, **17** (4), 685–689.
36   Shibata, K., Ito, T., Watanabe, S., and Inukai, A. 1969. A laboratory study on josamycin and its clinical use in the field of surgery. *Chemotherapy*, **17** (4), 690–693.
37   Kawashima, M., Sakai, K., and Nakao, J. 1969. Laboratory and clinical evaluation of josamycin. *Chemotherapy*, **17** (4), 694–700.

38   Ishigami, J., Hara, S., Fukuda, Y., and Hayami, S. 1969. Clinical application of josamycin in urological field. *Chemotherapy*, **17** (4), 701–704.

39   Namba, K. 1969. Clinical studies of josamycin. *Chemotherapy*, **17** (4), 705–708.

40   Takada, M., Mori, S., and Sano, S. 1969. Experimental and clinical studies on josamycin in the gynecological field. *Chemotherapy*, **17** (4), 709–716.

41   Tokuda, G., Yuasa, M., Mihara, S., and Kanao, M. 1969. On the study of josamycin in obstetric and gynecological fields. *Chemotherapy*, **17** (4), 717–720.

42   Iwasawa, T., and Kido, T. 1969. The clinical and experimental studies on josamycin. *Chemotherapy*, **17** (4), 721–731.

43   Hatano, H., Hariu, A., Kayaba, T., Saito, T., Takahashi, N., and Imai, K. 1969. Use of josamycin in ophthalmology. *Chemotherapy*, **17** (4), 732–738.

44   Mikuni, M., Ohishi, M., Suda, S., Imai, M., and Takahashi, T. 1969. Ophthalmic use of josamycin. *Chemotherapy*, **17** (4), 739–745.

45   Yoshimura, K. Experience in josamycin treatment of refractory complications in lung surgery, in preparation.

46   Stahl, E. 1956. Dünnschicht-Chromatographie. *Pharmazie*, **11**, 633–637; 1958. Dünnschicht-Chromatographie. II. Standardisierung, Sichtbarmachung, Dokumentation und Anwendung. *Chemiker-Ztg.*, **82**, 323–329; Stahl, E. 1962. *In* "Dünnschicht-Chromitographie," Springer-Verlag-Germany.

47   Tadokoro, I. 1967. Subcutaneous infection with staphylococci in mice. *Modern Media*, **13** (4), 110–118.

48   Omura, S., Ogura, H., and Hata, T. 1967. The chemistry of the leucomycins. I. Partial structure of leucomycin A_3. *Tetrahedron Letters*, (7), 609–613; 1967. II. Structure and stereochemistry of leucomycin A_3, *Tetrahedron Letters*, (14), 1267–1271. (presented at 151. Bimonthly Meeting of Japan Antibiot. Research Assoc., Sept. 22, 1966)

49   Omura, S., Katagiri, M., Umezawa, I., Komiyama, K., Maekawa, T,. Sekikawa, K., Matsumae, A., and Hata, T. 1968. Structure-biological activities relationships among leucomycins and their derivatives. *J. Antibiotics*, **21** (9), 532–538.

50   Ishiyama, S., Ueda, Y., Kuwabara, S., Kosakai, N., Koya, G., Konno, M., and Fujii, R. 1968. On the standardization of method for determination of minimum inhibitory concentrations. *Chemotherapy*, **16** (1), 98–99.

51   Nakazawa, S., Ono, H., Mekata, I., Gyoten, I., and Kubochi, J. 1969. Bacteriological study on clindamycin. *Chemotherapy*, **17** (5), 752–757.

52   Kono, M., Hashimoto, H., and Mitsuhashi, S. 1966. Drug resistance of staphylococci. III. Resistance to some macrolide antibiotics and inducible system. *Japan. J. Microbiol.*, **10** (1), 59–66; Kono, M., Kasuga, T., and

Mitsuhashi, S. 1966. IV. Resistance patterns to some macrolide antibiotics in *Staphylococcus aureus* isolated in the United States. *Japan. J. Microbiol.*, **10** (2), 109–113; Hashimoto, H., Oshima, H., and Mitsuhashi, S. 1968. IX. Inducible resistance to macrolide antibiotics in *Staphylococcus aureus. Japan. J. Microbiol.*, **12** (3), 321–327; Saito, T., Hashimoto, H., and Mitsuhashi, S. 1970. Macrolide resistance in *Staphylococcus aureus.* Isolation of a mutant in which leucomycin is an active inducer. *Japan. J. Microbiol.*, **14** (6), 473–478; Mitsuhashi, S. 1967. Epidemiological and genetical study of drug resistance in *Staphylococcus aureus* (review). *Japan. J. Microbiol.*, **11** (1), 49–68; Mitsuhashi, S., Mori, K., and Watanabe, K. 1970. Theoretical aspects of combined therapy. I. An application to the strains of staphylococci resistant to some macrolide antibiotics. *Chemotherapy*, **18** (3), 247–251.

53 Irwin, S. 1964. Drug screening and evaluation of new compounds in animals. *In* "Animal and Clinical Pharmacologic Techniques in Drug Evaluation," ed. by J. H. Nodine and P. E. Siegler, Year Book Medical Publishers, Chicago, p. 36–54.

54 Umezawa, H., Ishizuka, M., Hori, S., Chimura, H., and Takeuchi, T. 1968. The distribution of ³H-bleomycin in mouse tissue. *J. Antibiotics*, **21** (11), 638–642.

55 Mashimo, K., Kato, Y., Tanaka, K., and Matsui, K. 1968. Clinico-laboratory study on a new antibiotic, enduracidin, with special reference on the pharmacodynamic of the antibiotic. *Chemotherapy*, **16** (4), 523–529.

56 Welles, J. S., Anderson, R. C., and Chen, K. K. 1955. A metabolite of of erythromycin. *Antibiot. Annual—1954–1955*, 291–294.

57 Brodasky, T. F., Argoudelis, A. D., and Eble, T. E. 1968. The characterization and thin-layer chromatographic quantitation of the human metabolite of 7-deoxy-7(S)-chlorolincomycin (U-21, 251 F). *J. Antibiotics*, **21**, (5), 327–333.

58 Takahira, H., Kato, H., Sugiyama, N., Ishii, S., Haneda, T., Uzu, K,. Kumabe, K., and Kojima, R. 1966. Fundamental studies on acetyl spiramycin. *J. Antibiotics, Ser. B*, **19** (2), 95–100.

59 Furukawa, H. 1968. Studies on the metabolism of erythromycin base and its propionyl ester. *Chemotherapy*, **16** (6), 799–804.

60 Lee, C. C., Anderson, R. C., and Stephens, V. C. 1961. Further pharmacological studies on propionyl erythromycin ester lauryl sulfate. *Antibiot. and Chemoth.*, **11** (2), 110–117; Stephens, V. C., Pugh, C. T., Davis, N. E., Hoehn, M. M., Ralston, S., Sparks, M. C., and Thompkins, L. 1969. A study of the behavior of propionyl erythromycin in blood by a new chromatographic method. *J. Antibiotics*, **22** (11), 551–557.

61 Kato, R. 1968. *In* "Drug metabolism and drug effect," Chugai Igakusha,

Tokyo; 1965. The induction of drug-metabolizing enzymes in liver microsome. *Protein, Nucleic Acid and Enzyme*, **10** (9), 848–858; Gillette, J. R. 1963. Metabolism of drugs and other foreign compounds by enzymatic mechanisms. *Progress in Drug Research*, **6**, 11–73.

62   Osono, T., Abe, K., and Murakami, K. A new antibiotic, josamycin. IX. Metabolism of josamycin, in preparation.

63   Pattee, P. A., and Baldwin, J. N. 1962. Transduction of resistance to some macrolide antibiotics in *Staphylococcus aureus*. *J. Bacteriol.*, **84**, 1049–1055; Weaver, J. R., and Pattee, P. A. 1964. Inducible resistance to erythromycin in *Staphylococcus aureus*. *J. Bacteriol.*, **88**, 574–580.

64   Omura, S., Namiki, S., Shibata, M., Muro, T., and Sawada, J. 1970. On macrolide-resistance induction in staphylococci by neutral macrolides, kujimycins A and B. Proceedings of 23rd Conference of Kanto Branch of Japan. Bacteriol. Soc., June 25, 1970, Tokyo. *Japan. J. Bacteriol.*, **25** (12), 668–669.

65   Mitsuhashi, S., in preparation.

66   Ito, A, personal communication.

67   Osono, T. 1970. Studies on josamycin, a new antibiotic (review). *In* "Future Perspectives in Chemotherapy," University of Tokyo Press, Tokyo, p. 277–373.

68   Omura, S., Hironaka, Y., and Hata, T. 1970. Chemistry of leucomycin. IX. Identification of leucomycin A₃ with josamycin. *J. Antibiotics*, **23** (10), 511–513.

69   Fukushima, K. 1970. Clinical study on josamycin. *In* "Progress in Antimicrobial and Anticancer Chemotherapy (Proc. of 6th International Congress of Chemotherapy, Tokyo, 1969)," University of Tokyo Press, Tokyo, Vol. I, p. 750–754.

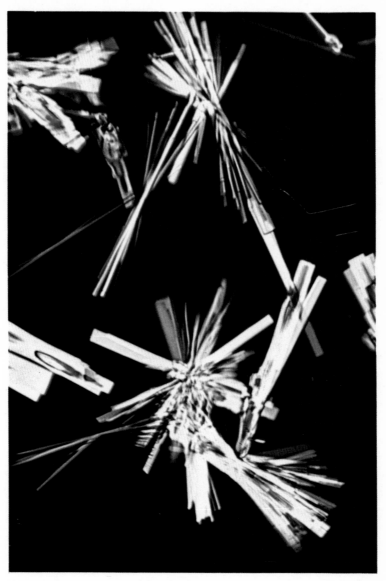

Photo 1.　Crystals of josamycin.

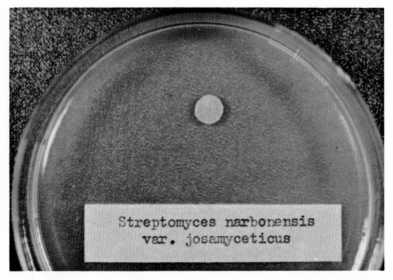

Photo 2. *Streptomyces narbonensis* var. *josamyceticus* (josamycin-producing organism).

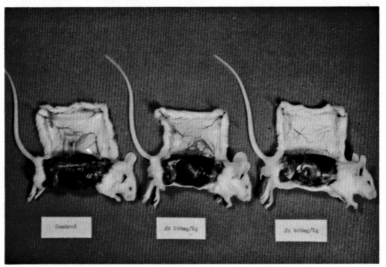

Photo 3. Effect of josamycin to subcutaneous staphylococcal infection in mice (oral administration).

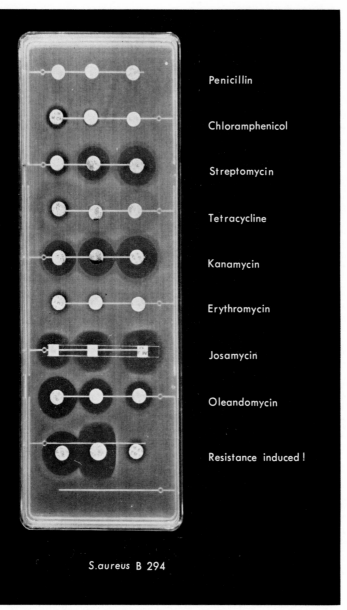

Penicillin

Chloramphenicol

Streptomycin

Tetracycline

Kanamycin

Erythromycin

Josamycin

Oleandomycin

Resistance induced!

S.aureus B 294

Photo 4. Inhibitory zones against *S. aureus* strain B 294 belonging to Group C inducible for macrolide resistance. Sensitivity discs containing antibiotics at three concentrations were placed on nutrient agar inoculated with 1% of overnight nutrient broth culture; incubated at 37°C for 16 hr.

II. ACTION AND RESISTANCE IN MACROLIDE ANTIBIOTICS AND LINCOMYCIN

THE CHEMISTRY AND CONFORMATION OF ERYTHROMYCIN

Thomas J. PERUN

Division of Experimental Therapy, Abbott Laboratories, North Chicago, Illinois, U.S.A.

Erythromycin (**1**) was not the first macrolide antibiotic discovered, nor was it the first to have its structure elucidated. It has become the most widely studied macrolide, however, because of its worldwide importance as a therapeutic agent against gram-positive bacteria and Mycoplasma. Chemical studies with erythromycin began with the structural elucidation (*20, 22, 27, 53, 61–63*) and continued with the determination of the relative and absolute configurations of its many asymmetric centers. Chemical modifications of erythromycin began before the configurational studies were completed but were given added impetus by the X-ray crystallographic determination of erythromycin A (*23*) and the configurational model proposed by Celmer (*5, 7*). The information obtained in the chemical studies along with the accumulated physical data obtained by spectroscopic studies ultimately led to the formulation of the solution conformation of the macrolide ring. Both the chemical modification studies and the conformational studies were helped greatly by the concurrent biosynthetic studies on erythromycin by Martin (38–40), which provided a number of novel macrolide structures amenable to chemical modification.

Structure and configuration

Erythromycin as elaborated in the fermentation broths of *Streptomyces erythreus* is a mixture of three closely related antibiotics, erythromycins A, B, and C. The major component produced by commercial high-yield strains is erythromycin A **(1a)**, the first component isolated, purified, and structurally defined. The second and third components isolated, erythromycins B **(1b)** and C **(1c)**, are less prevalent and the latter is present in only trace amounts.

1a R_1=H R_2=OH R_3=CH$_3$, 1b R_1=H R_2=H R_3=CH$_3$,
1c R_1=H R_2=OH R_3=H,   1d R_1=D-Rhodosamine
                                         R_2=OH R_3=H

Early studies on the erythromycin A molecule showed it to belong to a novel class of antibiotics containing a macrocyclic lactone ring to which were attached unique glycoside moieties. The presence of this macrocyclic lactone ring in erythromycin and other related antibiotics gave rise to the use of the term "macrolide" to describe an antibiotic belonging to this general class (67).

The glycosides were the first portions of the erythromycin molecule to be identified. It was found that erythromycins A and B both contained the same sugar moieties, desosamine **2** (a basic sugar) and cladinose **3a** (a neutral sugar) (8, 9, 20, 24). Both sugars were found to be 6-deoxypyranosides, with desosamine belonging to the D series (*25*), and cladinose being an L sugar (*26, 34*). The presence of a dimethylamino function on desosamine was responsible for its basic character. The most unusual feature of cladinose was the presence of a methyl group and a methoxyl attached to the same ring carbon.

CH_3-N-CH_3
HO.
HO   O CH_3

Desosamine 2

CH_3O CH_3
OH
HO   O CH_3

Cladinose 3a

HO CH_3
OH
HO   O CH_3

Mycarose 3b

Later it was found that erythromycin C contained desosamine and had the same aglycone present in erythromycin A (*63*). It differed only by the presence of the unmethylated neutral sugar mycarose, **3b** in place of cladinose (*27*). The anomeric configurations of the attached sugars have been determined by NMR (*4, 6, 23, 28*), molecular rotation (*4*), and X-ray crystallographic studies (*23*) to be β for desosamine and α in the case of cladinose. The regularity of β-D and α-L glycosidic linkages in the macrolide antibiotic series was recognized by Celmer (*4, 6*) as being an extension of Klyne's rule for glycosidic natural products (*51*).

Although it was recognized quite early that the aglycone portion of the erythromycins consisted of a large lactone ring containing a ketone function and numerous hydroxyl and methyl groups, the final structures were determined only after a lengthy series of chemical degradations by the Lilly investigators (*20, 22, 53, 61, 62*). Among the difficulties encountered in this work was the extreme lability of the aglycone system to acid or base treatment, preventing the isolation of the intact aglycone. The acid lability was overcome by the use of a dihydro derivative obtained by borohydride reduction of the ketone function. The presence of an alternating methyl and oxy functionality in the lactone ring system made determination of the specific location of degradative fragments somewhat difficult. This regular pattern of seven propionate-like units in the macrocyclic ring led to the recognition by Gerzon *et al.* (*22*) and by Woodward (*66*) of the existence of a "propionate rule" in the biogenesis of macrolide antibiotics.

The presence of 10 asymmetric centers in the erythromycin aglycone makes it theoretically possible to have over a thousand stereoisomeric combinations of carbons with the correct structural formula. The early degradative work by Gerzon *et al.* (*22*) and some by Djerassi *et al.* (*16*) identified the absolute configurations at C-8, C-10 and C-13, and the relative configurations of the C-2, C-3, C-4 unit. The total relative stereochemistry was obtained from the X-ray crystallographic study of erythromycin A hydro-iodide (*23*). This determination combined with the absolute con-figuration determined for C-8 (*16*) defines the total absolute con-figurations in the molecule. The result agrees with the configura-tional assignments predicted by Celmer (*5*). In his determination of the absolute configurations of aglycone carbons in the related macrolide antibiotic oleandomycin (*3*), Celmer noted a striking correspondence of stereochemistry for like asymmetric centers among the series of macrolide antibiotics whose configurational assignments had been partially determined. On the basis of a probable biogenetic similarity for all compounds belonging to the macrolide group, he proposed a configurational model which predicts the stereochemistry at each carbon in the macrocyclic lactones of all members of the series (*5*). The reliability of his configurational model has been complete in predicting the stereo-chemical assignments of all macrolide antibiotics so far determined.

Conformation of lactone ring

As biochemical and chemical modification studies began to pro-duce new erythromycins and erythromycin precursors, and mode of action studies began to determine the molecular events in the inhibition of protein synthesis by erythromycins (*37, 64*), knowl-edge of the three-dimensional shape of erythromycins in solution became increasingly important in attempting to explain some of the structure-activity relationships inherent in this family of derivatives.

Information about the conformation of the erythromycin molecule has been very useful in the determination of new erythromycin and erythronolide structures, and in the design of selective or specific chemical reactions for modification of these important compounds. There is some reason to speculate that the course of the biogenetic pathway leading to erythromycin is determined or controlled to some extent by the conformational requirements of such a large highly substituted ring system.

It is interesting to note the predominance of 14-membered and 16-membered ring systems among the known macrolide antibiotics (excluding the polyenes). In his determination of the conformations of macrocyclic hydrocarbons by the use of space-filling models (12), Dale has found that no hydrocarbon ring system from cycloheptane through cyclotridecane can exist in a strain-free conformation. This results from the fact that all ring sizes from 7 through 13 contain a number of internal interactions caused by intraannular (19) hydrogens attempting to occupy the same spatial positions in the "ideal" diamond-lattice arrangement of atoms.

Saunders (52) has reached the same conclusion using computer-determined conformations, but has noted that 10-membered ring systems can exist in a near-diamond-lattice arrangement by some distortion of the ring in order to reduce these "overlaps." Both the 14-membered and 16-membered hydrocarbon rings have one diamond-lattice conformation that contains no overlaps (52), although the 16-membered ring may prefer to exist in a non-diamond-lattice arrangement because of packing considerations. Presumably, the greater thermodynamic stability of 14- and 16-membered rings over that of smaller rings helps explain the preference for these two ring sizes among macrolide antibiotics. The presence of at least one double bond in the 16-membered macrolides probably confers greater stability to the conformation of this substituted ring system.

In some pioneering work on the conformation of the 14-membered macrolide oleandomycin, Celmer used the Dale diamond-lattice conformation of cyclotetradecane (4) as a model for the substituted ring system (7). Although there are 14 different theoretical modifications of the oleandomycin aglycone in this

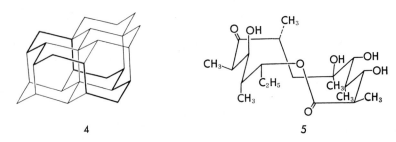

4   5

conformation (centrosymmetry reduces the number to seven), he found by using space-filling models that one modification appeared to be the most favorable because of the minimization of interactions from intraannular positioned substituents. This conformation can also be applied to the erythromycin aglycone because of the structural similarity and the configurational homogeneity. The resulting conformation for erythronolide B is shown as **5**.

In experimental studies of the conformation of erythronolide B **19** and its derivatives using nuclear magnetic resonance (*14, 15, 48–50*) and circular dichroism (*42*) techniques, it has been determined that the conformation, while very similar to that proposed by Celmer, is more closely related to the three-dimensional structure of erythromycin in the crystal state (*23*). Our proposed conformation is shown as **6**. The major points of difference between the previously proposed conformation **5** and the experimentally determined one are the orientations of the lactone function and the C-6 tertiary hydroxyl.

19   6

We have further proposed that the use of an alternate diamond-lattice arrangement of ring carbons (7) serves as a better conformational model for 14-membered ring macrolides (50). The theoretical conformation of erythronolide B using this alternate conformational model is shown as 8. In this conformation the lactone grouping is oriented correctly as it is shown in 6 and in the crystal structure. The presence of 1,3-diaxial interactions between the C-4, C-6 and C-8 methyls indicates that conformation 8 must not be the one with the lowest energy. In the Celmer model 5, the presence of the same interactions between methyls on C-4 and C-6 also indicates that there must be a better conformation which relieves these spatial interactions. A simple "upward" rotation of the C-6 atom in the conformational model 8 relieves these steric interactions and places the tertiary hydroxyl in a proximate relationship with the ketone at C-9 as shown in 6. The formation of a more stable arrangement of this highly substituted system presumably provides the driving force for deviation from the diamond-lattice arrangement.

7   8

Although this alternate conformational model is derived from the diamond-lattice arrangement of carbons, cyclotetradecane in this conformation would be thermodynamically less stable than in the diamond-lattice arrangement 4 because of the presence of "overlaps" at two spatial positions in the lattice (52). One of these overlaps is no longer possible in the case of the 14-membered macrolide lactones, because the presence of the lactone function removes the hydrogen involved in the overlap. The other overlap is removed when the C-6 to C-8 region is spatially repositioned into the conformation 6. It appears that because of the similarities in substitution patterns and stereochemistry among 14-membered macrolide rings this conformational model should provide an approximate solution to the conformation of other members of the series. Some evidence that this is correct in the case of lankamycin has been obtained in preliminary studies (R. S. Egan T. J. Perun, and J. R. Martin, unpublished results).

The nuclear magnetic resonance study of the erythromycin conformation was carried out with numerous derivatives of the aglycone erythronolide B. The variety of suitable derivatives obtained from chemical (47) and biogenetic studies (38–40) made it possible to carry out detailed analyses of this ring system on an HA-100 NMR spectrometer. The correspondence of coupling constants of nearly all identical proton combinations among the various derivatives indicated a conformational homogeneity throughout the series. Further evidence for a single stable conformation was obtained from NMR studies in solvents with differing polarity, and by variable temperature studies. The results showed an invariance of coupling constants under all these conditions.

The coupling constants were used to determine approximate vicinal proton dihedral angles using the Karplus equation (31), and the similarity of the experimental proton relationships to those present in a diamond-lattice arrangement was immediately apparent (48, 50). Even when compounds containing double bonds were included in the study, the coupling constants of protons in the saturated portion of the molecules did not change significantly (50). It has been shown that double bonds at the 6,7 and 10,11 positions can be accommodated easily by the conformation 6 because of the *trans* relationship of the eliminating groups and the production of no new internal interactions by the unsaturated grouping. The same circumstances presumably hold true in those macrolide antibiotics with naturally occurring double bonds.

Extension of the NMR studies to the parent antibiotics showed that the same proton relationships could be observed in these glycosidically substituted rings. This indicated that the conformation determined for the aglycone ring was the same in the complete molecule. The only coupling constant that was significantly different in the glycosides was that between protons on carbons 4 and 5. This was explained as due to the slight increase in the vicinal angle between H-4 and H-5, producing a relief in the interaction of the bulky sugar groups on C-3 and C-5. This change could be induced experimentally by the addition of other groups to the C-3 and C-5 ring hydroxyls (48).

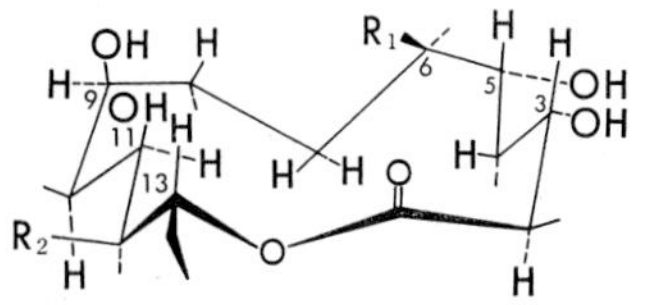

	R_1	R_2
9a	OH	H
9b	H	H
9c	OH	OH

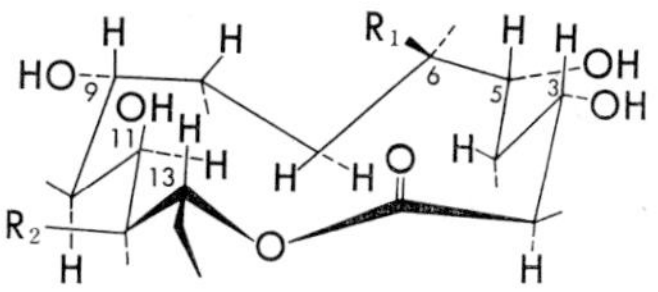

	R_1	R_2
10a	OH	H
10b	H	H

Another NMR technique which proved to be useful in the determination of substituent proximities in the macrolide ring was the aromatic solvent induced shift (ASIS) method as applied to hydroxylic compounds (13). This technique, which follows the chemical shift changes induced by solute-solvent association, proved to be most helpful with the 9-dihydroerythronolides 9 and 10, compounds obtained by sodium borohydride reduction of the ketone function (40, 49, 53, 62). Epimeric dihydro compounds

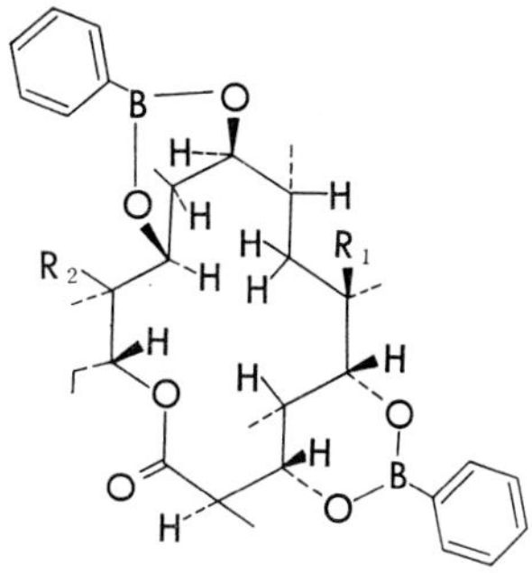

11

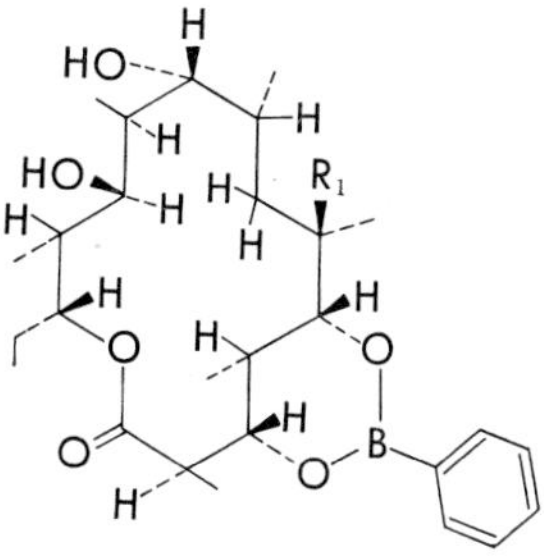

12

were obtained in the erythronolide B and 6-deoxyerythronolide B series whose stereochemistry at C-9 was determined (*14, 15, 49*) by comparison with 9S-dihydroerythronolide A, **9c**, a compound with a known configuration at C-9 (*4, 22*). The selective formation of cyclic esters **11** and **12** with benzeneboronic acid also proved to be very useful in the determination of relative configurations in this series of polyhydroxy compounds (*49*).

The preliminary conformational studies of these aglycone compounds by the two groups, while in substantial agreement, differed in their respective orientations of the C-11 hydroxyl group (*14, 15, 48*). The quasi-axial nature of this function was established by subsequent chemical, NMR, and circular dichroism studies (*42, 49, 50*). The preliminary communication also showed the lactone orientation as it was visualized in the Celmer conformation **5**. The current NMR techniques were not suitable for distinguishing between the two possible lactone orientations, although Demarco presented some preliminary evidence for the Celmer orientation from lactone carbonyl shielding effects (*14, 15*). Circular dichroism spectra are better suited for conformational studies of carbonyl functions, and we have obtained evidence from CD studies that the orientations of both the lactone and ketone carbonyls are oriented as shown in **6** (*42, 50*).

The macrolide ring of the erythromycins was well-suited for conformational analysis by circular dichroism techniques because of the presence of two separate chromophores in the molecule, each of which had a distinct absorption curve that could be analyzed using the existing theoretical rules. The similarity of the circular dichroism curves for most members in the series supported the previous evidence for conformational homogeneity. The standard curve in this series has a negative amplitude for both the ketone and the lactone portions. The negative ketone curve is explained readily by the use of the well-known octant rule as modified for moderately twisted systems (*17*). Figure 1 shows the ketone carbonyl octant projection derived from the conformation **6**. The methyl group on C-8 lying in a negative octant plays a dominant role in the sign determination. The negative amplitude of the lactone chromophore is most readily explained by use of the

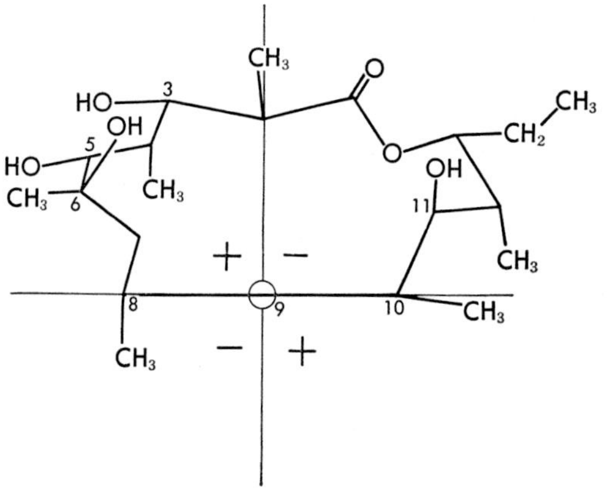

Fig. 1.   Carbonyl octant projection of the erythronolide conformation.

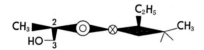

Fig. 2.   Partial lactone projection of the erythronolide conformation.

chirality rule as illustrated in Fig. 2. In this projection of **6** the lactone ring is considered as a twisted chromophore and the sign is determined by the helicity of the twist (*2, 46, 65*). The carbon β to the lactone carbonyl lies below the plane of the lactone function and is responsible for the negative amplitude. The alternate lactone orientation would be predictive of a positive curve (*42*).

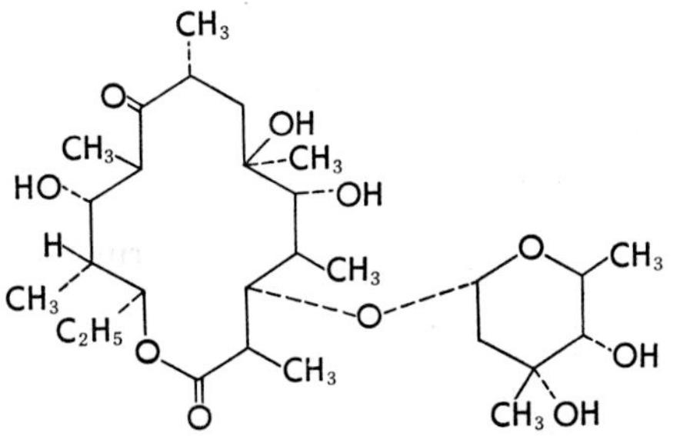

13

Although both the NMR studies and the circular dichroism curves gave evidence for a similar lactone ring conformation in both the erythromycin aglycones and the parent glycosides, further work on the monoglycosidic derivatives 3-α-L-mycarosylerythronolide B (13) (38) and 5-β-D-desosaminylerythronolide B (14) (62) as well as certain aglycone derivatives gives evidence of slight conformational changes in the C-6 to C-8 region (R. S. Egan, unpublished results).

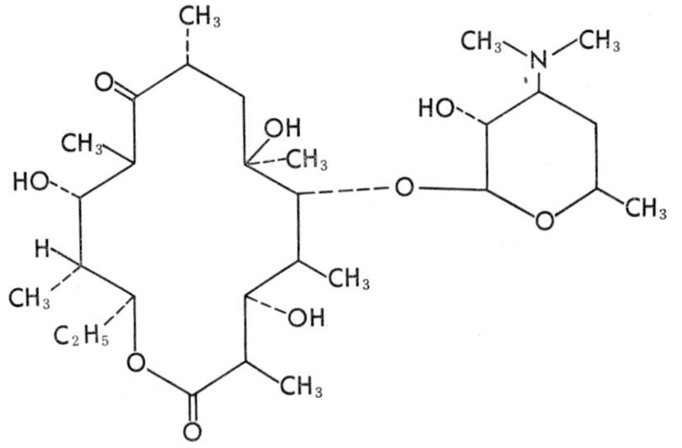

14

Orientation of sugars

An important conformational question that cannot be answered directly by either NMR or circular dichroism studies is the spatial orientation of the two sugar moieties relative to each other and relative to the plane of the lactone ring. The use of space-filling models shows that, because of the physical bulkiness of the two sugar groups attached to proximate ring carbons, these two groups must have nearly a parallel orientation with each other, which also is essentially perpendicular to the lactone ring. Further examination of these models indicates that in the complete di-glycoside molecule, the bulkiness of the two sugar groups does not permit a free rotation of either glycoside unit about the axis of the anomeric bond. This hindered rotation should thus permit the discrete existence of four geometrical isomers of the erythromycin molecule. Using the methyl group on C-5 of each sugar as a point of reference, isomers could exist with both methyls oriented toward the "upper" or hydrophilic face of the macrolide ring (see discussion of Fig. 3 below), both oriented toward the hydrophobic face, or with one "up" and one "down." There is some evidence in other systems that space-filling models do not always correctly predict the existence of hindered rotation, so the barrier toward interconversion of these geometrical isomers would have to be examined by experimental techniques.

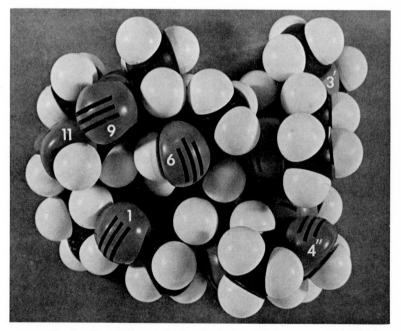

Fig. 3.   Space-filling model showing hydrophilic face of erythromycin A.

Plotting the coordinates* obtained in the X-ray crystallographic determination of erythromycin A (23) shows that in the crystal state the sugar groups have the chair conformation and exist in the geometrical form with the methyls oriented "up." If the barrier

* The coordinates were kindly supplied by Prof. D. R. Harris.

to rotation of the sugars does exist, then they should remain in the same orientation in solution. There is some evidence that chemical changes at the dimethylamino group of desosamine have an effect on the NMR chemical shift of the methoxyl on cladinose (L. A. Freiberg, unpublished results). This effect should only occur when the molecule exists in the geometrical arrangement present in the crystal state.

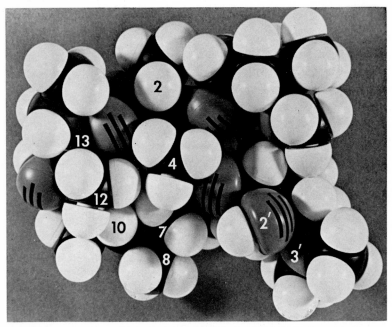

Fig. 4.   Space-filling model showing hydrophobic face of erythromycin A.

If this arrangement in solution is correct, it may be highly significant for the complexation of erythromycin with the ribosome. Previous communications (37, 49) have shown that in its most favorable conformation, the macrolide ring possesses a hydrophilic face and a hydrophobic face. The hydrophilic face is comprised of the lactone carbonyl, the ketone carbonyl and the hydroxyl groups at C-6 and C-11 (Fig. 3). The hydrophobic face is comprised of methyls on C-4, C-8, C-12 as well as hydrogens on

C-2, C-7, C-10, and some of those on the ethyl side chain at C-13 (Fig. 4). One might expect the sugars to be oriented such that their hydrophilic and hydrophobic groups would tend to reinforce like groups on the macrolide ring. Actually, the reverse is true; and of particular significance is the orientation of the dimethylamino group of desosamine and its adjacent hydroxyl away from the hydrophilic groups on the ring. Figure 3 is a photograph of the CPK model of erythromycin in this conformation, showing the hydrophilic face of the molecule and the projection of the dimethylamino group (3') away from the other polar groups in the molecule.

It, therefore, appears that the importance of the dimethylamino and adjacent hydroxyl function in the molecule is not directly related with the other polar groups present. It is known that the removal of the dimethylamino group from erythromycin causes essentially a complete loss in biological activity (37), and esterification of the adjacent hydroxyl also causes a substantial decrease in activity as measured by *in vitro* assay systems (59). Although changes in the other polar groups cause decreases in the activity of the molecule, complete loss of activity does not normally occur. The importance of the 3'-dimethylamino and 2'-hydroxyl on desosamine may be a result of the ability of this grouping to initiate complexation with the ribosomal surface through a strong hydrogen bond attachment. This could effectively anchor the erythromycin molecule to a portion of the binding site while the rest of the molecule completes its complexation with the ribosome through hydrophilic or hydrophobic bonding.

Chemical modifications—structure activity relationships

While the mechanism of action of erythromycin is best discussed by other investigators, some mention should be made of the effect of chemical changes on the whole-cell and cell-free activities of erythromycins. The importance of the nitrogen has been mentioned above and this is shown by the inactivity of derivatives modified at the dimethylamino function in both assays. Jones and Rowley (29) have developed a chemical method for removing the dimethylamino group in erythromycins A and B utilizing the N-oxide derivative (Fig. 5). The lack of ribosomal binding and the negligible whole-cell activity of 3'-de-(dimethylamino)-erythromycin A has been reported by Mao and Putterman (37). The similar inactivity of erythromycin A N-oxide (20, 29) is also reported (37). Thus, not only is the presence of the amino function important, but also the basicity must be unimpaired.

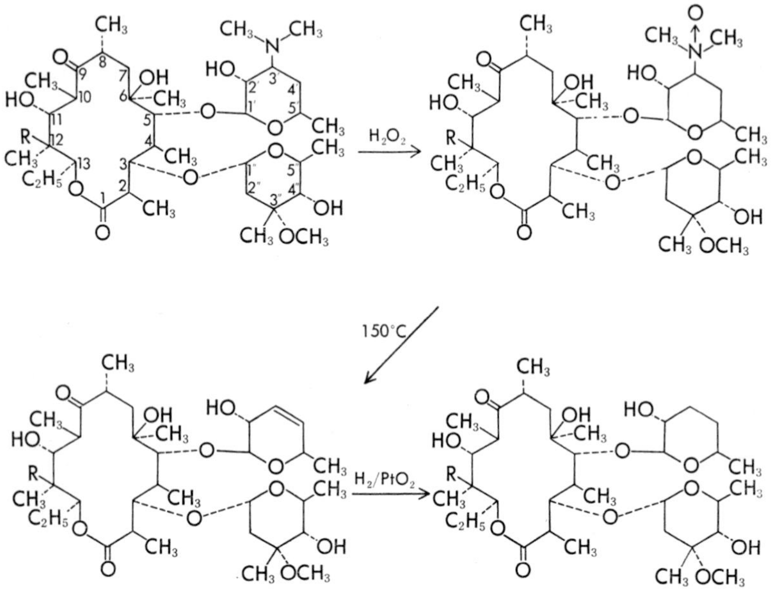

Fig. 5.   Synthesis of 3'-de-(dimethylamino)-erythromycins A and B.

Flynn and his co-workers reported a method of removing one of the methyl groups attached to the nitrogen by treatment with carbobenzoxy chloride, followed by hydrogenation (21). The des-N-methylerythromycin A was only 5% as active as erythromycin A in whole-cell assay. Clark and Freifelder used this compound to prepare a series of N-methyl-N-alkylerythromycins by a reductive alkylation technique (10). The biological results showed that the N-ethyl derivative had only 20% of the activity of erythromycin A and the activity decreased further through the series of higher homologues until it became negligible. Since the basicity of the amino function is not altered to any large degree by these alkyl substituents, the biological results imply that there is a strong steric factor associated with the importance of the dimethylamino function. Thus removal or replacement of one of the methyl groups on the nitrogen has a deleterious effect on its whole-cell activity. Mao has found that these decreases in activity can be correlated with the decrease in ribosomal binding (Fig. 1 in the paper by Mao, this volume). Thus, it appears that changes in the steric environment of the nitrogen reduce its ability to bind to the active site. The inactivity of the N-acetyl (*21*) derivative of des-N-methylerythromycin A could be predicted both by a steric effect and more importantly by the change in the basicity of the nitrogen.

The functionalization of the 2'-hydroxyl adjacent to the nitrogen also has a significant effect on the biological activity. A large number of 2'-esters of erythromycin have been synthesized (*11, 44, 54, 55*). Although the lower molecular weight esters appear to be active *in vivo* and give very good blood levels (*55*), their *in vitro* activity against whole cells is very low. This relative inactivity has been correlated with the greatly diminished ribosomal binding of 2'-esters (*59*). The activity of these compounds *in vivo* is reported to be a function of their hydrolysis rates (*59*). The esterifications of the 2'-hydroxyl of desosamine have the dual effect of removing a hydrogen-bonding site and decreasing the basicity of the amino function (*20*). Both of these effects may play a role in reducing the activity of 2'-esters.

An interesting effect on biological activity was observed with the 4'-hydroxy derivative of erythromycin A. In an elegant series of reactions shown in Fig. 6, Jones *et al.* (*30*) have synthesized this compound as well as a positional isomer where the 3'-dimethylamino and 4'-hydroxyl are interchanged. These compounds were prepared through the intermediary of the epoxide derivative obtained by the elimination of the N-oxide of erythromycin A followed by treatment with *m*-chloroperbenzoic acid. The stereospecific ring opening of the epoxide with the azide ion followed by reductive alkylation led to the exclusive formation of the two positional isomers. The antimicrobial spectrum of 4'-hydroxyerythromycin A was the same as that of erythromycin A, but it was only

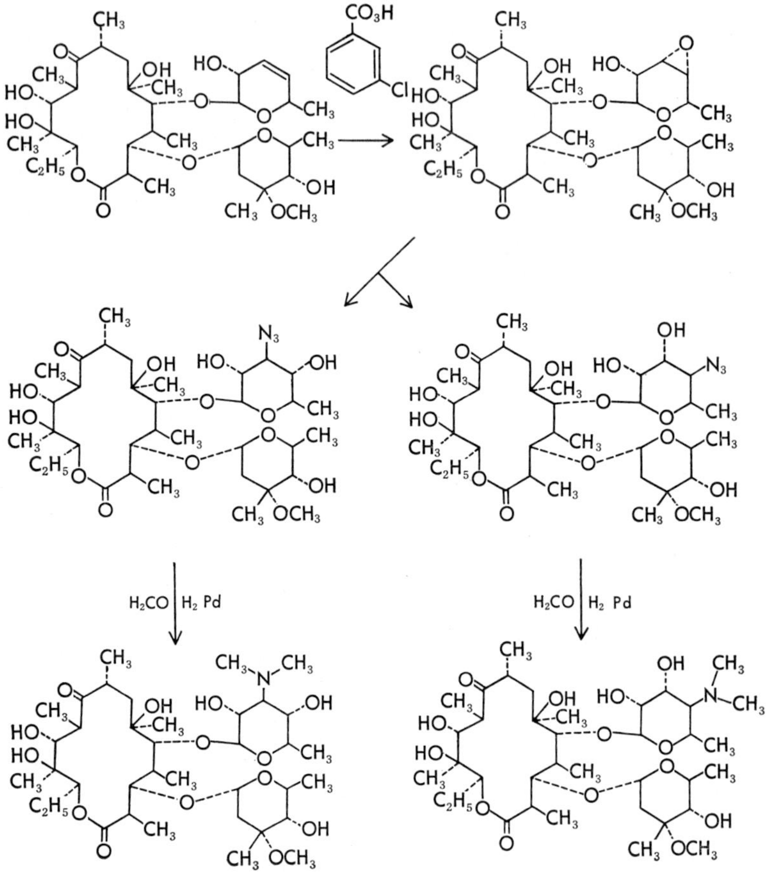

Fig. 6.   Synthesis of 4'-hydroxyerythromycin A.

60% as active in whole-cell assay. This was somewhat surprising since the chemical modification effected a conversion of desosamine to mycaminose, an amino sugar present in other macrolide antibiotics (43). A possible explanation for this result is that the presence of a second hydroxyl adjacent to the dimethylamino produces an ambiguity at this important site for ribosomal binding. Thus the molecule is able to initiate binding to the ribosome in two possible orientations, only one of which permits the rest of the molecule to complete the molecular complexation.

It is interesting to note the progressive decrease of activity in the erythromycin series, A, B and C. Erythromycin B **(1b)** is about two-thirds as active as erythromycin A. The slight decrease in activity must be related to the lack of a hydroxyl group at C-12, since conformational studies have shown these molecules to have similar shapes in solution. The conformational model shows the C-12 hydroxyl to be located on the periphery of the lactone ring and oriented away from either the hydrophilic or hydrophobic face of the molecule. Thus, the removal of this hydroxyl would not appear to have a large effect on the complexing ability of these two regions. In confirmation of this, the ribosomal binding of erythromycin B is only slightly less than that of erythromycin A (37, 64).

A more substantial decrease in antibacterial activity is observed with erythromycin C **(1c)** which is only 30% as active as erythromycin A. This activity difference is reflected by its decrease in ribosomal binding. Structurally, erythromycin C differs from erythromycin A only in the presence of a hydroxyl in place of the methoxyl at C-3″ of the neutral sugar. In the crystal structure of erythromycin A, the methoxyl group is the only polar group which lies in a region near that of the dimethylamino-hydroxyl grouping on desosamine. Thus, if the same relationship is present in solution, the presence of the hydrogen-donating hydroxyl in this position could produce an adverse effect on the electronic characteristics of the dimethylamino-hydroxyl grouping and its ribosomal-binding activity.

The recent structural determination of megalomicin A **(1d)** shows it to be a derivative of erythromycin C in which a new amino sugar, D-rhodosamine, is attached to the C-11 hydroxyl by a glycoside bond (35, 36). The *in vitro* activity of this compound against gram-positive bacteria is about 10% of that of erythromycin A (60). This is what would be expected for a compound structurally related to erythromycin C and containing a substituted hydroxyl group at C-11.

Monoglycosidic compounds have also been obtained in the erythromycin series and two of these, 3-α-L-mycarosylerythronolide B, **13** (38), and 5-β-D-desosaminylerythronolide B, **14** (62), have been studied extensively in both cell-free and whole-cell assays. Corcoran *et al.* (*64*) and Mao and Putterman (*37*) have reported that these compounds lack the ability to inhibit the binding of erythromycin A to ribosomes and do not inhibit protein synthesis. The whole-cell activity of either compound is negligible. This lack of biological activity is understandable in the case of **13** since it does not contain the dimethylamino-hydroxyl grouping, but this is not true with **14**. Corcoran has pointed out the importance of having two sugars present in the macrolide antibiotics, and has proposed that these compounds act by mimicking subunits of peptidyl-tRNA. The presence of sugars may be critical in the competition for a binding site because of their resemblance to the N-ribosyl groups in tRNA (*64*).

   Another possible explanation for the lack of biological activity of **14** is again related to the importance of the orientation of the dimethylamino-hydroxyl grouping. Whereas in the diglycosides there is the real possibility of steric inhibition to free rotation of the sugar groups, this is no longer true with the monoglycosides; and the amino sugar in **14** may not be constrained in the proper orientation for inhibition of erythromycin A binding to the ribosome. There is also some evidence for minor differences in the conformation of the lactone ring of the monoglycosides relative to the parent erythromycins (*50*) (R. S. Egan, unpublished results).

   In view of the lack of biological activity of either monoglycoside derivative of erythromycin B, **13** or **14**, it is not surprising that erythronolide B, **19** (*58*), the aglycone of erythromycin B has no activity in whole-cell or cell-free systems (*37, 64*).

   Although the dimethylamino group and its adjacent hydroxyl appear to be the most important functional unit in the erythromycins, chemical modifications of other parts of the molecule have provided useful compounds for determining structure-activity relationships. In a study of the importance of the other secondary hydroxyls in the molecule, a series of mono, di, and tri esters of erythromycins A and B have been synthesized at Abbott (P. H. Jones and T. J. Perun, unpublished results) and at the Polish Academy of Sciences (*1*). Both groups have found that the rate of esterification of the hydroxyl groups at C-2′, C-4″, and C-11 decreases in that order. The similar order of hydrolysis rates allowed the Polish workers to synthesize 4″-monoesters and 4″, 11-di-esters. Extension of this difference in hydrolysis rates by the Abbott group has permitted the synthesis of 11-monoesters.

The antibacterial activity of the 4″-monoacetate of erythromycin A is about 16% of that of the parent antibiotic (*1*). Mao has reported similar activity in the erythromycin B series and in addition he has reported the activity of the 11-monoacetyl derivative as 30% of the parent antibiotic (*37*). These results show that the antibacterial activity of monoesters of erythromycin decreases in the following order: C-11 ester>C-4″ ester>C-2′ ester. This would indicate that the 2′-hydroxyl plays a more important role in the mechanism of action than the 4″-hydroxyl, which in turn is more important than the 11-hydroxyl. A note of caution should be interjected here, however, because the activity of erythromycin derivatives against whole cells is not always correlated with the degree of ribosomal binding. Mao and Putterman (*37*) have shown that the 4″- and 11-monoesters are equally effective in competitive binding to the ribosome and the degree of binding indicates they should be nearly as effective as the parent erythromycin in antibacterial activity. Obviously, other factors such as cell permeability are also involved in the determination of whole-cell activity.

Another functional group in the erythromycins, which plays a key role in both the biological and chemical characteristics of the molecule, is the ketone at C-9. In the parent erythromycins, reduction of this carbonyl with borohydride effects the selective formation of the 9S-hydroxy compound. The reduction is practically stereospecific with only trace amounts of the 9R epimer being formed (K. Gerzon, personal communication; J. R. Martin, unpublished results). In the aglycone series a considerable amount of the 9R epimer is produced (*49*) and the relative amounts of the two epimers vary depending on the aglycone structure (T. J. Perun and J. R. Martin, unpublished results).

The whole-cell activities of the (9S)-9-dihydroerythromycins A and B are about 10% of that of the parent compounds, but the cell-free assays of these two compounds appear to show differences between them. Corcoran has reported that (9S)-9-dihydroerythromycin A (**15**) is able to inhibit cell-free protein synthesis although

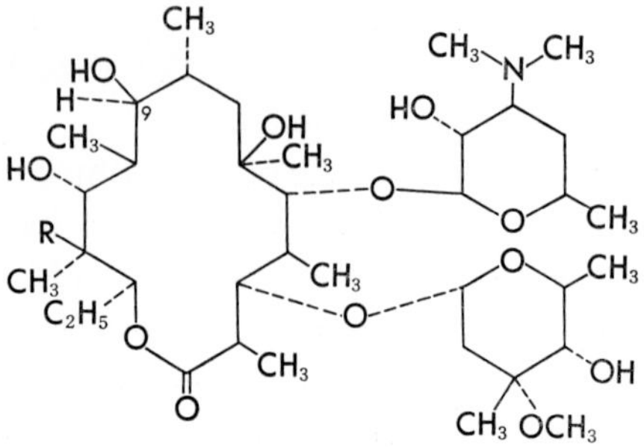

15 R=OH   16 R=H

not as effectively as the parent erythromycin (64). He also showed that **15** can compete with erythromycin A for the ribosomal binding site. Mao has confirmed that **15** inhibits erythromycin A binding (J. C.-H. Mao, unpublished results) and has found that (9S)-9-dihydroerythromycin B **(16)** is much less effective in ribosomal binding (37).

Acetic acid treatment of erythromycin A under conditions, which do not hydrolyze the sugars, converts it to a new compound reported to contain a hemiketal bond between the C-9 ketone and one of the tertiary hydroxyls at C-6 or C-12 (55). This compound is itself unstable in the presence of aqueous acid and is converted to anhydroerythromycin A **(17)** which contains a spiroketal grouping (61). This acid lability of the erythromycin A structure holds true even for substituted compounds. For instance, the 2'-esters of erythromycin A undergo an analogous reaction (55) as do the 4"-and 11-esters (1).

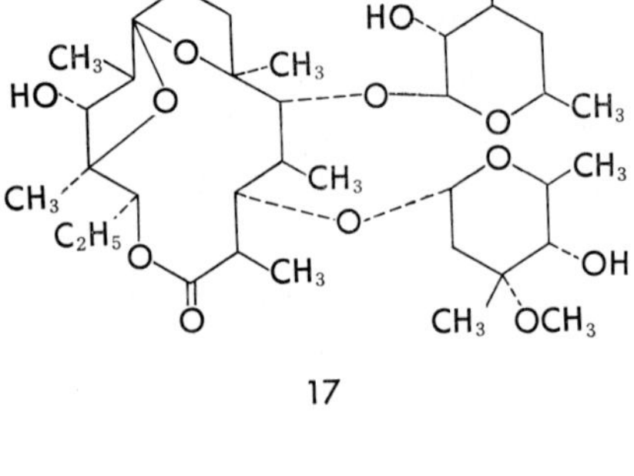

17

The biological characteristics of the hemiketal and spiroketal structures are somewhat analogous to the dihydroerythromycins. They show very low levels of activity against whole cells and also in ribosomal-binding studies, using amounts approximately equimolar with erythromycin A (37). At higher concentrations, however, inhibition of protein synthesis and ribosomal binding does occur (64).

A novel derivative of erythromycin A hemiketal has been reported recently (45), which is a cyclic carbonate ester of the C-9 and C-11 hydroxyls. Unlike the parent hemiketal compound, this structure (18) has activity against whole cells higher than erythromycin A.

18

Erythromycin B does not contain the C-12 hydroxyl and is consequently more acid stable than erythromycin A (9, 62). Experiments with the triacetate of erythronolide B (20) have shown that an equilibrium is established in aqueous acid between the hydroxy ketone structure and the enol ether derived from a hemiketal intermediate (47). For instance, 3,5,11-triacetylerythronolide B (20) is transformed by aqueous acid to its 6,9-enol ether derivative 21. With this triacetate compound, the equilibrium in aqueous acid lies on the side of the ring-closed structure; whereas with erythronolide B itself, the equilibrium lies on the side of the open structure, the hydroxy ketone. In the case of erythronolide derivatives containing a 10,11-double bond, hydrolysis of the enol ether structure (22) leads to the formation of two hydroxy ketone compounds 23 and 24 which are epimeric at C-8.

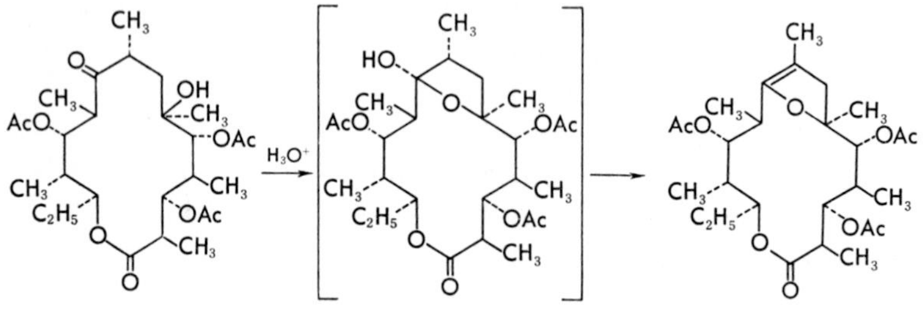

20   21

Recent work at Abbott (*32*) has determined that the supposed hemiketal obtained by acid treatment of erythromycin A (*55*) is in reality a 6,9-enol ether structurally related to the enol ethers obtained from erythronolide B (*33*) and its derivatives (*47*). The same work has shown that erythromycin B is converted to an analogous enol ether under the same conditions. Aqueous acid treatment of the erythromycin A enol ether leads to the spiroketal **17**, whereas

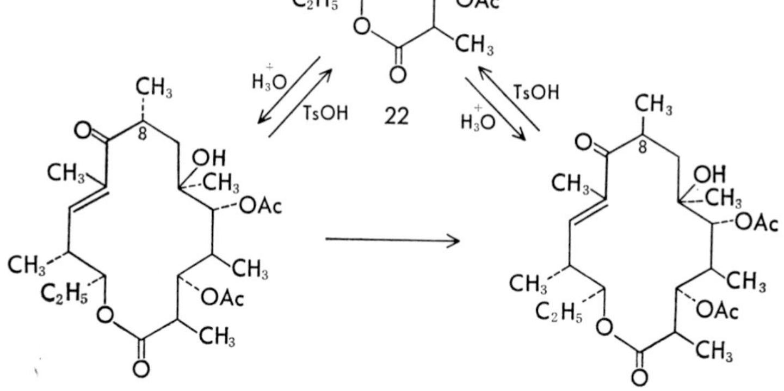

Kinetic product
23

Thermodynamic product
24

erythromycin B enol ether is stereospecifically hydrolyzed back to erythromycin B. In their work on the enol ether of erythronolide B, Kurath and Egan have determined unequivocally by NMR techniques the position of the double bond in these compounds.

The easy formation of enol ether structures in the erythromycin and erythronolide series is readily explained by examination of the conformation of the macrolide ring (6). The C-6 hydroxyl has a proximate relationship with the carbonyl at C-9 and a ring closure reaction between the two groups can occur without a major change in the conformation. This is not true in the case of a reaction between the C-12 hydroxyl and the ketone and it is surprising that the spiroketal formation should occur so readily. In the chemical transformation studies of erythronolide derivatives, a number of highly specific elimination reactions was found (47). The specificity of all such reactions in this series can now be explained by the use of the macrolide conformation 6 (50).

The ketone function in erythromycin A does not form normal carbonyl derivatives very readily (53). One of the few condensation products reported in the early chemical transformation work was

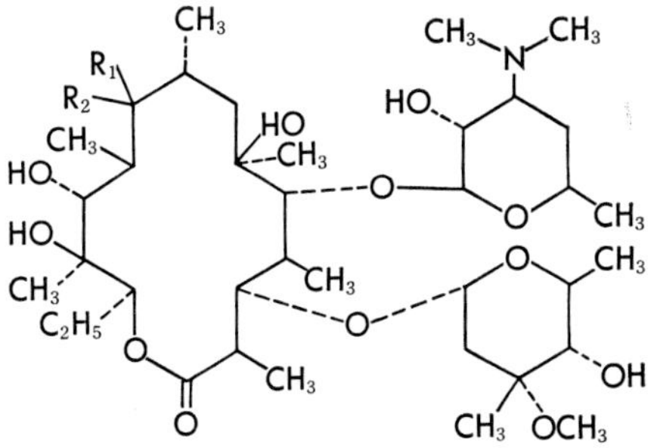

25   $R_1R_2=$ $=N-NH_2$

26   $R_1R_2=$ $=N-N=C\overset{\displaystyle CH_3}{\underset{\displaystyle CH_3}{<}}$

27   $R_1R_2=$ $=N-OH$

28   $R_1=NH_2$ $R_2=H$

the hydrazine adduct. A recent report on this early work showed that the hydrazine adduct **25** and its N'-isopropylidene derivative **26** could be converted to the 9-amino derivative **28** by catalytic reduction (*41*). This compound was also obtained by catalytic reduction of the oxime derivative **27**. Both 9-amino epimers appear to be formed in the reduction although one of these is the major product.

Other workers have also reported the preparation of the 9-oximino derivative **27** which appears to have approximately 50% of the activity of erythromycin A (*18*). These workers have also reported that the 9-amino derivative **28** can be obtained by sodium borohydride reduction of the oxime, but this has been disproved by the Lilly group (*41*). The oxime has been found to be reactive toward acylating agents and a number of active ester derivatives have been obtained (*56, 57*). The biological results of these ketone adducts of erythromycin show that while a reduction in activity is the usual case, moderate activity is retained with some derivatives. In general, it appears that compounds containing an sp^2 hybridized C-9 are more active than the sp^3 hybridized structures.

REFERENCES

1   Banaszek, A., Pyrek, J., and Zamojski, A. 1969. Esterification of erythromycin A. *Roczniki Chemii*, **43**, 763–774.
2   Beecham, A. F. 1968. Optical activity and lactone ring configurations. *Tetrahedron Letters*, 3591–3594.
3   Celmer, W. D. 1965. Macrolide stereochemistry. I. The total absolute configuration of oleandomycin. *J. Am. Chem. Soc.*, **87**, 1797–1799.
4   Celmer, W. D. 1965. Macrolide stereochemistry. II. Configurational assignments at certain centers in various macrolide antibiotics. *J. Am. Chem. Soc.*, **87**, 1799–1801.
5   Celmer, W. D. 1965. Macrolide stereochemistry. III. A configurational model for macrolide antibiotics. *J. Am. Chem. Soc.*, **87**, 1801–1802.
6   Celmer, W. D. 1965. Basic stereochemical research topics in the macrolide antibiotics. *In* "Biogenesis of Antibiotic Substances," ed. by Z. Vanek and Z. Hostalek, Academic Press, New York, p. 99–129.
7   Celmer, W. D. 1966. Biogenetic, constitutional, and stereochemical unitary principles in macrolide antibiotics. *Antimicrobial Agents and Chemotherapy—1965*, 144–156.
8   Clark, R. K., Jr. 1953. The chemistry of erythromycin. I. Acid degrada-

tion products. *Antibiotics and Chemotherapy*, **3**, 663–671.

9 Clark, R. K., Jr., and Taterka, M. 1955. The chemistry of erythromycin. III. Acid degradation products of erythromycin B. *Antibiotics and Chemotherapy*, **5**, 206–211.

10 Clark, R. K., Jr., and Freifelder, M. 1957. The synthesis of new erythromycins. *Antibiotics and Chemotherapy*, **7**, 483–486.

11 Clark, R. K., Jr., and Varner, E. L. 1957. New esters of erythromycin. *Antibiotics and Chemotherapy*, **7**, 487–489.

12 Dale, J. 1963. Macrocyclic compounds. III. Conformation of cycloalkanes and other flexible macrocycles. *J. Chem. Soc. (London)*, 93–111.

13 Demarco, P. V., Farkas, E., Doddrell, D., Mylari, B. L., and Wenkert, E. 1968. Pyridine induced solvent shifts in the nuclear magnetic resonance spectra of hydroxylic compounds. *J. Am. Chem. Soc.*, **90**, 5480–5486.

14 Demarco, P. V. 1969. Pyridine solvent shifts in the NMR analysis of erythromycin aglycones. *Tetrahedron Letters*, 383–386.

15 Demarco, P. V. 1969. NMR study of some erythromycin aglycones. A conformational and configurational analysis. *The Journal of Antibiotics*, **22**, 327–340.

16 Djerassi, C., Halpern, O., Wilkinson, D. I., and Eisenbraun, E. J. 1958. Macrolide antibiotics. VIII. The absolute configuration of certain centers in neomethymycin, erythromycin and related antibiotics. *Tetrahedron*, **4**, 369–381.

17 Djerassi, C., and Klyne, W. 1962. Optical rotatory dispersion: Application of the octant rule to some structural and stereochemical problems. *J. Chem. Soc. (London)*, 4929–4950.

18 Djokié, S., and Tamburašev, Z. 1967. Erythromycin study: 9-amino-3-O-cladinosyl-5-O-desosaminyl-6, 11, 12-trihydroxy-2, 4, 6, 8, 10, 12-hexamethylpentadecane-13-olide. *Tetrahedron Letters*, 1645–1647.

19 Dunitz, J. D., and Prelog, V. 1960. Röntgenographisch bestimmte Konformationen und Reaktivität mittlerer Ringe. *Angew. Chem.*, **72**, 896–902.

20 Flynn, E. H., Sigal, M. V., Jr., Wiley, P. F., and Gerzon, K. 1954. Erythromycin. I. Properties and degradation studies. *J. Am. Chem. Soc.*, **76**, 3121–3131.

21 Flynn, E. H., Murphy, H. W., and McMahon, R. E. 1955. Erythromycin. II. Des-N-methylerythromycin and N-methyl-^{14}C-erythromycin. *J. Am. Chem. Soc.*, **77**, 3104–3106.

22 Gerzon, K., Flynn, E. H., Sigal, M. V., Jr., Wiley, P. F., Monahan, R., and Quarck, U. C. 1956. Erythromycin. VIII. Structure of dihydroerythronolide. *J. Am. Chem. Soc.*, **78**, 6396–6408.

23 Harris, D. R., McGeachin, S. G., and Mills, H. H. 1965. The structure and stereochemistry of erythromycin A. *Tetrahedron Letters*, 679–685.

24 Hasbrouck, R. B., and Garven, F. C. 1953. The chemistry of erythro-

mycin. II. Acid degradation products. *Antibiotics and Chemotherapy*, **3**, 1040–1052.

25 Hofheinz, W., and Grisebach, H. 1962. Die Konfiguration des Deso-samins. *Tetrahedron Letters*, 377–379.

26 Hofheinz, W., Grisebach, H., and Friebolin, H. 1962. Zur Biogenese der Makrolide. VIII. Die Stereochemie der Mycarose und Cladinose. *Tetrahedron*, **18**, 1265–1274.

27 Hofheinz, W., and Grisebach, H. 1962. Zur Biogenese der Makrolide. X. Mitt.: Über das vorkommen von L-mycarose in Erythromycin C. *Z. Natur.*, **17b**, 852.

28 Hofheinz, W., and Grisebach, H. 1963. Die Konfiguration der Gly-kosidbindungen in Erythromycin und Magnamycin. *Chem. Ber.*, **96**, 2867–2869.

29 Jones, P. H., and Rowley, E. K. 1968. Chemical modifications of eryth-romycin antibiotics. I. 3'-De(dimethylamino)erythromycins A and B. *J. Org. Chem.*, **33**, 665–670.

30 Jones, P. H., Iyer, K. S., and Grundy, W. E. 1970. Chemical modifica-tions of erythromycin antibiotics. II. Synthesis of 4'-hydroxyerythro-mycin A. *Antimicrobial Agents and Chemotherapy—1969*, 123–130.

31 Karplus, M. 1963. Vicinal proton coupling in nuclear magnetic reso-nance. *J. Am. Chem. Soc.*, **85**, 2870–2871.

32 Kurath, P., Jones, P. H., Egan, R. S., and Perun, T. J. 1971. Acid de-gradation of erythromycin A and erythromycin B. *Experientia*, **27**, 362.

33 Kurath, P., and Egan, R.S. 1971. Oxidation and reduction of 8,9- anhydro-erythronolide B 6,9-hemiacetal. *Helv. Chim. Acta*, **54**, 523–532.

34 Lemal, D. M., Pacht, P. D., and Woodward, R. B. 1962. The synthesis of L-(−)-mycarose and L-(−)-cladinose. *Tetrahedron*, **18**, 1275–1293.

35 Mallams, A. K. 1969. The megalomicins. I. D-Rhodosamine, a new dimethylamino sugar. *J. Am. Chem. Soc.*, **91**, 7505–7506.

36 Mallams, A. K., Jaret, R. S., and Reimann, H. 1969. The megalomicins. II. The structure of megalomicin A. *J. Am. Chem. Soc.*, **91**, 7506–7508.

37 Mao, J. C.-H., and Putterman. M. 1969. The intramolecular complex of erythromycin and ribosome. *J. Mol. Biol.*, **44**, 347–361.

38 Martin, J. R., Perun, T. J., and Girolami, R. L. 1966. Studies on the biosynthesis of the erythromycins. I. Isolation and structure of an inter-mediate glycoside, 3-α-L-mycarosylerythronolide B. *Biochemistry*, **5**, 2852–2856.

39 Martin, J. R., and Rosenbrook, W. 1967. Studies on the biosynthesis of the erythromycins. II. Isolation and structure of a biosynthetic inter-mediate, 6-deoxyerythronolide B. *Biochemistry*, **6**, 435–440.

40 Martin, J. R., and Perun, T. J. 1968. Studies on the biosynthesis of the erythromycins. III. Isolation and structure of 5-deoxy-5-oxoerythronolide B, a shunt metabolite of erythromycin biosynthesis. *Biochemistry*, **7**, 1728–1733.

41 Massey, E. H., Kitchell, B., Martin, L. D., Gerzon, K., and Murphy, H. W. 1970. Erythromycylamine. *Tetrahedron Letters*, 157–160.
42 Mitscher, L. A., Slater, B. J., Perun, T. J., Jones, P. H., and Martin, J. R. 1969. The conformation of macrolide antibiotics. III. Circular dichroism and the conformation of erythromycins. *Tetrahedron Letters*, 4505–4508.
43 Morin, R., and Gorman, M. 1967. Macrolide antibiotics. *In* "Kirk-Othmer Encyclopedia of Chemical Technology, 2nd ed.," John Wiley & Sons, New York, p. 632–661.
44 Murphy, H. W. 1954. Esters of erythromycin. I. Some water-insoluble, substantially tasteless esters. *Antibiotics Annual 1953–1954*, 500–513.
45 Murphy, H. W., Stephens, V. C., and Conine, J. W. 1968. U. S. Patent 3,417,077.
46 Okuda, T., Harigaya, S., and Kiyomoto, A. 1964. Studies on optical rotatory dispersion of five-membered sugar lactones: Configuration and the sign of an optical rotatory dispersion curve. *Chem. Pharm. Bull. (Tokyo)*, **12**, 504–506.
47 Perun, T. J. 1967. Chemistry of erythronolide B. Acid-catalyzed transformations of the aglycone of erythromycin B. *J. Org. Chem.*, **32**, 2324–2330.
48 Perun, T. J., and Egan, R. S. 1969. The conformation of erythromycin aglycones. *Tetrahedron Letters*, 387–390.
49 Perun, T. J., Egan, R. S., and Martin, J. R. 1969. The conformation of macrolide antibiotics. II. Configurational and conformational studies of dihydroerythronolides. *Tetrahedron Letters*, 4501–4504.
50 Perun, T. J., Egan, R. S., Jones, P. H., Martin, J. R., Mitscher, L. A., and Slater, B. J. 1970. Conformation of macrolide antibiotics. IV. Nuclear magnetic resonance, circular dichroism, and chemical studies of erythromycin derivatives. *Antimicrobial Agents and Chemotherapy—1969*, 116–122.
51 Reichstein, T., and Weiss, E. 1962. The sugars of the cardiac glycosides. *In* "Advances in Carbohydrate Chemistry," ed. by M. L. Wolfrom Academic Press, New York, Vol. 17, 98.
52 Saunders, M. 1967. Medium and large rings superimposable with the diamond lattice. *Tetrahedron*, **23**, 2105–2113.
53 Sigal, M. V., Jr., Wiley, P. F., Gerzon, K., Flynn, E. H., Quarck, U. C., and Weaver, O. 1956. Erythromycin. VI. Degradation studies. *J. Am. Chem. Soc.*, **78**, 388–395.
54 Stephens, V. C. 1954. Esters of erythromycin. II. Derivatives of cyclic anhydrides. *Antibiotics Annual 1953–1954*, 514–521.
55 Stephens, V. C., and Conine, J. W. 1959. Esters of erythromycin. III. Esters of low molecular weight aliphatic acids. *Antibiotics Annual 1958–1959*, 346–353.

56 Tamburašev, Z., Vazdar, G., and Djokić, S. 1967. Erythromycin series
    II. Acylation of erythromycin oxime and 9-amino-3-O-cladinosyl-5-O-
    desosaminyl-6, 11, 12-trihydroxy-2, 4, 6, 8,10,12-hexamethylpentadecane-
    13-olide with ester-chlorides of dicarboxylic acids. *Croatica Chemica
    Acta*, **39**, 273–276.
57 Tamburašev, Z., and Djokić, S. 1968. Erythromycin series III. Acylation
    of erythromycin oxime and 9-amino-3-O-cladinosyl-5-O-desosaminyl-6,
    12-trihydroxy-2,4,6,8,10,12-hexamethylpentadecane-13-olide with chlo-
    rides of some aliphatic monocarboxylic acids. *Croatica Chemica Acta*,
    40, 93–95.
58 Tardrew, P. L., and Nyman, M. A. 1964. U. S. Patent 3,127,315.
59 Tardrew, P. L., Mao, J. C.-H., and Kenney, D. 1969. Antibacterial
    activity of 2′-esters of erythromycin. *Appl. Microbiol.*, **18**, 159–165.
60 Weinstein, M. J., Wagman, G. H., Marquez, J. A., Testa, R. T., Oden,
    E., and Waitz, J. A. 1969. Megalomicin, a new macrolide antibiotic
    complex produced by *Micromonospora*. *The Journal of Antibiotics*, **22**,
    253–258.
61 Wiley, P. F., Gerzon, K., Flynn, E. H., Sigal, M. V., Jr., Weaver, O.,
    Quarck, U. C., Chauvette, R. R., and Monahan, R. 1957. Erythromycin.
    X. Structure of erythromycin. *J. Am. Chem. Soc.*, **79**, 6062–6070.
62 Wiley, P. F., Sigal, M. V., Jr., Weaver, O., Monahan, R., and Gerzon,
    K. 1957. Erythromycin. XI. Structure of erythromycin B. *J. Am. Chem.
    Soc.*, **79**, 6070–6074.
63 Wiley, P. F., Gale, R., Pettinga, C. W., and Gerzon, K. 1957. Erythro-
    mycin. XII. The isolation, properties and partial structure of erythro-
    mycin C. *J. Am. Chem. Soc.*, **79**, 6074–6077.
64 Wilhelm, J. M., Oleinick, N. L., and Corcoran, J. W. 1968. Interaction
    of antibiotics with ribosomes: structure-function relationships and a
    possible common mechanism for the antibacterial action of the macro-
    lides and lincomycin. *Antimicrobial Agents and Chemotherapy—1967*,
    236–250.
65 Wolf, H. 1966. Cotton-Effekt und Konformation des δ-Lactonringes.
    Tetrahedron Letters, 5151–5156.
66 Woodward, R. B. 1956. Neuere Entwicklungen in der Chemie der
    Naturstoffe. *Angew. Chem.*, **68**, 13–20.
67 Woodward, R. B. 1957. Struktur und Biogenese der Makrolide. Eine
    neue Klasse von Naturstoffen. *Angew. Chem.*, **69**, 50–58.

MODE OF ACTION OF ERYTHROMYCIN

James C.-H. Mao

The Department of Chemical Pharmacology, Abbott Laboratories, North Chicago, Illinois, U.S.A.

Erythromycin A (EMA) has been shown to inhibit bacterial protein synthesis in intact cells (*1*) and in cell-free systems (*18, 19, 33, 34*). However, the specific step in the protein synthesis affected by EMA has not been identified. Two mechanisms of inhibition have been proposed. The first one is based on the inhibition of the formation of polylysyl-puromycin (*2*), the release of peptides by glycyl ApC (*25*) and the addition of a single lysine unit to the ribosome-bound polylysyl-tRNA (*9*). These data implied that EMA inhibits the peptide bond formation. In a recent paper, Teraoka *et al.* (*34*) indicated that the ribosomes of an EMA-resistant mutant of *Escherichia coli* have a lower peptidyl transferase activity, which also added some weight to this hypothesis. Evidence contradictory to this hypothesis is as follows. EMA stimulated N-acetylphenylalanyl-puromycin (Ac-Phe-puromycin) synthesis (*2*) did not inhibit the formation of N-formylmethionyl-puromycin (F-Met-puromycin) in a reaction mixture containing F-Met-hexanucleotide, 50S ribosomes and puromycin (*20*), and caused the accumulation of dilysine in a polylysine synthesizing system (18, 29).

The second mechanism is based on the inhibition of tRNA release (8); on the inhibition of Ac-triPhe, but not Ac-diPhe synthesis (4); and on the lack of inhibition of the puromycin induced release of nascent peptides in the presence of chlorotetracycline by EMA (5). These data suggested that EMA inhibits translocation. However, in a study of the movement of ribosomes on mRNA (messenger RNA), Gurgo et al. (7) found that chloramphenicol arrested peptide bond formation, but the movement of ribosomes on mRNA continued. They suggested that there are at least two ways that ribosomes can move on mRNA: one, "productive," makes protein; the other, "abortive," does not synthesize protein. The abortive movement is not totally inhibited by EMA (27). The earlier observation that EMA inhibited aminoacyl-tRNA binding to ribosomes (19) is most likely an artifact, resulting from the inhibition of peptide bond formation and/or translocation due to the use of unwashed ribosomes.

In this paper, the binding of EMA to the ribosomes is shown to be a prerequisite of its antibacterial activity; and some properties of the EMA-ribosome complexes are revealed. The effect of EMA on peptide bond formation and translocation was tested with various approaches. Finally, possible mechanisms of action are discussed.

Materials

The cell fractions were prepared from *Escherichia coli* Q13 by the procedure described previously (13). Washed ribosomes were prepared by repeated suspension and centrifugation of ribosomes in a solution containing 1M NH_4Cl, 0.01M Tris, pH 7.5, 0.01M $MgCl_2$ and 0.001M dithiothreitol. N-^{14}C-Methylerythromycin (^{14}C-EMA), which was synthesized by reductive methylation of Des-N-methylerythromycin, had a specific activity of 15 Ci/mole and had an antibiotic activity of 730 units/μmole (maximum activity is 734 units/μmole). ^{14}C-Lysine (271 Ci/mole), ^{14}C-phenylalanine (413 Ci/mole) and ^{14}C-methionine (187 Ci/mole) were purchased from the New England Nuclear Corp. and γ-^{32}P-GTP (4.6 Ci/mole), from the International Chemical & Nuclear Corp. F-^{14}C-Met-tRNA (3823 cpm/ODU) (ODU: Optical Density Unit), ^{14}C-Lys-tRNA (2676 or 4031 cpm/ODU) and ^{14}C-Phe-tRNA (3800 cpm/ODU) were prepared according to Leder and Bursztyn (10). ApUpG was prepared by the method of Leder et al. (12). The transfer factors T and G were prepared by the method of Ertel et al. (6).

Methods

1. Assay for the binding of ^{14}C-erythromycin to ribosomes
The reaction mixtures, in a total volume of 0.1 ml, contained ^{14}C-EMA (1.4×10^{-10} mole) and ribosomes (5 ODU) in the standard buffer (Tris, 0.01M, pH 7.6; NH$_4$Cl, 0.05M; MgCl$_2$, 0.016M and dithiothreitol, 0.001M). The binding of ^{12}C-analogues to ribosomes was determined by their ability to replace ^{14}C-EMA at a concentration five times higher than that of ^{14}C-EMA (32). After 15-minute incubation at 35°C, the reaction mixtures were diluted with a cold buffer, filtered, and washed as described in the previous paper (16).

2. Assay for the puromycin reaction with F-Met-tRNA
The reaction mixtures, in a total volume of 0.05 ml, contained unwashed ribosomes (5.5 ODU), ApUpG (0.66 ODU), F-Met-tRNA (2.6 ODU) and GTP (2.5×10^{-8} moles) in the standard buffer, except that the MgCl$_2$ concentration was 0.01M. The reaction mixtures were incubated for 5 min at 30°C. Then puromycin (5×10^{-8} moles) was added and the incubation was continued for 20 min. The F-Met-puromycin complex was measured by the ethylacetate extraction method (11).

3. Assay for polypeptide synthesis
The reaction mixture, in a total volume of 0.5 ml, contained washed ribosomes (5 ODU), ^{14}C-Lys-tRNA (10 ODU) or ^{14}C-Phe-tRNA (21 ODU), poly A (50 μg) or poly U (50 μg), 18 μg of T factor, 6.2 μg of G factor, and GTP (5×10^{-7} moles), in the standard

buffer. In some cases, the T and G factors were replaced by the S-100 fraction (0.8 mg protein per assay); ^{14}C-Lys-tRNA was replaced by ^{14}C-lysine (0.25 μc per assay) and GTP was replaced by a mixture, containing 1 mM ATP, 0.05 mM GTP, 5 mM phosphoenolpyruvate and 20 μg of pyruvate kinase (0.1 ml per assay). The incubation usually was 20 min at 35°C.

4. Analysis of lysine peptides

The polylysine-synthesizing reaction was stopped by adding KOH to 0.3 N and incubating for 30 min at 35°C. The mixtures were then neutralized with HCl, diluted to 3 ml with water. ^{12}C-Dilysine and trilysine were added as markers. $HClO_4$ was added to a final concentration of 0.3N, and the solutions were allowed to stand overnight in a refrigerator. The precipitates usually containing about 200 cpm were discarded. The supernatants were adjusted to pH 4–5 with KOH, and further diluted to 12 ml with H_2O. When the lysine peptides were separated into the ribosome-bound, tRNA-bound and free peptide fractions, the reaction mixtures were diluted with 3 ml of the standard buffer, filtered through three layers of membrane filter and washed with three 3-ml portions of the buffer. The ribosome-bound polyLys-tRNA was retained on the filters and was extracted with three 0.5-ml portions of 0.3 N KOH. The filtrates were further fractionated into 0.3N $HClO_4$ precipitable materials (tRNA-bound lysine peptides) and $HClO_4$ soluble materials (free lysine peptides). These fractions, after being treated as described above, were finally diluted to 12 ml. The separation of lysine peptides in the final solutions was done on a cellulose phosphate column according to Smith et al. (28), except that it was run at pH 5.0. In some experiments, lysine peptides were separated by descending paper chromatography. After the lysine peptides were cleaved from the tRNA by KOH, 0.1-ml samples were plotted on a paper strip (2.2 × 58 cm) and eluted with n-butanol: acetic acid: pyridine: water (36:6:20:24 by vol.) for 5 days (36).

5. Other assays

Phenylalanine peptides were separated by benzoylated DEAE-cellulose which could separate phenylalanine peptides into three fractions: 1) diphenylalanine, 2) tri- and tetraphenylalanine and 3) peptides longer than tetraphenylalanine (24). The G-dependent hydrolysis of γ-^{32}P-GTP was done according to Conway and Lipmann (3). Protein was measured by the Folin reagent with bovine serum albumin as a standard. Radioactivity was measured by the scintillation method with efficiency of 75% for ^{14}C and 38% for ^{32}P.

Results

1. The erythromycin-ribosome complex
It has been shown that EMA specifically binds to the 50S subunit of *Staphylococcus aureus* ribosomes, forming a 1:1 ratio complex (14, 16). The formation of this complex requires NH_4^+ or K^+ ions. The association constant of the erythromycin-ribosome complex determined by the membrane filtration method is 4.7×10^5 M^{-1} (16). For further study of the mode of action of EMA, we decided to use the *E. coli* cell-free system since the protein synthesis in *E. coli* has been more thoroughly studied than that of *S. aureus*. Also, we have demonstrated that although whole cell *E. coli* is insensitive to EMA, the cell-free protein synthesis system is just as sensitive as that of *S. aureus* because the impermeability of *E. coli* cells to EMA is the cause of their resistance (15). The association constant of EMA and *E. coli* ribosomes, determined by the membrane filtration method, is 6.3×10^5 M^{-1}.

Before determining the mechanism of action of EMA, it is of primary importance to establish that the binding of EMA to the ribosomes is related to its antibacterial activity, and to obtain more information about this complex.

a) Relationship of ribosomal binding and antibacterial activity of erythromycin and its analogues: The antibacterial activities of 15 EMA derivatives and 9 macrolides were determined by a turbidity assay with *S. aureus* 209P as the test organism. The antibacterial activity of EMA is arbitrarily assigned as 734 units per μmole (the molecular weight). The ability of EMA analogues to bind to the ribosomes was determined by the displacement of ^{14}C-EMA

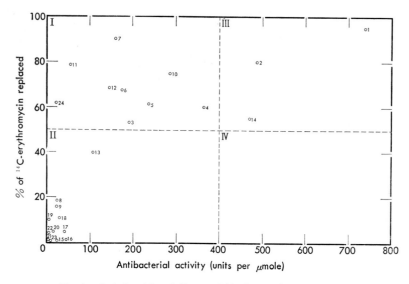

Fig. 1.   Relationship of ribosomal binding and antibacterial activity of erythromycin and its analogues. 1. erythromycin (EMA), 2. erythromycin B (EMB), 3. erythromycin C, 4. oleandomycin, 5. niddamycin, 6. spiramycin, 7. tylosin, 8. chalcomycin, 9. lankamycin, 10. 4″-formyl EMB, 11. 4″-acetyl EMB, 12. 11-acetyl EMB, 13. N-ethyl EMA, 14. 4′-hydroxyl EMA, 15. N-oxide EMA, 16. dihydro EMB, 17. Des-N-methyl EMA, 18. N-propyl EMA, 19. hemiketal EMA, 20. anhydro EMA, 21. erythronolide B, 22. 5-desosaminyl erythronolide B, 23. 3-mycarosyl erythronolide B and 24. 2′, 4″-diacetyl EMA.

on ribosomes. The results are shown in Fig. 1. The chart is divided into four equal areas. Those located in Quarter I have high binding ability but low antibacterial activity, those in Quarter II have both low binding and low antibacterial activity, those in Quarter III have both high binding and high antibacterial activity, and those in Quarter IV have low binding but high antibacterial activity. We concluded from this chart that compounds with low binding abilities always show low antibacterial activities. Compounds with high antibacterial activities always have high ribosome-binding abilities, but high binding ability does not necessarily correspond to high antibacterial activity.

b)   Thermal stability of ribosomes with respect to their protein synthesis function and binding of erythromycin: It is a common

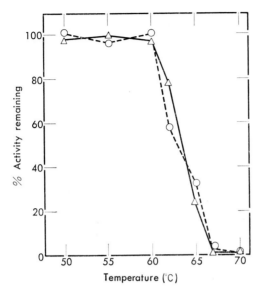

Fig. 2. Thermal stability of *E. coli* ribosomes. ○, poly U directed incorporation of phenylalanine; △, erythromycin bound to the ribosomes.

practice in the field of enzymology to show that a single enzyme acts on different substrates by determining the thermal denaturation of this enzyme with respect to different substrates. Although the ribosomes have a very complex structure, the thermal denaturation data could add some information about the relationship of EMA binding to protein synthesis. The ribosomes were incubated at various temperatures for 10 min, cooled in an ice bath, and tested for their ability to support the synthesis of polyphenylalanine and the binding of EMA. The results are shown in Fig. 2. The temperature profiles of these two functions are very similar with T_m values of 63.5°C and 63.0°C for EMA binding and protein synthesis, respectively.

c) Decrease of erythromycin binding to ribosomes by G and T factors: Factors G and T are supernatant proteins, but are also found on crude preparations of ribosomes and regarded as contaminants. Since their roles in protein synthesis are known, a study of their effect on EMA binding to the ribosomes may give

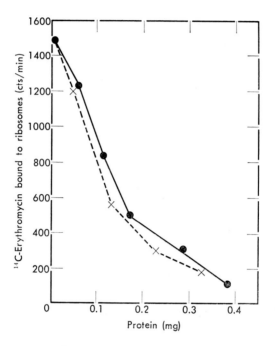

Fig. 3. Effect of G and T factors on the binding of erythromycin to the ribosomes. ●, G factor; ×, T factor.

some clue to the mode of action of EMA. G and T factors themselves cannot bind EMA as shown by equilibrium dialysis, yet they can decrease the binding of EMA to the ribosomes (Fig. 3).

d) Lack of competition between peptidyl-tRNA and erythromycin for ribosomal binding: It has been shown that EMA could not inhibit the coded binding of polyLys-tRNA, Ac-Phe-tRNA, Lys-tRNA and Phe-tRNA to ribosomes (*2, 30*). However, there is the possibility that they have a higher affinity than EMA for the ribosomes; and therefore, they can replace EMA, but EMA cannot replace them. To test this possibility various amounts of polyPhe-tRNA or polyLys-tRNA were added to the ribosomes and the corresponding mRNA; and after a 5-minute incubation period to complete the binding of peptidyl-tRNA to the ribosomes, ^{14}C-EMA was added. The results are shown in Table I. There is no

TABLE I

Binding of Erythromycin to Ribosomes in the Presence of Various Amounts of Peptidyl-tRNA

		^{14}C-Erythromycin bound to ribosomes
Ribosomes alone		1374 cpm
+poly U		1436
+poly U and polyPhe-tRNA	2.1 ODU	1423
+poly U and polyPhe-tRNA	4.2	1443
+poly U and polyPhe-tRNA	6.3	1421
Ribosomes alone		1328
+poly A		1349
+poly A and polyLys-tRNA	2.6 ODU	1339
+poly A and polyLys-tRNA	5.2	1397
+poly A and polyLys-tRNA	7.8	1384

indication that polyPhe-tRNA or polyLys-tRNA, at concentrations greater than those needed for saturation of the ribosomes, can decrease the binding of ^{14}C-EMA to the ribosomes.

2. Effect of erythromycin on the first peptide bond synthesis

Three different methods were used to determine the effect of EMA on the *first* peptide bond synthesis.

a) Dilysine synthesis in the absence of the G factor and GTP: Ribosomes, which were washed three times, were used in this experiment. The activity of the G factor in this ribosomal preparation was negligible as indicated by the low GTP hydrolysis and the slight amount of trilysine synthesized. The amount of dilysine synthesized in the presence of EMA was 6 to 15% above the control (Table II).

TABLE II

Effect of Erythromycin on Dilysine Synthesis in the Absence of G Factor and GTP

	Dilysine		Trilysine
Control	730 cpm	(100)	40 cpm
+EMA 10^{-3}M	788	(108)	27
+EMA 10^{-4}M	838	(115)	33
+EMA 10^{-5}M	794	(109)	19
+EMA 10^{-6}M	771	(106)	22

TABLE III

Effect of Erythromycin on Lysine Peptide Synthesis in the Presence of Fusidic Acid

	Dilysine		Trilysine	Tetralysine	Pentalysine	Hexalysine
Control	3344 cpm	(109)	2349 cpm	1864 cpm	1161 cpm	561 cpm
+fusidic acid 10^{-3}M	3056	(100)	76	0	0	0
+fusidic acid, +EMA 10^{-3}M	3354	(110)	0	0	0	0

b) Dilysine synthesis in the presence of fusidic acid: Fusidic acid is a translocation inhibitor (*31*). As shown in Table III, fusidic acid strongly inhibits trilysine synthesis but has little effect on dilysine synthesis. In the presence of both fusidic acid and EMA, trilysine is completely inhibited; yet the dilysine synthesis is increased about 10 % over the sample containing fusidic acid alone.

c) Formation of F-Met-puromycin: It may be argued that the synthesis of dilysine in the above experiments is an artificial test of peptidyl transferase activity because *in vivo* the action of this enzyme involves transferring an N-blocked aminoacyl moiety (F-Met or peptidyl) rather than transferring an N-free aminoacyl moiety as was the case in the previous experiments. However, the results of these experiments were made more valid by employing the F-Met-puromycin reaction. The data are shown in Table IV. EMA again stimulated the peptide bond formation about 20 %.

TABLE IV
Effect of Erythromycin on the Formation of F-Met-Puromycin

	F-Met-Puromycin formed	
Control	4517 cpm	(100)
+EMA 10^{-3}M	5061	(112)
+EMA 10^{-4}	5426	(120)
+EMA 10^{-5}	4654	(103)

3. Effect of erythromycin on translocation

Translocation is the most difficult to examine experimentally. The analysis of homopeptides may provide some information at this step, since formation of dipeptide is catalyzed by peptidyl transferase alone; and formation of tripeptide involves translocase in addition to the peptidyl transferase.

a) Static experiments: The final products of the poly A directed synthesis of lysine peptides were analyzed. When the reaction mixtures contained washed ribosomes, poly A, ^{14}C-Lys-tRNA, GTP, and G and T factors, EMA caused an accumulation of dilysine; but lysine peptides longer than dilysine were inhibited (Tables V-A, VI). Tanaka and Teraoka (*29*) have shown that EMA consistently caused the accumulation of di- and trilysine, sometimes even

TABLE V
Effect of Erythromycin on Peptide Synthesis

A.

	Dilysine	Trilysine	Tetralysine	Pentalysine	Hexalysine	Heptalysine
Control	3966 cpm	2528 cpm	2034 cpm	1039 cpm	891 cpm	662 cpm
+EMA 10^{-3}M	5790	933	0	0	0	0
+EMA 10^{-4}M	6923	1128	145	0	0	0
+EMA 10^{-5}M	7333	1488	475	0	0	0
+EMA 10^{-6}M	6904	1694	710	203	0	0
+EMA 10^{-7}M	4005	2150	1813	995	670	436

B.

	Dilysine	Trilysine	Tetralysine	Pentalysine	Hexalysine
Control	6180 cpm	2675 cpm	794 cpm	735 cpm	426 cpm
+EMA 10^{-4}M	8185	4454	904	0	0
+EMA 10^{-5}M	8344	4399	812	62	0
+EMA 10^{-6}M	6257	2786	710	91	0

C.

	Diphenylalanine	Tri- and Tetraphenylalanine	>	Tetraphenylalanine
Control	5615 cpm	2875 cpm		10742 cpm
+EMA 10^{-3}M	7311	3268		6406

TABLE VI
Lack of Effect of Erythromycin on Releasing Peptides from Ribosome

	Dilysine		Trilysine		Tetralysine		Pentalysine		Hexalysine	
	cpm	% of total	cpm	% of total	cpm	% of total	cpm	% of total	cpm	% of total
Control: Ribosome-bound	3129	(47)	2220	(54)	895	(48)	449	(68)	175	(100)
tRNA-bound	1702	(26)	678	(17)	249	(13)	47	(7)	0	
Free	1771	(27)	1189	(29)	719	(39)	164	(25)	0	
Total	6602	(100)	4087	(100)	1863	(100)	660	(100)	175	(100)
+EMA (1mM): Ribosome-bound	4006	(42)	2891	(66)	201	(71)	0		0	
tRNA-bound	3027	(32)	911	(20)	39	(14)	0		0	
Free	2610	(26)	614	(14)	43	(15)	0		0	
Total	9643	(100)	4416	(100)	283	(100)	0		0	

tetralysine. However, they used the S-100 fraction instead of the purified G and T factors. We ran a similar experiment, and indeed, tri- and tetralysine were also accumulated at higher concentrations of EMA (Table V-B). The accumulation of dilysine does not respond in a linear fashion to the concentration of EMA, the peak of accumulation being at 10^{-5} M EMA.

The effect of EMA on polyphenylalanine synthesis was also examined. In this experiment, although the purified G and T factors were used, EMA caused accumulation of di-, tri- and/or tetraphenylalanine but inhibited longer peptides (Table V-C).

b) Determination of ribosome-bound, tRNA-bound and free lysine peptides: The polylysine-synthesizing reaction mixtures were separated into three fractions: ribosome-bound, tRNA-bound and free lysine peptides, as described in "Methods." The lysine peptides in each fraction were analyzed. The results are shown in Table VI. In the control sample, 47% of dilysine, 54% of trilysine and 48% of tetralysine were bound to the ribosomes, as compared to the EMA-treated sample of 42, 66 and 71%, respectively. There is 5% less dilysine but 12% more trilysine and 23% more tetralysine bound to the ribosomes in the EMA-treated sample than in the control which rules out the possibility that the accumulation of short peptides is caused by the release of short peptides or peptidyl-tRNA from ribosomes.

c) Kinetic study of lysine peptide synthesis: The results from the analyses of homopeptide synthesis in static studies were rather confusing. No clear-cut mechanism could be proposed. The kinetic data, as shown in Fig. 4, clears up much of the confusion. At 3 min, EMA had already caused an accumulation of dilysine; and the accumulation became greater at 6 and 10 min. This phenomena can be explained by postulating that if EMA blocks a reaction after the synthesis of the first peptide bond, then the intermediate previous to this step will accumulate. EMA also caused the accumulation of trilysine in this experiment, but the accumulation of trilysine is much less than the accumulation of dilysine. This is probably due to the high amount of substrate (dilysine) which overcame the inhibitory effect of EMA. This explanation is consistent with the results of the inhibition of tetralysine by EMA

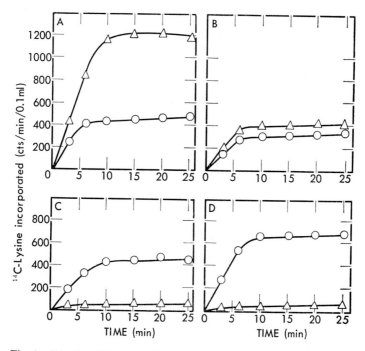

Fig. 4. Kinetics of lysine peptide synthesis. A, dilysine; B, trilysine; C, tetralysine; D, > tetralysine. O, control; △, in the presence of 1mM erythromycin.

TABLE VII
Effect of Erythromycin on G-Dependent GTP Hydrolysis

	γ-^{32}P-GTP-Hydrolyzed
Control	34326 cpm
+EMA 5× 10⁻³M	37551
+EMA 1× 10⁻³	36989
+EMA 1× 10⁻⁴	33387
+EMA 1× 10⁻⁵	32081
−G factor	1535

since the concentration of the substrate (trilysine) was only slightly higher than the control and it could not overcome the inhibition of EMA.

d) Effect of erythromycin on G-dependent GTP hydrolysis: The above data strongly suggest that EMA inhibits a reaction after the first peptide bond synthesis. The possibility of the inhibition of G-dependent GTP hydrolysis, a necessary reaction for the translocation, therefore was tested. The results showed that EMA has no effect on GTP hydrolysis (Table VII).

Discussion

The data presented in Fig. 1 showed that the correlation between binding affinity and antibacterial activity is poor. One of the possible reasons is that binding to the ribosomes was determined in a cell-free system, but the antibacterial activity was determined against whole cells. An EM derivative, unable to pass the bacterial cell wall or cell membrane, could show a low antibacterial activity, even though it may possess high binding affinity to the ribosomes.

   A direct comparison of the binding and inhibition of protein synthesis in the cell-free system is more meaningful. The inhibition of protein synthesis by several macrolides in the cell-free system has been reported (*19*). Niddamycin is about one hundred-fold and spiramycin and tylosin are about fifty-fold more potent than EMA, yet their binding affinity is no higher than EMA. This forces us to conclude that the binding affinity is not the only factor governing the potency of a macrolide. The binding affinity also seems to be related to the hydrophobic property of the derivatives, since most of the EMA derivatives in Fig. 1, Quarter I, are more lipid soluble than EMA. Nevertheless, it is safe to say that binding to the ribosomes is a prerequisite for antibacterial activity. The conclusion that it is necessary for EMA to be bound to the ribosomes before it exert an inhibitory effect on protein synthesis is further strengthened by the observations that ribosomes isolated from resistant strains of bacteria have a lower affinity for EMA (*21, 26, 34*); and ribosomes of animal origins cannot bind EMA, which makes their protein synthesis insensitive to this antibiotic (*17*).

   The thermal stability of ribosomes with respect to protein synthesis and to the binding of EMA is quite similar. Considering the complexity of ribosomal structure, it is not justifiable to say that denaturation of a single protein causes the diminution of both protein synthesis activity and EMA binding. Nevertheless, it does indicate that a similar gross structure is required for these two functions. It is interesting to observe that both the G and T factors can decrease the binding of EMA to ribosomes. It may mean that the G and T factors overlap the EMA binding site or both factors can change the conformation of the ribosomes to render it unfavorable for the binding of EMA. On the other hand, peptidyl-tRNA cannot decrease the binding of EMA to the ribosomes and EMA has no effect on the binding of peptidyl-tRNA and amino-acyl-tRNA (2, 30), which may indicate that the EMA binding site is neither at the peptidyl site nor at the aminoacyl site of the ribosomes.

The effect of EMA on the synthesis of the first peptide bond was examined by dilysine synthesis in the absence of the G factor and GTP, in the presence of fusidic acid and by the F-Met-puromycin reaction. EMA consistently showed slight stimulation of this step. Although the stimulation is rather weak, the maximal stimulation being about 20% over the control, we think this stimulative effect is real because not only was it consistently seen in three different assays as mentioned above, but it was also observed in another laboratory (Weisblum, this volume). The slight stimulation of the first peptide bond formation at high concentrations of EMA certainly cannot be regarded as the primary action of the antibiotic.

Analyses of lysine peptides in the complete protein synthesis reaction mixture yielded interesting information. The accumulation of dilysine was much more pronounced in the complete reaction mixture than in the reaction mixture which only allowed synthesis of dilysine. In some cases, the accumulation of trilysine and tetralysine was also observed; but in other cases, the inhibition of trilysine could be seen at a very low EMA concentration (10^{-7}M). A kinetic study showed that more dilysine was accumulated at the later stage of the reaction than at the earlier stage. There are at least three possible ways to cause the accumulation of short peptides. One way is by the intrinsic activity of EMA to stimulate short peptide synthesis. The results from the dipeptide synthesis indicated that EMA indeed can stimulate dipeptide synthesis, but the stimulation is too low to explain the drastic accumulation observed in the complete system. A second way is by the release of short peptides or peptidyl-tRNA from the ribosomes. This idea was dispelled by an experiment in which the ribosome-bound, tRNA-bound and free lysine peptides were separated and quantitatively measured, indicating that the ribosomes in the EMA-treated sample actually bound more di- and trilysine than those in the untreated sample. A third and more likely way is by blocking a reaction after the first peptide bond formation; and thus the product immediately preceding the block is accumulated. The accumulation of trilysine and sometimes tetralysine when the S-100 fraction was used instead of the purified G and T factors can be explained by the following: 1) the binding of EMA to ribosomes is reversible, 2) the accumulated diLys-tRNA pushes the reaction toward trilysine synthesis, and 3) probably the amount of S-100 fraction added to the reaction mixture contained more G factor than that added when the purified G factor was used, and the excess amount of G factor partially overcame the inhibition of EMA. This implies that the action of EMA is in some way related to the G factor or peptidyl-tRNA. In fact, we have observed that the G and T factors, but not peptidyl-tRNA, can decrease the binding of EMA to ribosomes. However, the high concentrations of G and T needed to decrease EMA binding cast some doubt on the importance of this phenomenon.

The question as to which step after the synthesis of the first peptide bond is inhibited by EMA has to be answered. There are several steps between the synthesis of the first and second peptide bonds: 1) the release of tRNA from the donor site, 2) the movement of the ribosome in relation to the dipeptidyl-tRNA-mRNA complex so that dipeptidyl-tRNA moves from the acceptor site on the ribosome to the donor site, 3) hydrolysis of GTP, 4) transmission of energy to the movement, 5) the binding of a third aminoacyl-tRNA to the acceptor site, and 6) the synthesis of a second peptide bond. Steps 1) to 4) should be covered under the term of translocation, but the binding of the third aminoacyl-tRNA and the synthesis of the second peptide bond are not. The inhibition of any step listed above could result in the inhibition of tripeptide synthesis. Igarashi *et al.* (*8*) have shown that EMA inhibited the release of tRNA. Cundliffe and McQuillen (*5*) have suggested that EMA caused the peptidyl-tRNA to stick in the acceptor site. Those suggestions are consistent with our findings but inconsistent with Schlessinger's observation (*27*) that the movement of ribosomes on mRNA continues in the presence of EMA, unless there is an unknown mechanism in which tRNA remains on the donor site and peptidyl-tRNA remains on the acceptor site but ribosomes can move along mRNA.

We have shown that the G-dependent hydrolysis of GTP is not inhibited by EMA, but we don't know whether EMA can uncouple the transmission of energy to the translocation. The possibility that the inhibition of tripeptide synthesis due to the inhibition of the binding of a third aminoacyl-tRNA is unlikely, since both enzymic and non-enzymic binding of aminoacyl-tRNA could not be inhibited by EMA (*18*).

If indeed EMA inhibits translocation, the mechanism of action is entirely different from that of fusidic acid since EMA cannot inhibit G-dependent GTP hydrolysis. Another distinction between EMA and fusidic acid is that EMA causes the accumulation of dipeptides but fusidic acid does not. The manner in which ribosomes are attached to artificial mRNA (poly A or poly U) is not known. If the ribosomes attach to the artificial mRNA randomly, fusidic acid, although it blocks translocation, should cause an accumulation of dipeptides. If, however, the ribosomes enter the mRNA from the 5'-end in an orderly fashion, then the blockage of translocation would not cause an accumulation of dipeptides if there is a saturating amount of aminoacyl-tRNA. Our data as well as data from another laboratory (*22, 23*) showed that fusidic acid does not cause the accumulation of dipeptides, indicating that the ribosomes enter the artificial mRNA from the 5'-end. Consequently, the accumulation of dipeptides in the presence of EMA requires the movement of the ribosome on mRNA to be continued. This argument and the observation that EMA did not stop the movement of ribosomes on mRNA (*27*) prompted us to give an alternative hypothesis, namely; EMA binds to the 50S ribosomes and changes the activity of peptidyl transferase, most likely through an allosteric effect, and thus stimulates the first peptide bond formation and inhibits the second and subsequent peptide bond formations. This implies that the formation of the first peptide bond and the second peptide bond is somewhat different, a theory which remains to be proven experimentally. The virtue of the second hypothesis is that it accommodates all seemingly contradictory data reported from various laboratories. For instance, the addition of one lysine to polyLys-tRNA and the formation of polyLys-puromycin, which test the synthesis of peptide bonds beyond the first one, were inhibited by EMA. On the other hand, the puromycin reaction with Ac-Phe-tRNA and F-Met-tRNA, which tests the synthesis of the first peptide bond, was not inhibited. This hypothesis is similar to the mechanism of action of chloramphenicol which inhibits peptide bond formation but allows the movement of ribosomes on mRNA to continue (7). This is reasonable because EMA competes with chloramphenicol for a binding site on the 50S ribosome.

SUMMARY

Twenty-four erythromycin congeners were tested for their binding affinity to the bacterial ribosomes and antibacterial activity. Results showed that binding to the ribosomes is a prerequisite for their activity. However, a high binding affinity does not necessarily correspond to a high antibacterial activity. Permeability and the hydrophobic property of a compound also have influence on its activity and affinity to binding to the ribosomes. Erythromycin did not inhibit the first peptide bond formation when tested with three different assays, namely, N-formylmethionyl-puromycin formation, dilysine synthesis in the absence of the G factor and GTP and dilysine synthesis in the presence of fusidic acid. In fact, erythromycin may be slightly stimulative to this step (the maximal stimulation being 20% over the control). In the complete protein synthesis system, the apparent stimulation of the first peptide synthesis was much more pronounced (two- to three-fold over the control); and the inhibition of trilysine was seen at extremely low concentrations of erythromycin. However, in some cases the inhibition of trilysine was overcome by some unknown factor, possibly the G factor and peptidyl-tRNA; and therefore, the accumulation of trilysine and even tetralysine was observed. The kinetic data on lysine peptide synthesis indicated that the step after the first peptide bond formation was inhibited by erythromycin. Two alternative mechanisms were discussed: 1) Erythromycin inhibits some phase of translocation; and 2) erythromycin distorts the conformation of the peptidyl transferase region through allosteric effect and thus slightly stimulates the first peptide bond synthesis and inhibits the second and subsequent peptide bond synthesis.

Acknowledgments
The author is greatly indebted to Miss E. E. Robishaw for her help in researching and preparing of this manuscript, to Mrs. M. Putterman who participated in some of the experiments reported here, and to Dr. R. G. Wiegand for discussions and for reviewing the manuscript.

REFERENCES

1 Brock, T. D., and Brock, M. L. 1959. Similarity in mode of action of chloramphenicol and erythromycin. *Biochim. Biophys. Acta*, **33**, 274–275.

2 Cerná, J., Rychlík, I., and Pulkrábek, P. 1969. The effect of antibiotics on the coded binding of peptidyl-tRNA to the ribosome and on the transfer of the peptidyl residue to puromycin. *European J. Biochem.*, **9**, 27–35.

3 Conway, T. W., and Lipmann, F. 1964. Characterization of a ribosome-linked guanosine triphosphatase in *Escherichia coli* extracts. *Proc. Natl. Acad. Sci. U. S.*, **52**, 1462–1469.

4 Corcoran, J. W., and Oleinick, N. L. 1969. Abstr. on the mechanism of inhibition of bacterial protein synthesis by erythromycin. *6th Intern. Congr. Chemotherapy*, 47.

5 Cundliffe, E., and McQuillen, K. 1967. Bacterial protein synthesis: the effects of antibiotics. *J. Mol. Biol.*, **30**, 137–146.

6 Ertel, R., Brat, N., Redfield, B., Allende, J. E., and Weissbach, H. 1968. Binding of guanosine 5′-triphosphate by soluble factors required by polypeptide synthesis. *Proc. Natl. Acad. Sci. U. S.*, **59**, 861–868.

7 Gurgo, C., Apirion, D., and Schlessinger, D. 1969. Polyribosome metabolism in *Escherichia coli* treated with chloramphenicol, neomycin, spectinomycin or tetracycline. *J. Mol. Biol.*, **45**, 205–220.

8 Igarashi, K., Ishitsuka, H., and Kaji, A. 1969. Comparative studies on the mechanism of action of lincomycin, streptomycin, and erythromycin. *Biochem. Biophys. Res. Commun.*, **37**, 499–504.

9 Jayaraman, J., and Goldberg, I. G. 1968. Localization of sparsomycin action to the peptide-bond-forming step. *Biochemistry*, **7**, 418–421.

10 Leder, P., and Bursztyn, H. 1966. Initiation of protein synthesis. I. Effect of formylation of methionyl-tRNA on codon recognition. *Proc. Natl. Acad. Sci. U. S.*, **56**, 1579–1585.

11 Leder, P., and Bursztyn, H. 1966. Initiation of protein synthesis. II. A convenient assay for the ribosome-dependent synthesis of N-formyl-^{14}C-methionyl-puromycin. *Biochem. Biophys. Res. Commun.*, **25**, 233–238.

12 Leder, P., Singer, M. F., and Brimacombe, R. L. C. 1965. Synthesis of trinucleoside diphosphates with polynucleotide phosphorylase. *Biochemistry*, **4**, 1561–1567.

13 Mao, J. C.-H. 1967. Protein synthesis in a cell-free extract from *Staphylococcus aureus*. *J. Bacteriol.*, **94**, 80–86.

14 Mao, J. C.-H. 1967. The stoichiometry of erythromycin binding to ribosomal particles of *Staphylococcus aureus*. *Biochem. Pharmacol.*, **16**, 2441–2443.

15 Mao, J. C.-H., and Putterman, M. 1968. Accumulation in gram-positive and gram-negative bacteria as a mechanism of resistance to erythromycin. *J. Bacteriol.*, **95**, 1111–1117.

16 Mao, J. C.-H., and Putterman, M. 1969. The intermolecular complex of erythromycin and ribosome. *J. Mol. Biol.*, **46**, 347–361.

17 Mao, J. C.-H., Putterman, M., and Wiegand, R. G. 1970. Biochemical basis for the selective toxicity of erythromycin. *Biochem. Pharmacol.*, **19**, 391–399.

18 Mao, J. C.-H., and Robishaw, E. E. 1971. Effect of macrolides on peptide-bond formation and translocation. *Biochemistry*, **10**, 2054–2061.

19 Mao, J. C.-H., and Wiegand, R. G. 1968. Mode of action of macrolides. *Biochim. Biophys. Acta*, **157**, 404–413.

20 Monro, R.E., and Vazquez, D. 1967. Ribosome-catalyzed peptidyl transfer: effect of some inhibitors of protein synthesis. *J. Mol. Biol.*, **28**, 161–165.

21 Oleinick, N. L., and Corcoran, J. W. 1969. Two types of binding of erythromycin to ribosomes from antibiotic-sensitive and-resistant *Bacillus subtilis* 168. *J. Biol. Chem.*, **244**, 727–735.

22 Pestka, S. 1970. Studies on the formation of tRNA-ribosome complexes. V. Survey of the effect of antibiotics on N-acetyl-phenylalanyl-puromycin formation: possible mechanism of chloramphenicol action. *Arch. Biochem. Biophys.*, **136**, 80–88.

23 Pestka, S. 1970. Studies on the formation of tRNA-ribosome complexes. IX. Effect of antibiotics on translocation and peptide bond formation. *Arch. Biochem. Biophys.*, **136**, 89–96.

24 Pestka, S., Scolnick, E. M., and Heck, B. H. 1969. A convenient assay for mono-, di-, and oligo-phenylalanines. *Anal. Biochem.*, **28**, 376–384.

25 Rychlík, I., Chládek, S., and Žemlička, J. 1967. Release of peptide chains from the polylysyl-tRNA ribosome complex by cytidylyl-(3′→5′)-2′(3′)-O-glycyladenosine. *Biochim. Biophys. Acta*, **138**, 640–642.

26 Saito, T., Hashimoto, H., and Mitsuhashi, S. 1968. Drug resistance of *Staphylococci*: decrease in formation of erythromycin-ribosome complex in erythromycin resistant strains of *S. aureus*. *Japan J. Microbiol.*, **13**, 119–121.

27 Schlessinger, D. 1969. Ribosomes: development of some current ideas. *Bacteriol. Rev.*, **33**, 445–453.

28 Smith, J. D., Traut, R. R., Blackburn, G. M., and Monro, R. E. 1965. Action of puromycin in polyadenylic acid—directed polylysine synthesis. *J. Mol. Biol.*, **13**, 617–628.

29 Tanaka, K., and Teraoka, H. 1968. Effect of erythromycin on polylysine synthesis directed by polyadenylic acid in an *Escherichia coli* cell-free system. *J. Biochem.*, **64**, 635–648.

30 Tanaka, K., Teraoka, H., Nagira, T., and Tamaki, M. 1966. Erythromycin-ribosome complex formation and non-enzymatic binding of aminoacyl-tRNA to ribosome-mRNA complex. *Biochim. Biophys. Acta*, **123**, 435–437.

31 Tanaka, N., Kinoshita, T., and Masukawa, H. 1968. Mechanism of protein synthesis inhibition by fusidic acid and related antibiotics. *Biochem. Biophys. Res. Commun.*, **30**, 278–283.

32 Tardrew, P. L., Mao, J. C.-H., and Kenney, D. 1969. Antibacterial activity of 2′-esters of erythromycin. *Appl. Microbiol.*, **18**, 159–165.

33 Taubman, S. B., So, A. G., Young, F. E., Dovie, E. W., and Corcoran, J. W. 1964. Effect of erythromycin on protein bio-synthesis in *Bacillus subtilis*. *Antimicrobial Agents and Chemotherapy—1963*, 395–401.

34 Teraoka, H., Tamaki, M., and Tanaka, K. 1970. Peptide transferase activity of *Escherichia coli* ribosomes having an altered protein component in the 50S subunit. *Biochem. Biophys. Res. Commun.*, **38**, 328–332.

35 Vazquez, D. 1966. Antibiotics effect chloramphenicol uptake by bacteria. Their effect on amino acid incorporation in a cell-free system. *Biochim. Biophys. Acta*, **114**, 289–295.

36 Waley, S. G., and Watson, J. 1953. The action of trypsin on polylysine. *Biochim. J.*, **55**, 328–337.

ERYTHROMYCIN AND THE BACTERIAL RIBOSOME
A Study of the Mechanism of Sensitivity and Resistance to Macrolide Antibiotics and Lincomycin in *Bacillus subtilis* 168

John W. Corcoran

Department of Biochemistry, Northwestern University Medical School Chicago, Illinois, U.S.A.

In the fall of 1961, studies on the biogenesis of the clinically useful antibiotic erythromycin A had developed to the point where we were planning an extensive characterization of the enzymes in the cell-free and pure state (*3*). This effort, still in progress, reflects our desire to develop a model system, employing the producing actinomycete, *Streptomyces erythreus*, from which we can learn as much as possible about the biochemistry of the erythromycins. It is our intention to learn why these so-called secondary metabolites are produced in the first place and to understand the comparative biochemistry of the synthetic apparatus and other enzyme-catalyzed activities of *S. erythreus*. This effort which results from a curiosity about the relationship of the erythromycins to the producing organism was matched by an equal curiosity as to the interaction of the secondary metabolites (antibiotics) with foreign cells—especially those for which they are toxic agents. In this regard, erythromycin is a very useful clinical agent with broad spectrum bacteriostatic activity towards many Gram-positive bacteria, but with generally little activity towards Gram-negative and eucaryotic cells (1).

When we started our work in 1962, very little was known about the mode of action of erythromycin A (erythromycin). Brock and Brock (2) studying a rather insensitive strain of *Escherichia coli* had provided some data indicating that erythromycin was an inhibitor of protein synthesis, but the high concentrations of antibiotic required might also have caused this inhibition by secondary means. Nothing at all had been reported concerning the mechanism of bacterial resistance to erythromycin. Thus it seemed important to define a bacterial system in which both problems could be studied.

For this purpose we started with a strain of *Bacillus subtilis* 168 which was well described from the genetic point of view (12). In order to provide for a comparison between nucleic acid and protein metabolism in this strain, the particular strain of *B. subtilis* used was a double auxotroph requiring both indole (tryptophan) and adenine for growth. The strain of bacteria selected was also extremely sensitive to erythromycin, being reduced in its multiplication rate by 50% (ID_{50}) when the antibiotic concentration was about 5×10^{-8}M (0.04 μg/ml). A considerable number of spontaneous mutants of the parent strain of *B. subtilis* 168 were obtained when the culture was cultivated on agar plates containing erythromycin. These new strains were stable and quite similar both to the parent strain and each other. All had about the same degree of relative resistance to erythromycin when this was determined by the serial tube dilution method. One of the strains was chosen for our work and it was about 125-fold more resistant to erythromycin ($ID_{50} = 4 \times 10^{-6}$M or 3.0 μg/ml). It should be emphasized that this strain, which together with subcellular parts will be referred to in this review as "resistant," is still quite sensitive to erythromycin.

The genetic nature of the mutation leading to the "resistant" strain of *B. subtilis* 168 was demonstrated by studies in which DNA isolated from the mutant was shown to transform the parent or "sensitive" bacterial strain to resistance at a rate comparable to that for the transformation of nutritional markers. According to this evidence, the other mutants obtained were similar to the one selected for further study, since their DNA transformed the "sensitive" strain at comparable rates. All the data mentioned (*13*) served to support the conclusion that the class of spontaneous mutants represented by our erythromycin-resistant strain of *B. subtilis* 168 had suffered a single nucleotide base change in its chromosomal DNA and that the expression of this alteration should lead to a bacterium having only a single primary chemical difference from its parent. Naturally, the physiological expression of a single chemical difference between two bacterial strains may lead to many differences in both cell chemistry and function; and for this reason, it was anticipated that it might be difficult to define exactly the target of erythromycin action.

The first experimental approach (*13*) using the two strains of *B. subtilis* 168 was aimed at defining the mechanism of the acquired resistance to erythromycin. The question asked was whether the resistance had anything to do with a biochemical change at the target site. If so, then the study of the mechanism of action and of resistance would be the same. It was soon suspected that the resistance to erythromycin shown by the mutant form of *B. subtilis* was indeed related to some change associated with the site of drug action, since neither strain of bacteria was able to destroy the antibiotic and both strains accumulated large amounts of it in their interior (Fig. 1). The amounts of erythromycin taken up were sufficient to suggest active transport of some sort, but this explanation may be incorrect in view of our later observation (below) that the antibiotic binds to subcellular particles (ribosomes). The amount of erythromycin taken up by the "resistant" *B. subtilis* was somewhat less than that taken up by the "sensitive" strain, but the difference (2–2.5-fold) is insufficient to explain the 125-fold difference in sensitivity shown by these cells. The studies also demonstrated that the entry of erythromycin into the bacterial cells is readily reversible (Fig. 2). Finally, a study of the utilization of adenine-^{14}C and tryptophan-^{3}H by the two bacterial strains showed that both substrates are utilized, and when erythromycin is added in sub-lethal amounts it is a potent inhibitor of protein synthesis (tryptophan utilization is blocked) but not of nucleic acid formation (adenine utilization continued).

Subsequent studies have for the most part employed cell-free systems derived from the "sensitive" and "resistant" strains of *B. subtilis* 168, and they have confirmed this preliminary finding that protein synthesis is the target of erythromycin action and that at least one class of antibiotic resistant mutants is biochemically different at this site of action. The work of Taubman *et al.* (*13, 14*) showed that erythromycin could inhibit protein synthesis in cell-free systems and demonstrated significantly that the amount required was higher in the preparation made from the "resistant" bacteria. The step in protein synthesis affected by erythromycin was identified as that in which activated amino acids (amino acyl-tRNA's) are joined in peptide linkage in a monosome (mRNA-70S ribosome complex) dependent process.

Wilhelm and Corcoran (*16*) extended the previous findings by fractionating the crude systems and then making reconstituted cell-free systems. The "message" RNA (mRNA) upon which these reconstituted systems depended was either endogenous material which was retained on a fraction of the purified ribosomes or was a synthetic homopolyribonucleotide like polyadenylic (poly A),

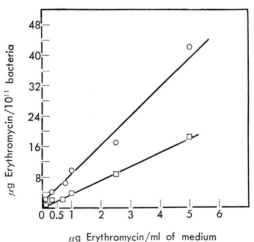

Fig. 1.   Uptake of erythromycin by erythromycin-sensitive and erythromycin-resistant *B. subtilis* as a function of extracellular antibiotic concentration. ○, sensitive; □, resistant (*13*).

polycytidylic (poly C) or polyuridylic (poly U) acid. The latter mRNA's are coded for a single amino acid each and thus promote the formation of homooligopeptides (polylysines, polyprolines and polyphenylalanines, respectively). The properties of the synthesis depending on the endogenous mRNA's will be discussed below, but the incorporation of L-lysine, L-proline and L-phenylalanine into the respective homooligopeptides was qualitatively similar and permitted a definition of the component in the cell-free extracts which determined their sensitivity to erythromycin.

The reconstituted systems with and without erythromycin utilized the amino acids for peptide synthesis at a linear rate (after a short lag period) for about 20 min and then ceased to function (Fig. 3). No explanation for either the lag or the cessation of synthesis is available, but the behavior of the systems was similar to that described by others. The reconstituted systems were similar to the crude extracts in that more erythromycin was required for equivalent inhibition of polypeptide synthesis when the whole

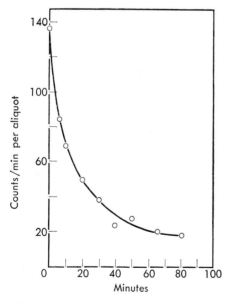

Fig. 2.   Exchange of intracellular and extracellular erythromycin on incubation of *B. subtilis*. ○, erythromycin-sensitive (*13*).

system was derived from the "resistant" strain of *B. subtilis* (Fig. 4). When reconstituted systems were made in which the components were "cross matched" (for instance, when the soluble enzyme fraction was taken from the "sensitive" bacteria and the ribosomes from the "resistant" mutant strain), it became evident that the single factor which defines the amount of erythromycin required for equivalent inhibition of polypeptide synthesis is the bacterial ribosome—in particular the 50S subunit (Fig. 5). On the basis of a functional criterion, our studies had implicated the 50S ribosomal subunit as being involved in the action of erythromycin; and in addition, they had indicated that the 50S ribosomal unit from the "resistant" strain of *B. subtilis* is functionally different from that present in the "sensitive" parent bacterium.

A dramatic confirmation of the conclusion that both erythro-

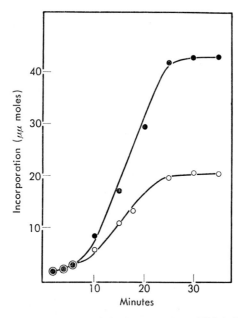

Fig. 3.   Kinetics of the incorporation of ^{14}C-lysine into polypeptides with ribosomes from EaDC-sensitive *B. subtilis*. ●, standard reaction mixture plus poly A and ^{14}C-lysine (aliquots were taken at times indicated after addition of the enzyme fraction); ○, as above, but with 2.0×10^{-6}M erythromycin.

mycin sensitivity and resistance are related to the 50S ribosomal particle came from studies of the physical behavior of the antibiotic. Tritiated erythromycin had been added to crude extracts of both strains of *B. subtilis* by Taubman *et al.* (*15*); and upon physical fractionation of the system by centrifugation through a density gradient of sucrose, it was observed that erythromycin was specifically bound to the 50S ribosomal particles derived from the "sensitive" strain. Under the conditions used there was no observable binding to 50S particles derived from the "resistant" bacteria. Since the "resistant" bacteria are really quite sensitive to the action of erythromycin, this "all-or-none" behavior had seemed to argue against a direct correlation between the binding of the antibiotic to the 50S ribosomal unit and its inhibitory action on protein synthesis involving these same ribosomal particles. However, the

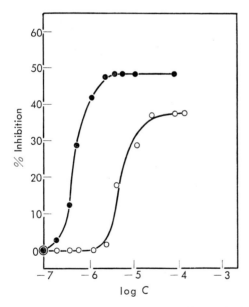

Fig. 4. Comparison of EaDC-sensitive and EaDC-resistant ribosomes and the inhibitory effect of EaDC on incorporation of ^{14}C-lysine into polypeptides. ●, standard reaction mixture employing ribosomes from the EaDC-sensitive strain of *B. subtilis* plus poly A and ^{14}C-lysine; ○, as above, but with ribosomes from the EaDC-resistant strain.

possibility of some direct relationship was strong, especially in the light of genetic mapping experiments which had also correlated the acquisition of resistance to erythromycin by *B. subtilis* with a chemical change in the 50S ribosomal subunit (*4, 5*). Accordingly, a more detailed examination was made of the interaction of erythromycin with ribosomes derived from our two bacterial strains.

When purified ribosomes and ribosomal subunits from both the "sensitive" and "resistant" strains of *B. subtilis* were incubated with varying concentrations of tritiated erythromycin, it was found that both types of ribosome have a strong affinity for the antibiotic with the "sensitive" units binding it most tightly (*9, 10*). Two types of binding were observed (Fig. 6): one at low concentra-

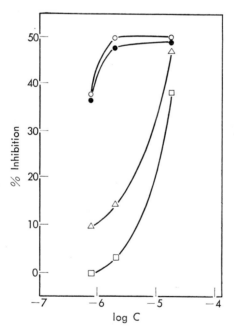

Fig. 5.   Inhibition of polylysine synthesis; incubations contained ribosomes, enzyme fraction, and erythromycin plus poly A and ^{14}C-lysine. ●, sensitive ribosomes and sensitive enzyme fraction; ○, sensitive ribosomes and resistant enzyme fraction; △, resistant ribosomes and resistant enzyme fraction; □, resistant ribosomes and sensitive enzyme fraction.

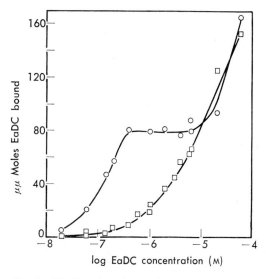

Fig. 6.   Binding of erythromycin to sensitive and resistant ribosomes as a function of erythromycin concentration. The standard incubation mixtures contained Tris-HCl, magnesium acetate, ammonium chloride, erythromycin, consisting of combinations of ^{3}H-erythromycin and unlabeled erythromycin, and ribosomes. ○, sensitive ribosomes; □, resistant ribosomes.

tions of the drug and the other when the amount of erythromycin is very high. The former binding is stoichiometric (one molecule of erythromycin per 50S ribosomal unit), reversible and dependent on the presence of monovalent cations (40mM NH_4^+ or K^+). The stoichiometry of the binding is easily seen in the case of the "sensitive" 50S ribosomal units; but with the "resistant" ribosomes, analysis of the data was required to confirm the presence of a unique binding site for one erythromycin molecule (*cf. 10*). In both cases, the association constant is very high (2.6×10^7 M^{-1} for the "sensitive" ribosomal unit and $8 \times 10^5 M^{-1}$ for the "resistant" particle).

Knowing that erythromycin interacts with both species of 50S ribosomal particles with a different association constant and that something about these same 50S units differs when their function in promoting peptide synthesis is measured, it was tempting to

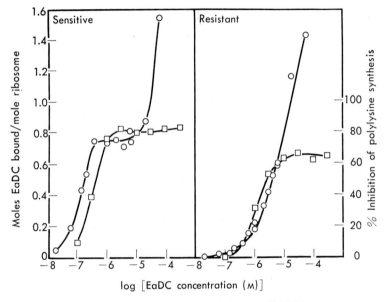

Fig. 7. Correlation of erythromycin binding and inhibition of poly-peptide synthesis. The curves for binding of erythromycin to sensitive and resistant ribosomes are those of Fig. 6. ○, binding; □, inhibition.

propose that the binding of the antibiotic to the ribosome is a prerequisite for the inhibitory action. The concentration depend-encies of the two phenomena are roughly similar (Fig. 7) and it is of interest to note that the multiple site binding of the antibiotic which occurs at very high concentrations of the drug is not ac-companied by any additional inhibition of protein synthesis. Another observation, although at first quite perplexing, seemed to offer support for linking the binding step with inhibitory action. This was an observation made by Wilhelm *et al.* (*17*) that protein synthesis, in reconstituted cell-free systems, which depends on endogenous mRNA, is completely insensitive to erythromycin. Further work (*10*) has confirmed the general nature of this observa-tion and demonstrated that the same extracts and ribosomes, when assayed for their ability to form homooligopeptides in response to poly A, *etc.*, are very sensitive to erythromycin (Table I). Only one explanation seemed to make sense. Perhaps, those ribosomes associated with some parts of the "natural" mRNA's which were being translated at the time cell growth that was interrupted have their binding site for erythromycin blocked. If this explanation could be verified, there would be some convincing proof of an obligatory relationship between the binding of erythromycin to some "site" on the 50S ribosomal unit and the observed inhibition of polypeptide synthesis.

TABLE I

Comparison of Erythromycin Sensitivity of Poly A- and Endogenous mRNA-Directed Amino Acid Incorporation

Conditions		Incorporation system (cpm incorporated)	
		^{14}C-Lys+Poly A	^{14}C-Amino acid mixture
Complete		7172	832
Complete+erythromycin,	10^{-7}M	5926	820
	10^{-6}M	1617	698
	3×10^{-6}M		810
Complete+rifamycin SV,	2×10^{-6}M		642
	10^{-5}M		882

The reaction mixtures contained in 0.25 ml: 2.5 μmoles Tris-HCl buffer at pH 7.6, 3 μmoles Mg(OAc)$_2$, 10 μmoles NH$_4$Cl, 1.5 μmoles β-mercaptoethanol, 0.25 μmoles Na$_2$ATP, 0.02 μmoles GTP, 12.5 μmoles phosphoenolpyruvate, 12.5 μg pyruvate kinase, 50 μg B. subtilis tRNA, 150 μg protein from the dialyzed S-100 supernatant fraction, 2.5 $A_{260m\mu}$ units of ribosomes from a sensitive strain of B. subtilis, and the indicated concentrations of erythromycin or rifamycin SV. In addition, either 50 μg poly A, 0.4 μCi ^{14}C-lysine, and a mixture of 19 ^{12}C-amino acids minus lysine, or 0.125 μCi ^{14}C-amino acid mixture and a mixture of 6 ^{12}C-amino acids (asparagine, glutamine, cysteine, tryptophan, methionine and histidine, those which are absent or limiting in the ^{14}C-amino acid mixture each at a final concentration of 8×10^{-5} M) were added. After incubation at 37°C for 30 min, a 50 μl aliquot was transferred to a filter paper disk and treated with hot trichloroacetic acid.

A series of experiments were performed by Oleinick which employed a strain of E. coli sensitive to erythromycin and possessing low endogenous amounts of ribonuclease (MRE 600). The reason for using this strain rather than either of our strains of B. subtilis was that the stability of the 30S ribosomal subunits from the latter is low. Stability was important because the goal of the study was to make functional 70S monosome complexes in a stepwise fashion and measure the effect of erythromycin on these at each stage. For this purpose, a procedure reported from Lipmann's laboratory was followed (6) in which N-acetylated phenylalanyl-tRNA (N-Ac-Phe-tRNA) is used as a substitute for the normal initiator of bacterial protein synthesis (N-formyl-methioninyl-tRNA) and phenylalanyl-tRNA for the amino acyl-tRNA's required for completion of the polypeptide chain. The system is somewhat artificial in that the homo ribonucleotide poly U is the mRNA upon which the synthesis depends. However, in many ways the system mimics normal protein synthesis. For instance, the ribosome/poly U/N-Ac-Phe-tRNA complex is formed with the initiation factors and energy sources (GTP) required for "normal" protein synthesis and the formation of N-acetylated oligophenylalanines by this complex requires not only the Phe-tRNA substrate molecules but GTP and the soluble factors involved in the translocation process, again typical of more normal protein synthesis.

The experiments employing the 30S and 50S ribosomal units from E. coli MRE 600 are reported on in Table II (10). The initiation complex formed from the 30S ribosomal unit, poly U and N-Ac-Phe-tRNA-^{14}C (System A), was mixed with 50S ribosomal particles which had been separately treated with ^{14}C-Phe-tRNA and also either had been treated with erythromycin (System C) or had not (System B). The ^{14}C-N-Ac-Phe-tRNA is bound stably to the 30S/poly U complex, but the radioactive Phe-tRNA is stably bound to the 50S ribosomal subunit only when the latter is incorporated into the monosome (70S) complex (Table II-1 and -2). When GTP and soluble enzymes are not supplied, the synthetic potential of such a mixture is limited to the production of dipeptides (some tripeptides are formed, but the mechanism seems not to involve the normal "translocation" step (11)). The enzymatic activity catalyzing the peptide bond formation, peptidyl synthase, is believed to be a constitutive part of the ribosomal complex. It is interesting to note (Table II-2) that the presence or absence of erythromycin in the complex has no effect on the amount of di- and tripeptides produced. When the same complexes are provided with GTP, the pattern remains similar; but when soluble enzyme factors (supernatant after centrifugation of the cell-free extract at $100,000 \times g$) are also added, the picture changes dramatically.

TABLE II
Limited Access of Erythromycin to Preformed Peptide Synthesizing Complexes

1. Preincubation mixtures (20 min, 25°C)	dpm bound
A=30S subunit+initiation factors+poly U+^{14}C-acetyl-Phe-tRNA	2100
B=50S subunit+^{14}C-Phe-tRNA	140
C=50S subunit+erythromycin+^{14}C-Phe-tRNA	183

2. Combined mixtures (20 min, 25°C)	dpm bound	% of total dpm on chromatogram		%inhibition
		Dimers and trimers	Polymers	
A+B	4580	7.5	1.0	
A+C	4700	7.9	1.3	
3. Additions (20 min, 30°C)				
A+B+GTP	6750	12.3	1.4	
A+C+GTP	6780	13.3	1.9	
A+B+GTP+S-100	15274	19.1	8.3	0
A+B+GTP+S-100 +erythromycin	14442	18.6	7.1	14
A+C+GTP+S-100	13912	21.8	4.5	46

Three preincubation mixtures were prepared. Mixture A contained in 1.0 ml: 12 $A_{260m\mu}$ units of purified 30S ribosomal subunits from E. coli MRE-600, 0.1 M Tris-HCl buffer at pH 7.2, 40 mM NH$_4$Cl, 5 mM Mg(OAc)$_2$, 500 μg poly U, 1 mg E. coli B tRNA charged with 296 μmoles acetyl- ^{14}C-phenylalanine (1100 dpm/μmole), and 224 μg initiation factor protein. Mixtures B and C each contained in 0.6 ml: 0.1 M Tris-HCl buffer at pH 7.2, 40 mM NH$_4$Cl, 10 mM Mg(OAc)$_2$, 0.6 mg E. coli B tRNA charged with 230 μmoles ^{14}C-phenylalanyl-tRNA, and 14.4 $A_{260m\mu}$ units purified E. coli MRE-600 50S ribosomal subunits. In addition, Mixture C contained 0.4 mM erythromycin A. The three mixtures were incubated for 20 min at 25°C after which a 50 μl aliquot of each was assayed for bound substrate by millipore filtration (Part A). Next, 50 μl aliquots of Mixture A were combined with 50 μl aliquots of either B or C and incubated for another 20 min at 25°C (Part B). Samples were taken for the binding assay and for chromatography. Finally, 5×10^{-5} M GTP, 38 μg dialyzed E. coli supernatant protein (S-100), and 2×10^{-4} M erythromycin were added as indicated and the reaction mixtures were given a further 20-minute-incubation at 30°C. After which, samples were treated with KOH to hydrolyze the amino acyl-tRNA bond.

Much more utilization of the radioactive substrates is seen and a large amount of polymeric material is formed (Table II-3). Erythromycin present in the preformed 50S complex (A+C+GTP+S-100 (Table II-3, line 5)) inhibited oligopeptide formation (tetra and higher) by nearly 50%.

The control system which possessed no bound erythromycin (A+B+GTP+S-100) functioned very much like the same system to which erythromycin was added at the time of assay (Table II-3, lines 3 and 4). The amount of erythromycin added was equivalent to that used in preparing the 50S ribosome-erythromycin complex used in readying the companion system (A+C+GTP+S-100), and clearly erythromycin added after formation of the 70S/N-Ac-Phe-tRNA complex has no significant inhibitory action on the formation of oligopeptides (tetra and higher). This result showed that a model system which presumably mirrors a "natural protein synthesis" behaves exactly as does our system from *B. subtilis* when it is assayed for the elongation of nascent peptide chains in response to retained "natural" mRNA. In both cases erythromycin fails to act as an inhibitor of oligopeptide synthesis. The same set of experiments, however, also provide proof that erythromycin, which has been incorporated into the ribosomal complex at the time of its formation, has the ability to inhibit amino acid polymerization (Table II-3, line 5). The sole difference between the system in which this effect was demonstrated and that which failed to show a similarly large inhibition (Table II-3, line 4) was that in the former the erythromycin was allowed to interact with the 50S ribosomal particle *before* the 30S/poly U/N-Ac-Phe-tRNA complex was formed and in the latter the erythromycin was added *after* the formation of the 70S/poly U/N-Ac-Phe-tRNA/Phe-tRNA complex.

From the experiment just discussed, it appears that we have provided evidence which proves that erythromycin must bind to its "site" on the 50S ribosomal subunit before it can act as an inhibitor of protein synthesis and also that this same binding "site" is at least partially blocked by even the first substrate initiating this synthesis (N-Ac-Phe-tRNA).

A different sort of experimental verification for this interpretation is available. The aminoacyl nucleoside antibiotic puromycin acts by substituting for normal amino acyl-tRNA moieties. When it does so, a covalent bond (peptide) is formed with the nascent peptide chain, which formally was attached to the ribosome complex at the "donor" site *via* the tRNA specie specific for the last

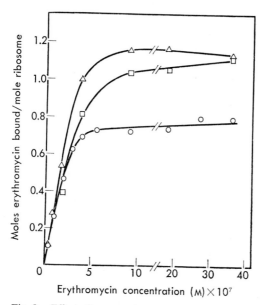

Fig. 8.   Effect of puromycin on the binding of erythromycin to sensitive *B. subtilis* ribosomes. Reaction mixtures contained Tris-HCl buffer,
$Mg(OAc)_2$, NH_4Cl, β-mercaptoethanol, *B. subtilis* (sensitive) ribosomes, ^{14}C-erythromycin and puromycin. $\triangle$, 10^{-4}M puromycin; $\square$,
10^{-5}M puromycin; $\bigcirc$, no puromycin.

amino acid utilized. The puromycyl radical is not associated with
a tRNA molecule and once it has reacted with the nascent protein
chain the puromycyl-protein molecule dissociates from the complex. Thus, in effect, puromycin removes nascent peptide chains
from ribosomes which are still associated with mRNA molecules.
Puromycin should, if the hypothesis developed above is correct,
remove peptidyl-tRNA molecules from any ribosome bearing
them in the extract from *B. subtilis* and increase the total number
of binding sites available to erythromycin.

When puromycin was added to a fresh extract of *B. subtilis*, one
which had a reasonable ability to utilize an amino acid mixture in
response to nascent peptides and "endogenous" mRNA, a considerable increase in the number of erythromycin binding sites was
observed (Fig. 8). When the same system was aged, a procedure
which permits natural dissociation of the peptidyl-tRNA chains,

the effect of puromycin largely disappeared (Fig. 9). Thus, these observations also are evidence that peptidyl-tRNA somehow blocks the 50S ribosomal binding site for erythromycin.

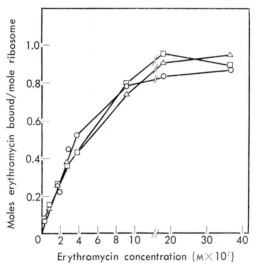

Fig. 9.   Effect of puromycin on the binding of erythromycin to dialyzed ribosomes. Reaction conditions are similar to those of Fig. 8. △, 10^{-4}M puromycin; □, 10^{-5}M puromycin; ○, no puromycin.

The peptidyl-tRNA molecule occupies a site on the ribosomal complex which is often termed the "donor" site, because the growing peptide chain occupies this location at the time the peptidyl radical is donated to the incoming amino acyl-tRNA moiety. A result of the attack by this amino acyl-tRNA molecule is that the new peptide chain is now attached to the second or "acceptor" site which binds this most recent amino acyl-tRNA molecule and the entire polypeptide chain is attached to the ribosomal complex *via* the tRNA molecule peculiar to this amino acid. The shifting of this new peptidyl-tRNA chain back to the first site mentioned, the "donor" site, requires both GTP and the soluble enzymes (S-100 fraction). This part of the synthetic cycle is what is referred to as the "translocation" process and is distinct from the first half of the cycle, which is catalyzed by the constitutive "peptidyl synthase."

We had clearly shown (Table II) that bound erythromycin affects polypeptide synthesis, and our data also support the idea that the antibiotic either bound or unbound has no effect on peptidyl synthase (*17*), (Table II). However, before it could be safely concluded that bound erythromycin is a specific inhibitor of the "translocation" half of peptide synthesis, it was necessary to answer one additional question.

From the experiments reported on in Table II, it seems evident that "translocation" begins occurring when polymeric N-acetylated oligophenylalanines are produced. However, in the experiments with the *B. subtilis* system where erythromycin failed to inhibit elongation of nascent peptides, there was no proof that any "translocation" was taking place. It could be that no given nascent peptide chain was reacting more than once, and then only in the case of those ribosomes which by chance had their peptidyl-tRNA chains in the "donor" site at the time of preparation of the cell-free extracts. If this is true, the observed utilization of amino acids would merely reflect the single addition of the appropriate amino acyl-tRNA moiety to these ribosomal complexes. It would also show that only peptidyl-synthase activity was being assayed. This, as already demonstrated, is not sensitive to erythromycin.

Proof that at least a significant number of the nascent protein chains was reacting with more than a single amino acid came from degradation of the polypeptides after utilization of a mixture of radioactive amino acids. Degradation of such a mixture was done according to the method of Dakin and West (C-terminal amino acids are converted to amino ketones). If only the C-terminal position was radioactive, as would be the case if only a single amino acid was added to any nascent peptide chain, the amino acids produced after the Dakin-West treatment and acid hydrolysis would be free of radioactivity. In our experiments (*10*), the C-terminal positions possessed less than half of the radioactivity that was incorporated into the nascent peptide chains, and thus at least a significant number of the chains was able to go completely through several cycles of amino acid addition.

Taken together with the previous data, this last experiment provides convincing evidence for the hypothesis that erythromycin is a specific inhibitor of the translocation step in bacterial protein synthesis. It must be stressed that the data cited are a reflection of slow assay procedures, in which we can see only the rate-limiting step and this only in a case where the inhibition is so severe that a small amount of product accumulates than in a control assay. Some evidence exists (8), suggesting that erythromycin does not completely block any of the reactions of protein synthesis and that at the most it merely retards a part of the machinery involved. None of the data mentioned above prove or disprove this possibility, but are compatible with it.

After defining the site and something of the nature of erythromycin action in the systems derived from B. subtilis, and having learned that the consequence of the genetic mutation conferring relative resistance is some change in the nature of the 50S ribosomal unit in the mutant, it became of interest to learn what the change might be. According to genetic mapping data, the mutation is located in a region of the chromosome related both to the expression of 50S ribosomal proteins and ribosomal RNA. On the chance (later predicted by better mapping data) that a ribosomal protein is altered in the 50S ribosomal particle of the mutant, an experiment was designed to permit a comparison of the proteins in both types of 50S unit. The "sensitive" strain of B. subtilis was grown in the presence of ^{14}C-lysine and the "resistant" strain in the presence of tritiated lysine. After growth, the two cultures were combined and the total population of 50S ribosomal particles was isolated and purified by differential centrifugation. The RNA in the 50S units was destroyed by RNase digestion in the presence of 6 M urea. The resulting mixture of ribosomal proteins was chromatographed on a carboxymethylcellulose-column and the proteins eluted with a gradient of lithium chloride in 6 M urea. The eluted protein-containing fractions were examined for radioactivity. A plot of radioactivity and of the ^{14}C/^{3}H ratio was made (Fig. 10). As can be seen, there is a constant ratio of the two different isotopic markers except for the last peak eluted from the column which shows the presence of radiocarbon but not of any tritium. Thus, there apparently is a protein present in the "sensitive" strain of B. subtilis which is lacking in the mutant or so altered as to be hidden under one of the other peaks present in both bacterial types of the 50S unit (7). This finding must be regarded as preliminary but a second experiment in which the administration of the isotopically-labeled L-lysines was inverted (tritium labeled to the "sensitive" strain and carbon-fourteen, to the "resistant" bacteria) gave the same picture.

In summary, the series of investigations described above have led to a considerable understanding of both the mode of action of erythromycin and of the mechanism of bacterial resistance to the antibiotics. Erythromycin binds to some "unique site" on the 50S ribosomal subunit and once bound is an inhibitor of the reactions involved in peptidyl-tRNA and amino acyl-tRNA polymerization into proteins. Erythromycin is blocked from its binding site by previously attached peptidyl-tRNA molecules. The rate-limiting step in erythromycin action seems to be that of the so-called translocation process.

Perhaps, the most fascinating question about erythromycin action remaining to be answered is that of what is the structural basis for both the binding to 50S ribosomal subunits and the

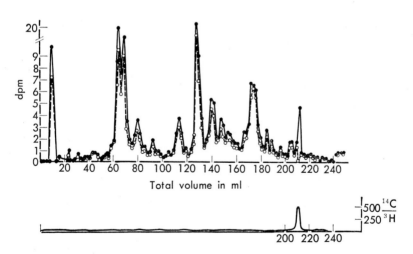

Fig. 10.   Chromatographic profile of 50S ribosomal proteins from sensitive and resistant strains of *B. subtilis* 168 (ordinates are ^{14}C and ^{3}H as indicated and the ^{14}C/^{3}H ratio is plotted below). O, ^{3}H× 10^{-3} resistant; ●, ^{14}C× 10^{-2} sensitive.

inhibitory effect shown by the bound drug. Relatively little information is available, but the studies reported to date (*17*) have
emphasized the importance of the sugar moieties present in the
erythromycin group of antibiotics.

The macrolide antibiotics which possess either a single basic
sugar-like D-desosamine (*e.g.*, methymycin) and those having two
neutral sugars (*e.g.*, lankamycin) were studied, as were several
erythromycin derivatives which have a single sugar (mycarosyl
erythronolide B and desosaminyl erythronolide B (Fig. 11)). When
compared with the bis glycosides, either of the erythromycin type
in which the two sugars are attached separately to the macrocylic
lactone (Fig. 11A) or of the magnamycin (carbomycin) type (Fig.
11D) in which a disaccharide between the amino and neutral sugars
is so attached, these monoglycosides and neutral bis glycosides
(Fig. 11B, C and F) had very low biological activity. Furthermore,
when the activity shown toward the "erythromycin-resistant"

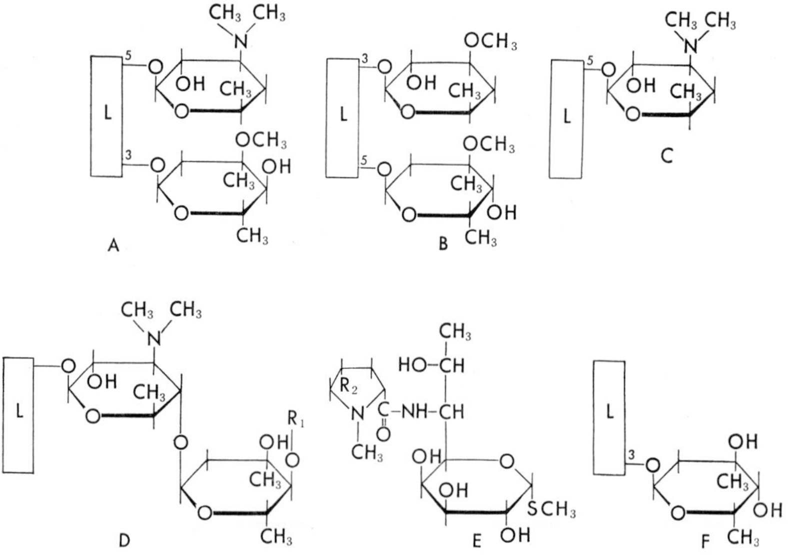

Fig. 11. Schematic representation of several antibiotic structures.
A, erythromycin; B, lankamycin; C, methymycin; D, niddamycin;
E, lincomycin; F, mycarosyl erythronolide B. L=various lactone
moieties. R_1=isovaleryl residue. R_2=*n*-propyl residue.

B. subtilis mutant was measured, it was seen that all structures lacking a neutral sugar were just as effective with this strain as with the parent "sensitive" bacterium.

It may be that the mutation leading to relative resistance to erythromycin affects some region on the 50S ribosomal unit which interacts with the neutral sugar (L-cladinose in the case of erythromycins A and B). The non-macrolide antibiotic lincomycin (Fig. 11E) has a mode of action very similar to that of erythromycin and we have reported (*17*) that the two antibiotics compete for at least some common binding region on the 50S ribosomal particle. Erythromycin binds more tightly but is somewhat less effective as an inhibitor once bound, so that mixtures of the two antibiotics may be less effective than lincomycin alone. The structure of lincomycin may be viewed as that of a monoglycoside attached to an amino acid-like residue. Lincomycin like the basic macrolide monoglycosides is just as effective an inhibitor of the "resistant" strain of *B. subtilis* as it is of the "sensitive" strain.

The data referred to indicate very little about the importance of the lactone structure for the biological activity of the erythromycin (macrolide) group of antibiotics. A few structures with chemically altered lactones have been examined (9-dihydro erythromycins A and B, hemi- and full-ketal derived from erythromycin A, *etc.*). It is evident that these are fully active when measured in the cell-free assay systems in which binding to 50S ribosomal subunits or inhibition of protein synthesis are measured ((*17*), J. Majer and J. W. Corcoran, unpublished results).

Many more structures derived from the erythromycins by chemical or biological means must be examined before any solid hypothesis can be proposed for the intimate mode of action of the macrolide antibiotics and lincomycin. However, on the basis of the limited data cited above, Wilhelm *et al.* (*17*) proposed that the erythromycins may act as structural analogues of peptidyl-tRNA. It is conceivable that the erythromycin lactone joined to the basic sugar D-desosamine is similar in some way to the neutral peptide joined in ester linkage to the terminal adenosyl moiety of each peptidyl-tRNA. The latter must be positioned accurately on the 50S part of the 70S ribosomal complex in order that a rapid chemical reaction can occur with the amino group of the charged amino acyl-tRNA when it is positioned close-by. If the erythromycin molecule resembles the region of the peptidyl-tRNA which is involved in this attachment to the ribosome (distinct from the codon-anticodon interaction which involves the 30S/mRNA region of the 70S complex), it may bind instead and thus prevent the close approach of this part of the peptidyl-tRNA molecule. Such a possibility is consistent with our finding that erythromycin cannot reach its binding site once a peptidyl-tRNA molecule is positioned on the 70S ribosomal complex. It is also in accord with the probability that erythromycin even if bound to the 50S part of the ribosomal complex does not prevent peptide bond formation. Within certain spacial limits a slight displacement of the peptidyl-tRNA molecule, such as might be caused by the binding of a molecule of erythromycin, at a site which normally attracts the reactive end of the growing peptide chain, might not prevent a new peptide bond from being formed with the incoming amino acid, but the rate of the reaction could be dramatically reduced. It will be interesting to see if any part of this suggestion proves to be correct, for at the first glance, the macrolide group of antibiotics seems to have little structural similarity to peptidyl-tRNA molecules.

In conclusion, the work summarized above which has been carried out using two strains of *B. subtilis* 168 has given answers to many of the questions concerning the mechanism of action of erythromycin (a macrolide antibiotic) and of lincomycin. The results described have been confirmed and extended by other workers (*cf.* chapters by J. Mao, K. Tanaka and B. Weisblum in this volume). The studies of erythromycin and lincomycin action have aided greatly in the still incomplete definition of the mechanism of bacterial protein synthesis.

Acknowledgments
The author gratefully acknowledges the collaboration of his former associates: Drs. Nancy L. Oleinick, Sheldon B. Taubman and James M. Wilhelm, Mr. Arden Hanson, Mrs. Helen Coady and Miss Allison Whitehead. He also has benefited from discussions

with Dr. James C.-H. Mao and Dr. Kentaro Tanaka. Research support was provided by Abbott Laboratories, the American Heart Association, Inc. (No. 65 G 126, 68–799); National Institutes of Health, Institutes of Allergy and Infectious Diseases (No. AI 06758, AI 09158) and General Medical Studies (GM 2545); National Science Foundation (No. GB 18157); Northwestern University Medical School (Dean Richard H. Young).

REFERENCES

1 Abbott Laboratories. 1966. Erythromycin, a review of its properties and clinical status. Abbott Laboratories Scientific Divisions, North Chicago, Ill.

2 Brock, T. D., and Brock, M. L. 1959. Similarity in mode of action of chloramphenicol and erythromycin. *Biochim. Biophys. Acta*, **33**, 274.

3 Corcoran, J. W., and Chick, M. 1966. Biochemistry of the macrolide antibiotics. *In* "Biosynthesis of antibiotics," ed. by J. F. Snell, Academic Press, New York, p. 159.

4 Dubnau, D., Smith, I., Morell, P., and Marmur, J. 1965a. Gene conservation in *Bacillus* species, I. Conserved genetic and nucleic acid base sequence homologies. *Proc. Natl. Acad. Sci. U.S.*, **54**, 491.

5 Dubnau, D., Smith, I., and Marmur, J. 1965b. Gene conservation in *Bacillus* species, II. The location of genes concerned with the synthesis of ribosomal components and soluble RNA. *Proc. Natl. Acad. Sci. U.S.*, **54**, 724.

6 Haenni, A. L., and Chapeville, F. 1966. The behavior of acetylphenylalanyl soluble ribonucleic acid in polyphenylalanine synthesis. *Biochim. Biophys. Acta*, **114**, 135.

7 Hanson, A., and Corcoran, J. W. 1969. Alteration in a ribosomal protein of *Bacillus subtilis* 168 associated with sensitivity to erythromycin. *Federation Proc.*, **28**, 725.

8 Kaempfer, R. O. R., Meselson, M., and Raskas, H. J. 1968. Cyclic dissociation into stable subunits and reformation of ribosomes during bacterial growth. *J. Mol. Biol.*, **31**, 277.

9 Oleinick, N. L., and Corcoran, J. W. 1968. Two types of binding of erythromycin to ribosomes from antibiotic-sensitive and -resistant *Bacillus subtilis* 168. *J. Biol. Chem.*, **244**, 727.

10 Oleinick, N. L., and Corcoran, J. W. 1970. Evidence of a limited access of erythromycin A to functional polysomes and its action on bacterial translocation. *In* "Progress in antimicrobial and anticancer chemotherapy (Proceedings of the 6th International Congress of Chemotherapy)," University of Tokyo Press, Tokyo, Vol. I, p. 202.

11 Pestka, S. 1968. Studies on the formation of transfer ribonucleic acid-ribosome complexes. III. The formation of peptide bonds by ribosomes in the absence of supernatant enzymes. *J. Biol. Chem.*, **243**, 2810.

12 Spizizen, J. 1958. Transformation of biochemically deficient strains of *Bacillus subtilis* by deoxyribonucleate. *Proc. Natl. Acad. Sci. U.S.*, **44**, 1072.

13 Taubman, S. B., Young, F. E., and Corcoran, J. W. 1963. Antibiotic Glycosides. IV. Studies in the mechanism of erythromycin resistance in *Bacillus subtilis*. *Proc. Natl. Acad. Sci. U.S.*, **50**, 955.

14 Taubman, S. B., So, A. G., Young, F. E., Davie, E. W., and Corcoran, J. W. 1963. Effect of erythromycin on protein synthesis in *Bacillus subtilis*. *In* "Antimicrobial Agents and Chemotherapy," ed. by G. L. Hobby American Society for Microbiology, Bethesda, p. 395.

15 Taubman, S. B., Jones, N. R., Young, F. E., and Corcoran, J. W. 1966. Sensitivity and resistance to erythromycin in *Bacillus subtilis* 168: the ribosomal binding of erythromycin and chloramphenicol. *Biochim. Biophys. Acta*, **123**, 438.

16 Wilhelm, J. M., and Corcoran, J. W. 1967. Antibiotic glycosides. VI. Definition of the 50S ribosomal subunit of *Bacillus subtilis* 168 as a major determinant of sensitivity to erythromycin A. *Biochemistry*, **6**, 2578.

17 Wilhelm, J. M., Oleinick, N. L., and Corcoran, J. W. 1968. Interaction of antibiotics with ribosomes: structure-function relationships and a possible common mechanism for the antibacterial action of the macrolides and lincomycin. *In* "Antimicrobial agents and chemotherapy," American Society for Microbiology, Bethesda, p. 236.

MUTANTS OF *ESCHERICHIA COLI* RESISTANT TO MACROLIDE ANTIBIOTICS

Kentaro Tanaka, Hiroshi Teraoka, Mikio Tamaki and Sachihiko Watanabe, and Syozo Osawa, Eiko Otaka and Renkichi Takata

Shionogi Research Laboratory, Shionogi & Co., Ltd., Osaka, Japan and Research Institute for Nuclear Medicine and Biology, Hiroshima University, Hiroshima, Japan

The group of antibiotics having a macrocyclic lactone ring was classified by Woodward in 1957 as macrolide antibiotics. A number of common features have been shown for these antibiotics, but they also have some different properties.

Erythromycin, one of the most important antibiotics in this group, has been shown to stop the growth of sensitive bacteria by inhibiting protein synthesis in the cells (*1, 20, 27*). We have shown that the antibiotic binds to *Escherichia coli* ribosomes and induces characteristic changes in the ability of the ribosome to participate in cell-free protein biosynthesis (*14, 17*). Using radioactive erythromycin, it was confirmed that an equimolar amount of this antibiotic combines with the 50S subunits of the ribosomes from *E. coli* (*15, 16, 18*) from *Bacillus subtilis* (*21*) and from *Staphylococcus aureus* (*6*).

Ribosomes from resistant mutants

By treating *Escherichia coli* Q13 cells with N-methyl-N'-nitro-N-nitrosoguanidine or 2-aminopurine, we have isolated a number of mutants which are highly resistant to erythromycin. Ribosome preparations obtained from these mutant cells, except those from a single exceptional mutant (QE114), were found to have a reduced ability to bind erythromycin and to carry out peptide synthesis in a cell-free system (*19*). In the following descriptions, the ribosomes which have a reduced affinity for erythromycin will be referred to as erythromycin resistant ribosomes. The ribosomes from QE114 cells had almost the same ability to bind erythromycin and to synthesize peptide as those from the parent Q13 cells. Thus, the resistance of this mutant to the antibiotic may be due to reason(s) other than a mutational change in the ribosomal character.

The binding of erythromycin to ribosomes has been shown to require a monovalent cation such as K^+ or NH_4^+ (*7, 9, 23*). Detailed studies on the role of these monovalent cations indicated that the conformation of *E. coli* ribosomes is reversibly converted from one favorable for the binding of erythromycin to one unfavorable for such binding, with decreases in the concentration of K^+ or NH_4^+, and that the rate of this conversion depends largely upon the incubation temperature (*23*). Compared with the ribosomes from *E. coli* Q13 (*ery^s*), the erythromycin-resistant ribosomes require a much higher concentration of K^+ or NH_4^+ before they can bind an equimolar amount of erythromycin (*11*).

Puromycin, whose structure had been considered as an analogue to the aminoacyl end of aminoacyl-tRNA, inhibits protein synthesis by forming peptidyl-puromycin (*28*). Lucas-Lenard and Lipmann found that N-acetylphenylalanyl-puromycin was synthesized from N-acetylphenylalanyl-tRNA and puromycin on ribosomes in the absence of supernatant factors. This puromycin reaction has been considered to be a useful analogue of peptide bond formation (*5*). This reaction has also been proved to be largely dependent upon the conformation of ribosomes, regulated by the concentration of monovalent cations such as K^+ or NH_4^+ (*8*). The erythromycin-resistant ribosomes described above needed a much higher concentration of K^+ or NH_4^+ compared with the erythromycin-sensitive Q13 ribosomes for this puromycin reaction, as found for the binding of erythromycin (22).

Protein components of erythromycin-resistant ribosomes

To examine possible alterations in the ribosomal protein structure of erythromycin-resistant ribosomes, ribosomal protein of 30S and 50S subunits from ³H-lysine labelled Q13 cells and from ¹⁴C-lysine labelled erythromycin-resistant mutant cells were mixed, respectively, and simultaneously chromatographed on a carboxymethylcellulose-column (2, 11, 18).

In the chromatographic patterns of the protein components from the 30S ribosomal subunits, no difference was detected between those from erythromycin-resistant and erythromycin-sensitive ribosomes. However, a distinct difference in a specific protein component (50-8 component) of the 50S ribosomal subunits was detected between these two ribosome preparations. With the erythromycin-resistant ribosome preparations, no significant radioactive peak was found at the position (50-8 position) where the 50-8 protein of Q13 ribosomes was eluted, while the amount of the protein detected at the position 50-7 was generally twice that observed for the Q13 50-7 protein peak.

It has been reported that the 50-7 and 50-8 peaks of the Q13 ribosomes each contain only a single protein component, and that these two proteins are chemically distinct (10). The 50-8 protein contains tryptophan as a constituent while the 50-7 protein has no tryptophan (18). Analyzing the ribosomal protein of ³H-tryptophan labelled erythromycin-resistant ribosomes on a carboxymethylcellulose-column, the radioactivity of the ³H-tryptophan of protein from erythromycin-resistant ribosomes was generally found at around the 50-7 protein peak of Q13 ribosomes.

By treating 50S ribosomal subunits of *E. coli* with 1.25 M 40S LiCl, some protein components are released and 40S particles (LiCl-particles) are formed. During this treatment, the 50-7 protein is lost, while the 50-8 protein still remains in the 40S LiCl-particles (4). We thus prepared the 40S LiCl-particles by treating ¹⁴C-lysine labelled 50S subunits of the resistant strain with 1.25 M LiCl and their protein composition was chromatographically analyzed together with that of ³H-lysine labelled 50S subunit protein from the Q13 cells. In the 40S LiCl-particles, the amount of protein at the 50-7 position was reduced to about one half of that in the original 50S subunits from erythromycin-resistant ribosomes. These results indicated that the true 50-7 component had been released during the treatment with LiCl, while the remaining protein found at the 50-7 position may well be the mutationally altered counterpart of the 50-8 protein of the Q13 ribosomes.

These experimental evidences strongly suggested that in the erythromycin-resistant ribosomes, the structure of the 50-8 protein component was mutationally altered, and eluted earlier than the corresponding component from the parent strain Q13. In this analysis, the protein components of ribosomes from two strains labelled with different kinds of isotopes were chromatographically compared simultaneously on a carboxymethylcellulose-column. This allowed direct comparison of the elution profiles of the protein components from these two strains. When the elution profiles of the protein components of ³H-tryptophan labelled erythromycin-resistant ribosomes were carefully compared with those of ¹⁴C-lysine labelled Q13 ribosomes, definite differences in the elution positions of mutationally altered 50-8 protein components were observed among the erythromycin-resistant ribosome preparations from independently isolated mutants. Although most of the altered 50-8 proteins of these mutants were found around the position at which the 50-7 protein of the Q13 ribosome was eluted, the altered 50-8 protein of the ribosomes from the QE201 strain was found between the 50-5 and 50-6 positions. Compared with other erythromycin-resistant ribosomes, the ribosome preparation from the QE201 strain has a remarkably lower affinity for erythromycin and a reduced peptide bond synthesizing activity (*11, 22*). This may indicate that the structural alteration of the 50-8 protein of QE201 ribosomes differs greatly from those of other erythromycin-resistant ribosomes. This difference is reflected not only in the erythromycin binding affinity, but also in the peptidyl transferase activity.

These findings can best be explained by assuming that this type of mutation of *E. coli*, from an erythromycin-sensitive to a resistant form, is actually a mutation of the 50-8 protein of the ribosomes, which consequently induces an alteration in the conformation of the ribosomes, causing a decrease in the affinity for erythromycin and in activity for peptide synthesis.

Genetic analysis of erythromycin resistance

Although, so far, the only distinct difference was that found in the 50-8 protein of the 50S ribosomal subunits in all the erythromycin-resistant mutants with altered ribosomes, it was still open to question whether the mutation caused by the mutagens induced a change, not only on the 50-8 protein cistron, but also on the cistrons for other components, which might effect the sensitivity of *E. coli* ribosomes for this antibiotic.

To examine this point, genetic analyses on this type of mutation have been carried out (*13*). When erythromycin resistance was transduced by Plkc phage from QE107 (ery^r_{107}, str^s) to JC411 (ery^s, str^r), out of three erythromycin-resistant transductants, two were found to be streptomycin-sensitive. This fact indicated that *ery* and *str* are closely linked on the chromosome. This linkage of *ery* to *str* was further examined by transduction of str^r from AB313 (ery^s, str^r) to QE004, QE005, QE105, QE107 and QE201 (all ery^r, str^s). In each case, the frequencies of co-transduction of ery^s and str^r were found to be around 70%.

Mapping of the *ery* marker on the chromosome was performed by the mating of AB313 (*Hfr*, ery^s, str^r) with JC411E01 (F^-, ery^r_{107}, str^s), which is the ery^r_{107} transductant of JC411 from QE107 by Plkc phage. The experiments revealed a gene order: *mal A-str-ery-arg G*, with recombination frequencies of 30.5% between *mal A* and *str*, 7.4% between *str* and *ery*, and 22.2% between *ery* and *arg G*.

By the transduction of str^r by Plkc phage from AB313 (ery^s, str^r) to JC411E01 (ery^r_{107}, str^s), two types of streptomycin-resistant transductants, one to which ery^s was co-transduced (*e.g.*, ES01, ES02) and the other retaining ery^r (*e.g.*, ER04, ER05), were ob-

tained. The protein components of ribosomes from these transductants were analyzed, as well as those from JC411 and JC411-
E01 cells. The results indicated that the transduction of ery^r or
ery^s from the donor to the recipient bacteria was always accompanied by a corresponding change in the 50-8 protein component.
The characteristic properties of ribosomes, such as erythromycin
binding activity and the ability for peptidyl transfer reaction, were
also changed in parallel with the transduction of ery^r or ery^s.

The results of these genetic studies demonstrated that the character of the 50-8 protein component was always co-transduced
with the *ery* marker, which is located in the *str* region on the *E.
coli* chromosome map. This suggests that the alteration of the
50-8 protein component and the acquisition of erythromycin
resistance by ribosomes are due to one mutational event.

TABLE I

Peptidyl Transferase Activity of the Ribosomes from Various Transductants

Ribosomes from	N-Acetyl-Phe release by puromycin from N-acetyl-Phe-tRNA	
	Maximum activity	Activity at 0.04 M KCl
JC411	1093 cpm	39%
JC411E01	807	7
AB313	534	34
ES01	706	43
ES02	847	37
ER04	867	5
ER05	912	0

The maximum activities were obtained at 0.16 M NH_4Cl. The assays were carried out
as previously reported (*22*).

Cross-resistance between erythromycin and other macrolides

Cross-resistance between erythromycin and other macrolide antibiotics has been reported (*3*). Vazquez demonstrated that all the
macrolide antibiotics tested (spiramycin, carbomycin, angolamy-
cin, lankamycin, erythromycin and oleandomycin) inhibited the
binding of ^{14}C-chloramphenicol to ribosomes. Since it has been
shown that chloramphenicol binds to 50S ribosomal subunits (*24*),
these macrolides were also considered to bind with the 50S subunit
of ribosomes (*25*). Thus it would be quite interesting to know

TABLE II

Susceptibilities of Various Mutants and Transductants to Macrolide Antibiotics

	Strain	Leucomycin (μg/ml)	Oleandomycin (μg/ml)	Spiramycin (μg/ml)	Tylosin (μg/ml)
Exp. 1	Q13	200–350	250–440	100–300	75–200
	QE004	>1400	>850	>2000	>1500
	QE005	>1400	>850	>2000	>1500
	QE105	700–1400	>850	>2000	>1500
	QE107	>1400	>850	>2000	>1500
	QE114	700–1400	>850	>2000	>1500
	QE201	>1400	>850	>2000	>1500
Exp. 2	JC411	<500	<500	<500	<500
	JC411E01	>1000	>1000	>1000	>1000
	ES01	<500	<500	<500	<500
	ES02	<500	<500	<500	<500
	ER04	>1000	>1000	>1000	>1000
	ER05	>1000	>1000	>1000	>1000
	AB313	<500	<500	<500	<500

In the data, > shows that the colonies were observed on the agar plate containing a given concentration of the antibiotic, < shows that no colony was detected on the agar plate containing a given concentration of the antibiotic, and 200–350 means that colonies were observable at 200 μg/ml but not at 350 μg/ml of the antibiotic. The agar plate (pH 7) contained 1% Bacto-peptone, 0.5% beef extract, 0.5% NaCl and 1.5% agar.

whether the alteration of the 50-8 protein component induces changes in the susceptibility to macrolide antibiotics other than erythromycin. As shown in Table II, all the erythromycin-resistant mutants were found to be highly resistant to leucomycin, oleandomycin, spiramycin and tylosin. Further, all the ery^r_{107} transductants were found to be highly resistant to these macrolide antibiotics. On the other hand, erythromycin-sensitive transductants were all sensitive to these macrolides, as was the AB313 strain from which ery^s was co-transduced with str^r. These facts, considered together with those described above, strongly suggest that the chemical structure of the 50-8 protein component is closely correlated with the affinity of ribosomes not only to erythromycin but also to other macrolides.

Ribosomes from the mutant resistant to specific macrolides

As shown in Table III, when N-methyl-N'-nitro-N-nitrosoguanidine treated *E. coli* cells were first selected for their resistance to a

TABLE III
Cross-Resistance to Macrolide Antibiotics by Various Mutants

Antibiotics in agar plates (µg/ml)		Resistant to TY (300 µg/ml)										Resistant to SP (300 µg/ml)										Resistant to LE (300 µg/ml)									
Mutant number		1	2	3	4	5	6	7	8	9	10	1	2	3	4	5	6[a]	7	8[b]	9	10	1	2	3	4	5	6	7	8	9	10
EM	500	–	+	–	–	+	–	–	+	+	+	–	+	+	–	+	–	+	–	+	+	+	+	–	+	+	+	+	+	+	+
	700	–	–	–	+	+	–	+	+	+	+	–	+	+	–	–	–	+	–	+	+	+	+	–	+	+	+	+	–	+	+
	1000	–	–	–	–	+	+	+	+	–	+	–	+	+	–	–	–	+	–	+	+	+	+	–	–	–	+	+	–	+	+
TY	500	+	+	+	+	+	+	+	+	+	+	+	+	+	+	+	+	+	+	+	+	+	+	+	+	+	+	+	+	+	+
	700	+	+	+	–	+	+	+	+	+	+	+	+	–	+	+	–	+	+	+	+	+	+	+	+	+	+	+	+	+	+
	1000	–	+	+	–	–	+	+	+	–	+	+	+	+	+	+	–	–	+	+	+	+	+	+	+	+	+	+	+	+	+
LE	500	+	+	+	+	+	+	+	+	+	+	+	–	+	+	+	–	+	+	+	+	+	+	+	+	+	+	+	+	+	+
	700	+	+	+	–	+	+	+	+	+	+	–	–	+	+	+	–	+	+	+	+	+	+	+	+	+	+	+	+	+	+
	1000	–	–	+	–	–	+	+	+	–	+	–	–	–	+	+	–	+	+	+	+	+	+	+	+	+	+	+	+	+	+
SP	500	+	+	+	+	+	+	+	+	+	+	+	+	+	+	+	+	+	+	+	+	+	+	+	+	+	+	+	+	+	+
	700	+	+	+	–	+	+	+	+	+	+	+	+	+	+	+	+	+	+	+	+	+	+	+	+	+	+	+	+	+	+
	1000	–	+	+	–	–	+	+	+	–	–	+	+	+	+	+	+	+	+	+	+	+	+	+	+	+	+	+	+	+	+

+ indicates that colonies were observed on the agar plate (see legend of Table II). – indicates that no colony was observed.
EM, erythromycin; TY, tylosin; LE, leucomycin; SP, spiramycin. [a] This strain was named QSP006. [b] This was named QSP008.

particular macrolide antibiotic other than erythromycin, most of the mutants selected were found to also be resistant to the other macrolide antibiotics. Among these mutants, however, we found some which were less resistant to erythromycin, *e.g.*, QSP008; and we discovered a particular spiramycin-resistant mutant, QSP006, which was less resistant to other macrolides, such as erythromycin, tylosin and leucomycin.

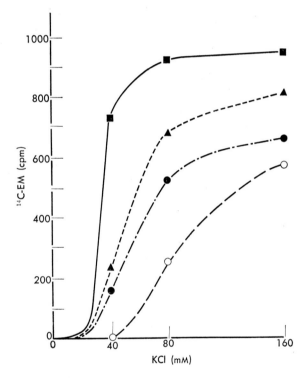

Fig. 1. The binding of ^{14}C-erythromycin to ribosomes from the spiramycin-resistant mutants. The binding of ^{14}C-erythromycin to ribosomes was measured by the adsorption of the ^{14}C-erythromycin-ribosome complex on Millipore filters as described by Teraoka (*23*). The reaction mixture (125 μl) contained 3.0 A_{260} units of ribosomes, 2,700 counts/min (175 μμmoles) of ^{14}C-erythromycin, 50 mM Tris-HCl (pH 7.8), 16 mM magnesium acetate and the indicated amounts of monovalent cations. The incubation was carried out at 37°C for 15 min. ■, Q13; ▲, QSP006; ●, QSP008; ○, QE005.

The ribosome preparations from these mutants showed only a mediocre binding affinity to ^{14}C-erythromycin as indicated in Fig. 1. The binding of ^{14}C-erythromycin to ribosomes was competitively inhibited by other macrolide antibiotics (26). This suggests that the binding sites of these macrolides are, if not the same site, so closely located on the 50S subunits that the binding of one macrolide is affected by the concomitant addition of other macrolide(s). If the resistance for a certain macrolide is due to the reduced affinity of ribosomes for this antibiotic as found for erythromycin resistance, then the inhibitory effect of this macrolide on erythromycin binding may also be reduced when the ribosomes have a selective resistance to this macrolide.

As shown in Fig. 2, the binding of ^{14}C-erythromycin to the ribosomes from QSP006 and QSP008, both resistant to spiramycin,

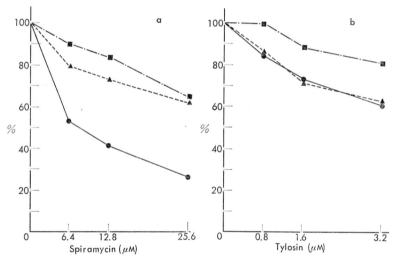

Fig. 2.　(a) Effect of spiramycin on the binding of ^{14}C-erythromycin to the ribosomes from spiramycin-resistant mutants. ■, QSP008; ▲, QSP006; ●, Q13. (b) Effect of tylosin on the binding of ^{14}C-erythromycin to the ribosomes from spiramycin-resistant mutants. As a spiramycin-sensitive control, the ribosome preparation from parent Q13 cells was employed. The reactions were carried out at varying concentrations of spiramycin (a) or tylosin (b) at 60 mM KCl, using 2.5 A_{260} units of ribosomes. Other experimental conditions were the same as described in the legend of Fig. 1. ■, QSP008; ▲, QSP006; ●, Q13.

was effected to a lesser degree by the concomitant addition of spiramycin than were spiramycin-sensitive ribosomes from the parent Q13 cells. The inhibitory effect of tylosin on the binding of ^{14}C-erythromycin to the ribosomes from the QSP008 strain, which is resistant to tylosin, was distinctly less than that on ribosomes from QSP006 or Q13 cells which are sensitive to this antibiotic.

Since the genetic studies on the macrolide resistance described above indicated that the alteration of the 50-8 protein component and the resistance to at least erythromycin, tylosin, oleandomycin, leucomycin and spiramycin, if not to all macrolide antibiotics, were caused by one mutation, the protein components of the 50S ribosomal subunits from QSP006 and QSP008 mutants were analyzed chromatographically on a carboxymethylcellulose-column.

As illustrated in Fig. 3, a distinct difference in the elution pattern was observed between the 50-8 component from Q13 ribosomes and that from QSP008 ribosomes.

The chromatographic profile of the protein components from QSP006 50S ribosomal subunits, however, coincided with that from the Q13 ribosomes. This chromatographic analysis on a carboxymethylcellulose-column is considered to be quite sensitive for detecting any structural change in a protein which induces an alteration of the electrostatic properties of the protein, but less sensitive for other types of structural alterations. Thus, it is conceivable that not all alterations in the structure of the 50-8 protein component, which induce changes in biological activity, are detectable by this method. It is, therefore, logical to consider that the failure to detect the expected alteration of the 50-8 component of QSP006 might be due to such a technical reason.

Although the present study is not entirely conclusive—the final proof for the alteration of the 50-8 protein component of QSP006 ribosomes must await an exhaustive chemical analysis of this protein component—the findings reported here do permit a logical interpretation of the mechanism of cross-resistance found among this class of antibiotics. It is quite possible that the mutational change in the cistron for the 50-8 ribosomal protein component induces an alteration of the chemical structure of this protein and

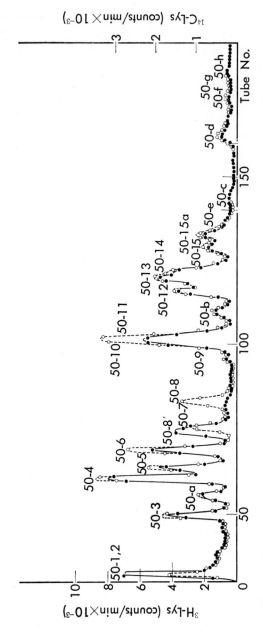

Fig. 3. Chromatography on the carboxymethylcellulose-column of protein components of 50S ribosomal subunits from *E. coli* Q13 and from the spiramycin-resistant mutant QSP008 of *E. coli*. The preparation and fractionation of ribosomal protein were carried out as previously reported (*10*). ○, ¹⁴C-lysine-labeled Q13 protein; ●, ³H-lysine-labeled QSP008 protein.

consequent changes in the conformation of the ribosomes, and that the changes in the affinity of ribosomes for macrolide antibiotics are largely dependent upon the particular type of alteration of the 50-8 protein.

Macrolide-resistant mutant with unaltered ribosomes

At present, very little is understood concerning the other type of macrolide-resistant mutant of *E. coli*, QE114. This mutant showed no significant difference in the character of its ribosomes. Preliminary results of the genetic study indicated that the location of the gene responsible for the character of this type of mutation is far from the *str* region, and that it is distinct from the gene for the 50-8 ribosomal protein component (unpublished data).

Sekiguchi and Iida have isolated two cell-wall mutants of *E. coli* which were highly sensitive to actinomycin and lysozyme (*12*). A recent study in our laboratory showed that one of these mutants, *E. coli* AS19, has a much higher sensitivity to erythromycin than the parent *E. coli* B cells (unpublished data). This fact may indicate that the natural resistance of *E. coli* is due to an impermeability of the cells to this antibiotic, and that the mutation of the character which influences the permeability of this group of antibiotics may largely affect the susceptibility of the cells to these antibiotics. The possibility that the macrolide resistance of QE114 is originated by the mutational change in the permeability of the cell to these antibiotics may be considered, but further work is required to clarify the nature of this type of mutation.

SUMMARY

Two different types of erythromycin-resistant *E. coli* mutants were isolated by treatment of *E. coli* with N-methyl-N'-nitro-N-nitrosoguanidine or 2-aminopurine. In the majority of cases, the mutants had altered ribosomes which showed a lowered affinity for erythromycin. Chromatographic analyses of the protein components of the ribosomes from these mutants demonstrated that a specific component of the 50S ribosomal subunit (50-8) had been mutationally altered in these mutants. Genetic analyses indicated that the gene responsible for the character of this type of erythromycin resistance is located in the *str* region, and that the alteration of the 50-8 protein component with the concomitant acquisition of erythromycin resistance by ribosomes is due to one mutational event. Studies on the sensitivity of the erythromycin-resistant mutant (QE107) and of the erythromycin-resistant and -sensitive transductants to other macrolides such as leucomycin, oleandomycin, spiramycin and tylosin clearly indicated that the chemical structure of the 50-8 ribosomal protein component is closely correlated with a sensitivity not only to erythromycin but also to the other macrolide antibiotics.

Only one macrolide resistant mutant having no significant alteration of ribosomal character was isolated. Although only little is understood at present about this mutant, this mutation is genetically distinguished from one which leads to an alteration of the ribosomal protein component.

Acknowledgments

We thank Dr. N. Otsuji of Kyushu University for his interest and help. Thanks are also due to Dr. M. Sekiguchi of Kyushu University who kindly provided us the *E. coli* AS19 strain. This work was supported in part by a grant from the Jane Coffin Childs Memorial Fund for Medical Research (project No. 233) and a grant from the Ministry of Education of Japan.

REFERENCES

1   Brock, T. D., and Brock, M. L. 1959. Similarity in mode of action of chloramphenicol and erythromycin. *Biochim. Biophys. Acta,* **33,** 274.
2   Dekio, S., Takata, R., Osawa, S., Tanaka, K., and Tamaki, M. 1970. Genetic studies of the ribosomal proteins in *Escherichia coli.* IV. Pattern of the alteration of ribosomal protein components in mutants resistant to spectinomycin or erythromycin in different strains of *Escherichia coli. Mol. Gen. Genetics,* **107,** 39.
3   Grundy, W. E. 1964. The macrolides (erythromycin group). *In* "Experimental Chemotherapy," ed. by R. T. Schnitzer and F. Hawking, Academic Press, New York, Vol. III, p. 39.
4   Itoh, T., Otaka, E., and Osawa, S. 1968. Release of ribosomal proteins

from *Escherichia coli* ribosomes with high concentrations of lithium chloride. *J. Mol. Biol.*, **33**, 109.

5 Lucas-Lenard, J., and Lipmann, F. 1967. Initiation of polyphenylalanine synthesis by N-acetylphenylalanyl-sRNA. *Proc. Natl. Acad. Sci. U.S.*, **57**, 1050.

6 Mao, J. C.-H. 1967. The stoichiometry of erythromycin binding to ribosomal particles of *Staphylococcus aureus*. *Biochem. Pharmacol.*, **16**, 2441.

7 Mao, J. C.-H., and Putterman, M. 1969. The intermolecular complex of erythromycin and ribosome. *J. Mol. Biol.*, **44**, 347.

8 Miskin, R., Zamir, A., and Elson, D. 1968. The inactivation and reactivation of ribosomal-peptidyl transferase of *E. coli*. *Biochem. Biophys. Res. Commun.*, **33**, 551.

9 Oleinick, N. L., and Corcoran, J. W. 1969. Two types of binding of erythromycin to ribosomes from antibiotic-sensitive and-resistant *Bacillus subtilis* 168. *J. Biol. Chem.*, **244**, 727.

10 Otaka, E., Itoh, T., and Osawa, S. 1968. Ribosomal proteins of bacterial cells: strain and species specificity. *J. Mol. Biol.*, **33**, 93.

11 Otaka, E., Teraoka, H., Tamaki, M., Tanaka, K., and Osawa, S. 1970. Ribosomes from erythromycin-resistant mutants of *Escherichia coli*, *J. Mol. Biol.*, **48**, 499.

12 Sekiguchi, M. and Iida, S. 1967. Mutants of *Escherichia coli* permeable to actinomycin. *Proc. Natl. Acad. Sci. U.S.*, **58**, 2315.

13 Takata, R., Osawa, S., Tanaka, K., Teraoka, H., and Tamaki, M. 1970. Genetic studies of the ribosomal proteins in *Escherichia coli*. V. Mapping of erythromycin resistance mutations which lead to alteration of a 50S ribosomal protein component. *Mol. Gen. Genetics*, **109**, 123.

14 Tanaka, K., and Teraoka, H. 1966. Binding of erythromycin to *Escherichia coli* ribosomes. *Biochim. Biophys. Acta*, **114**, 204.

15 Tanaka, K., Teraoka, H., Nagira, T., and Tamaki, M. 1966. ¹⁴C-Erythromycin ribosome complex formation and non-enzymatic binding of aminoacyl-transfer RNA to ribosome-messenger RNA complex. *Biochim. Biophys. Acta*, **123**, 435.

16 Tanaka, K., Teraoka, H., Nagira, T., and Tamaki, M. 1966. Formation of ¹⁴C-erythromycin-ribosome complex. *J. Biochem.*, **59**, 632.

17 Tanaka, K., and Teraoka, H. 1968. Effect of erythromycin on polylysine synthesis directed by polyadenylic acid in an *Escherichia coli* cell-free system. *J. Biochem.*, **64**, 635.

18 Tanaka, K., Teraoka, H., Tamaki, M., Otaka, E., and Osawa, S. 1968. Erythromycin-resistant mutant of *Escherichia coli* with altered ribosomal protein component. *Science*, **162**, 576.

19 Tanaka, K., Teraoka, H., Tamaki, M., Otaka, E., and Osawa, S. 1970. Studies on ribosomes from erythromycin resistant mutant of *Escherichia*

coli with altered ribosomal protein component. *In* "Progress in Antimicrobial and Anticancer Chemothrapy (Proceedings of the 6th International Congress of Chemotherapy)," University of Tokyo Press. Tokyo, Vol. II, p. 499.

20   Taubman, S. B., So, A. G., Young, F. E., Davie, E. W., and Corcoran, J. W. 1964. Effect of erythromycin on protein biosynthesis in *Bacillus subtilis. Antimicrobial Agents and Chemotherapy—1963*, 395.

21   Taubman, S. B., Jones, N. R., Young, F. E., and Corcoran, J. W., 1966. Sensitivity and resistance to erythromycin in *Bacillus subtilis* 168: the ribosomal binding of erythromycin and chrolamphenicol. *Biochim. Biophys. Acta*, **123**, 438.

22   Teraoka, H., Tamaki, M., and Tanaka, K. 1970. Peptidyl transferase activity of *Escherichia coli* ribosomes having an altered protein component in the 50S subunit. *Biochem. Biophys. Res. Commun.*, **38**, 328.

23   Teraoka, H. 1970. A reversible change in the ability of *Escherichia coli* ribosomes to bind to erythromycin. *J. Mol. Biol.*, **48**, 511.

24   Vazquez, D. 1964. The binding of chloramphenicol by ribosomes from *Bacillus megaterium. Biochem. Biophys. Res. Commun.*, **15**, 464.

25   Vazquez, D. 1966. Binding of chloramphenicol to ribosomes. The effect of a number of antibiotics. *Biochim. Biophys. Acta*, **114**, 277.

26   Wilhelm, J. M., Oleinick, N. L., and Corcoran, J. W. 1968. Interaction of antibiotics with ribosomes: structure-function relationships and a possible common mechanism for the antibacterial action of macrolides and lincomycin. *Antimicrobial Agents and Chemotherapy—1967*, 236.

27   Wolfe, A. D., and Hahn, F. E. 1964. Erythromycin: mode of action. *Science*, **143**, 1445.

28   Yarmolinsky, M. B., and Haba, G. L. de la. 1959. Inhibition of puromycin of amino acid incorporation into protein. *Proc. Natl. Acad. Sci. U.S.*, **45**, 1721.

MACROLIDE RESISTANCE IN *STAPHYLOCOCCUS AUREUS*

Bernard WEISBLUM

Department of Pharmacology, University of Wisconsin Medical School, Madison, Wisconsin, U.S.A.

Two major patterns of resistance to erythromycin have been described. One appears to involve the alteration of some ribosomal component presumably by mutation of a structural gene corresponding to ribosomal protein(s). The other pattern involves an inducible change such that cells become resistant only after 30- to 40-minute exposure to low concentrations of erythromycin. In this work, I would like to review ways in which resistance to erythromycin as well as to other macrolide antibiotics can be expressed, and the methods in which they can be studied.

Comparison of various forms of erythromycin resistance

Strains of *Staphylococcus aureus* showing "dissociated" resistance to erythromycin were first described by Chabbert (*3*). Such strains, it was noted, remained sensitive to spiramycin, another macrolide antibiotic, and the term "dissociated" was employed in order to denote the lack of co-resistance to other macrolides. A second feature of these strains noted by Chabbert was that erythromycin could antagonize the action of spiramycin, that is, the zone of inhibition by spiramycin was distorted so that bacterial growth on the side proximal to erythromycin approached the spiramycin disc. This type of deformity of the inhibition zone is illustrated in Fig. 1 c, d, e.

In subsequent studies by Pattee and co-workers (14, 20), the inducible nature of this resistance and its transducibility by phage were first described. On the basis of our present knowledge, we can say that, in fact, such strains are initially sensitive to both erythromycin and spiramycin. However, erythromycin acts as an inducer; and resistance is induced by the low levels initially attained as it diffuses out of the disc. By the time a toxic erythromycin concentration is reached the cells have become induced and they grow well near the erythromycin disc. Because spiramycin is inactive as an inducer, it produces a clear zone of inhibition, except where the cells have been previously induced by erythromycin. On the basis of evidence described in more detail below, this explains the mechanism of deformation of the inhibitory zone.

In contrast, other strains selected in the laboratory for resistance to erythromycin were found to be co-resistant to spiramycin; the name applied by Garrod (6) to this form of resistance was "nondissociated" or "double" resistance. This latter form of resistance may be easier to understand intuitively in terms of a receptor altered by mutation in a gene which specifies some structural element of the ribosome, so that the ribosome binds macrolide antibiotics with decreased affinity. This type of resistant mutant can be isolated in other bacterial species as described elsewhere in this volume. One such strain of S. aureus, which we selected for resistance to erythromycin, was found to be co-resistant to other macrolides such as spiramycin, carbomycin and triacetyloleandomycin, but not to niddamycin (21) (Fig. 1). It would appear that the terminology "double resistance" only reflects the fact that a limited number of macrolides was used in the initial resistance assays. In such a strain as illustrated in Fig. 1b, erythromycin does not induce resistance to niddamycin or to any of the other antibiotics shown.

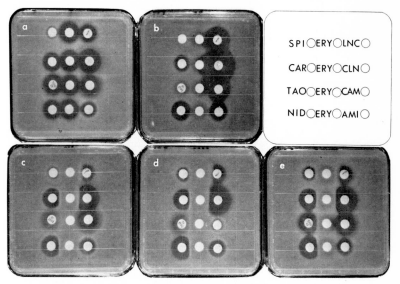

Fig. 1. Effect of erythromycin on the sensitivity of five *S. aureus* strains to antibiotics. The antibiotics used and their disposition on each plate correspond to the pattern given (upper right). Abbreviations and antibiotics which they represent are summarized in Table I. The antibiotics surveyed are known to be inhibitors of the 50S ribosomal subunit function. a, COPEN⁺; b, COPEN ERY-R; c, 1206; d, CR-51; e, CR-27 (C⁻).

By the use of the disc method, Barber and Waterworth (*1*) as well as Griffith *et al.* (*7*) found that erythromycin could induce resistance to lincomycin in strains which show dissociated resistance. Later, Bourse and Monnier (*2*) reported that erythromycin could similarly induce resistance to pristinamycin I, a streptogramin B antibiotic, but not to pristinamycin II, a streptogramin A antibiotic. Some properties of the streptogramin family of antibiotics have been reviewed recently by Vazquez (*19*).

In our approach to this question, we performed a survey of many antibiotics and asked the following question: what generalizations can be made as to the specificity of the antibiotics to which erythromycin induced resistance? We had recently characterized lincomycin as an inhibitor of the 50S ribosome subunit (*4,5*) and so we asked whether this feature might be common to other anti-

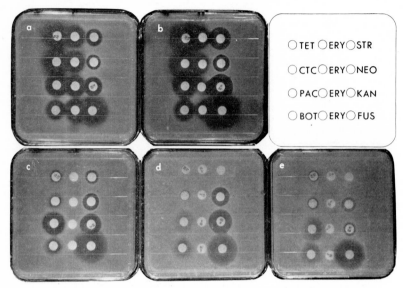

Fig. 2. Effect of erythromycin on the sensitivity of five *S. aureus* strains to antibiotics. The antibiotics used and their disposition on each plate correspond to the pattern given (upper right). Abbreviations and the antibiotics which they represent are summarized in Table I. The antibiotics surveyed include two members each from the streptogramin A and streptogramin B families, as well as a repeat test of spiramycin. a, COPEN+; b, COPEN ERY-R; c, 1206; d, CR-51; e, CR-27 (C⁻).

biotics which affect this subunit. We therefore performed a survey in which a total of about 30 different antibiotics which affect 30S and 50S ribosome subunit function, as well as some which affect DNA, RNA, or cell wall synthesis, were tested by the disc method.

The results of this survey, shown in Figs. 1, 2 and 3, are summarized in Table I. Erythromycin could only induce resistance to inhibitors of the 50S (but not 30S) ribosome subunit function, and only three (out of eight) different classes which act on the 50S subunit appear to be involved (*21,22*). We have also noted that erythromycin does not induce resistance to thiostrepton, an inhibitor of the 50S subunit function.Moreover, erythromycin appears to induce resistance to *all* members of each of the three classes involved.

In contrast, erythromycin-resistant mutants of the non-dis-

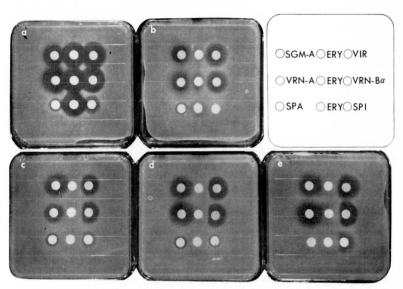

Fig. 3. Effect of erythromycin on the sensitivity of five *S. aureus* strains to antibiotics. The antibiotics used and their disposition on each plate correspond to the pattern given (upper right). Abbreviations and the antibiotics which they represent are summarized in Table I. The antibiotics surveyed include known inhibitors of the 30S ribosomal sub-unit (aminoglycosides, pactamycin and tetracyclines), as well as fusidic acid which inhibits a function requiring both ribosomal subunits and bottromycin. a, COPEN⁺; b, COPEN ERY-R; c, 1206; d, CR-51; e, CR-27 (C⁻).

sociated type do not show this strict pattern of co-resistance. For example (see Fig. 1a), the strain of *S. aureus* Copenhagen selected for resistance to 10 μgm/ml erythromycin was found to be co-resistant to carbomycin and triacetyloleandomycin but sensitive to niddamycin and lincomycin. The presence of the erythromycin disc did not deform the zone of inhibition due to lincomycin or niddamycin.

Inducible strains grown in a nutrient growth medium acquire high level resistance (100 μg/ml) to macrolide antibiotics after prior treatment with subinhibitory concentrations of erythromycin (0.01 to 0.1 μg/ml). Kono *et al.* (*10*) showed that if a known concentration of erythromycin is mixed with induced cells or with a crude extract from induced cells which had acquired high level

TABLE I

Summary of Antibiotics Which are Inhibitors of Ribosomal Function[a]

Abbreviation	Full name	Amt (μg/disc)	Class	Subunit specificity	Erythromycin-antagonizable
AMI	amicetin	20	aminoacylamino nucleoside	50S	−
BOT	bottromycin	5	—[b]	nd[c]	−
CAM	chloramphenicol	10	—[b]	50S	−
CAR	carbomycin	10	macrolide	50S	+
CLN	7-chloro-7-deoxylincomycin	2.5	lincosaminide	50S	+
CTC	chlortetracycline	20	tetracycline	30S	−
ERY	erythromycin	10	macrolide	50S	+
FUS	fusidic acid	0.5	—[b]	30S and 50S	−
KAN	kanamycin	30	aminoglycoside	30S	+
LNC	lincomycin	2	lincosaminide	50S	−
NEO	neomycin	20	aminoglycoside	30S	+
NID	niddamycin	10	macrolide	50S	−
PAC	pactamycin	5	—[b]	nd[c]	−
SGM-A	streptogramin A	5	streptogramin A	50S	−
SPA	sparsomycin	20	—[b]	50S	−
SPI	spiramycin	10	macrolide	50S	+
STR	streptomycin	25	aminoglycoside	30S	−
TAO	triacetyl oleandomycin	15	macrolide	50S	+
TET	tetracycline	30	tetracycline	30S	−
VIR	viridogrisein	5	streptogramin B	50S	+
VRN-A	vernamycin A	5	streptogramin A	50S	−
VRN-Bα	vernamycin Bα	40	streptogramin B	50S	+

Weisblum and Demohn (22). [a] At the concentrations listed (μg/disc) the following antibiotics, which are inhibitors of nonribosomal functions, were not erythromycin-antagonizable: Bacitracin (BAC), 10; cephalosporin (CPH), 15; cycloserine (CSR), 20; nitrofurantoin (NFR), 50; novobiocin (NOV), 15; rifamycin SV (RIF), 0.5; sulfisoxazole (SXL), 30; vancomycin (VAN), 30. [b] Single member of its chemical class tested. [c] Not determined.

resistance macrolide antibiotics, no loss of erythromycin could be detected within the limits of sensitivity of the bioassay which they used. It was also reported, subsequently, by Nakajima *et al.* (*12*) that both sensitive and uninduced resistant cells accumulated a larger amount of erythromycin if an exponentially growing culture was exposed to erythromycin (100 μg/ml) for one hour. In contrast, both constitutive and induced resistant cells were found to accumulate one tenth or less the amount of erythromycin as the sensitive cells did. It was found, furthermore, that decreased erythromycin accumulation in an induced population of erythromycin-inducible strain could be related to an apparent decreased affinity between erythromycin and the ribosome (*15*).

Studies by Shimizu *et al.* (16–18) have shown that induced and constitutively resistant strains of *S. aureus* take up less spiramycin and that ribosomes from these strains also have a decreased affinity for spiramycin. We were able, subsequently, to rule out in a more rigorous fashion the possibility that enzymatic inactivation of erythromycin might in any way be involved (*23*). Upon mixing the 50S ribosome subunits obtained from an uninduced, sensitive strain with those obtained from an induced or constitutively resistant strain, we noted that the amount of erythromycin or lincomycin bound was additive at limiting ligand concentrations (Figs. 4 and 5).

Thus far, erythromycin-inducible resistance has only been described in *S. aureus*, and only in strains isolated from natural sources. Passage of erythromycin-sensitive strains in media containing erythromycin has not yet made it possible to select inducibly resistant strains. This observation is consistent with the possibility that a plasmid may play a role in inducible resistance. Mitsuhashi *et al.* (*11*) showed that penicillinase production and macrolide resistance could be jointly transduced by phage or eliminated by acridine, which provided presumptive evidence that these characteristics were carried as a single unit. More recently, Novick (personal communication) has been able to transduce erythromycin-inducible resistance into a "rec⁻" strain of *S. aureus*. Because such rec⁻ strains are unable to repair or to integrate DNA, only DNA which does not require integration into the host genome will be expressed. Novick (*13*) has also studied a form of erythromycin resistance in *S. aureus* localizable on a plasmid and linked to penicillinase production. One such strain, provided by Novick, was tested and found to be constitutively resistant, *i.e.*, it was resistant to macrolides, lincosamides and streptogramin B antibiotics. These observations provide further presumptive evidence that an extrachromosomal element could specify inducible resistance, at least in part.

Studies of erythromycin-induced resistance

1. Methods for studying induced resistance
a) Disc method: In this technique, one determines whether erythromycin diffusing out of one filter paper disc will antagonize

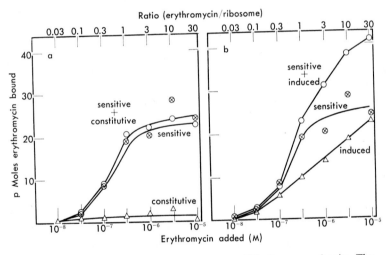

Fig. 4. Binding of ^{14}C-erythromycin to 50S ribosome subunits. The antibiotic/ribosome input ratio indicated above the figure and the 100% binding level indicated on the right-hand ordinate refer to the uninduced, induced, or constitutively resistant strains tested alone. a: Effect of 50S subunits obtained from a constitutively resistant strain on erythromycin binding to 50S subunits from the sensitive uninduced strain, 1206$^+$. b: Effect of 50S subunits obtained from induced cells of 1206$^+$ on erythromycin binding to 50S subunits from the sensitive uninduced strain, 1206$^+$.

the inhibitory effect of another test antibiotic such as spiramycin or lincomycin which has been used to impregnate a second disc. As described above, this technique has been useful mainly in determining qualitatively whether erythromycin can induce resistance to a particular test antibiotic (2, 3, 6, 7, 22).

b) *Turbidimetric method:* A test inoculum is exposed to different inducing conditions such as a variable inducer concentration, a variable time of induction, presence or absence of other antibiotics during induction. The test inoculum is inoculated into a broth culture containing 50 μgm/ml erythromycin, turbidity is determined, and a growth curve is plotted. If the test inoculum has been efficiently induced, growth in a medium containing 50 μgm/ml erythromycin begins immediately. If the test inoculum has been induced to a lesser degree, progressively longer lag periods lasting up to several hours are seen (*20*).

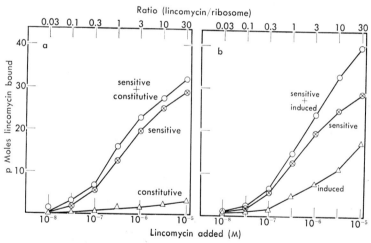

Fig. 5. Binding of ^{14}C-lincomycin to 50S ribosome subunits. The antibiotic/ribosome input ratio indicated above the figure and the 100% binding level indicated on the right-hand ordinate refer to the uninduced, induced, or constitutively resistant strains tested alone. a: Effect of 50S subunits obtained from a constitutively resistant strain on lincomycin binding to 50S subunits from the sensitive uninduced strain, 1206[+]. b: Effect of 50S subunits obtained from induced cells of 1206[+] on lincomycin binding to 50S subunits from the sensitive uninduced strain, 1206[+].

c) Clone-formation method: A broth culture of uninduced cells is subjected to various conditions of induction as mentioned above. Aliquots, suitably diluted, are plated on a solid medium containing either no antibiotic to determine the number of viable cells or on a medium containing 50 μgm/ml erythromycin to determine the number of resistant cells. In the latter case, erythromycin in the medium simultaneously selects and maintains in the resistant state those cells which are induced (*20, 23*).

2. Requirements for induction

In our own work described below (*22, 23*), we have found it useful to employ the first and last technique.

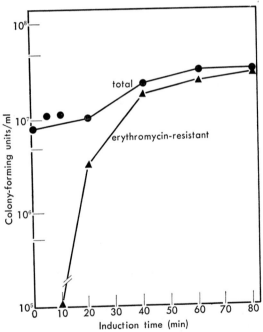

Fig. 6.   Kinetics of induction, colony-forming units per ml as a function of time. Erythromycin, 10^{-7} M, was added to a culture of *S. aureus* 1206⁺. At various times, as indicated, aliquots were withdrawn and tested by plating on an antibiotic-free medium and on a medium containing 5×10^{-5} M erythromycin.

By determining time-course and concentration-dependence for the appearance of erythromycin-resistant clones, we could determine that: 1) more than 95% was induced within 1-hour exposure to optimal inducing concentrations of erythromycin (Fig. 6), and 2) the optimal concentration for induction during 1-hour exposure to the inducer was in the range from 0.01 to 0.1 μgm erythromycin/ml (10^{-8} to 10^{-7} M) (Fig. 7). Over this range, nearly complete induction of the culture was seen. Even at a concentration as low as 0.001 μgm/ml or 10^{-9} M, a significant number of inductants, 10 to 20-fold over the background level, was seen (Fig. 8).

While these conclusions are essentially similar to those previ-

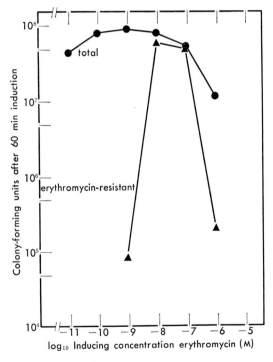

Fig. 7. Colony-forming units per ml as a function of erythromycin concentration used for induction. Cells were induced with erythromycin at concentrations between 10^{-9} and 10^{-6} M as indicated. After a 60-minute incubation period, aliquots were withdrawn and plated as in Fig. 6.

ously arrived at by Weaver and Pattee (*20*), the determination of the actual number of cells capable of forming colonies allows one to rule out a model proposed by Garrod (*6*), according to which a small highly resistant fraction of the population retained the ability to grow in erythromycin-containing medium and that the outgrowth of a resistant population merely represented a selection of this fully resistant fraction. The all-or-none aspect of this assay for induction increases the sensitivity and extends the range of detectible induction. If induced cells are diluted away from erythromycin into an antibiotic-free medium, the induced state is found to persist for 90 min after which time the cells become

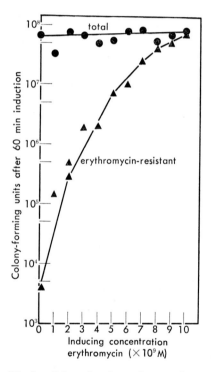

Fig. 8.   Colony-forming units per ml as a function of erythromycin concentration used for induction. Cells were induced with erythromycin at concentrations between 0 and 10^{-8} M as indicated. After a 60-minute incubation period, aliquots were withdrawn and plated as in Fig. 6.

sensitive. A 30-minute interval is required for more than 99% of the culture to become sensitive again (Fig. 9).

In order to determine whether a given system is inducible in the classical sense, it would be desirable to show that RNA and protein synthesis are directly required, whereas DNA synthesis, on the other hand, is not. Also, it must be shown that the uninduced cells are still viable. As test antibiotics, we used novobiocin, streptovaricin and chloramphenicol as inhibitors of DNA, RNA, and protein synthesis, respectively. We found that the process of induction was sensitive to the latter two antibiotics (Fig. 10b, c). Novobiocin, however, was not seen to have an inhibitory effect

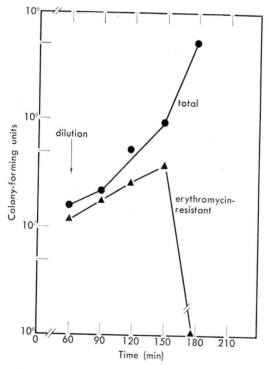

Fig. 9. Kinetics of deinduction, colony-forming units per ml as a function of time. Cells were induced for 1 hr with 10^{-7} M erythromycin. The induced culture was diluted 10^4-fold into an erythromycin-free medium and incubated further. At various times as indicated, aliquots were withdrawn and plated as in Fig. 6.

on induction independent of its effect on viability (Fig. 10a). These observations are consistent with those made earlier by Weaver and Pattee (20). In view of the coupling between DNA, RNA, and protein synthesis, these results are only suggestive and not conclusive in regard to the macromolecular requirements for induction.

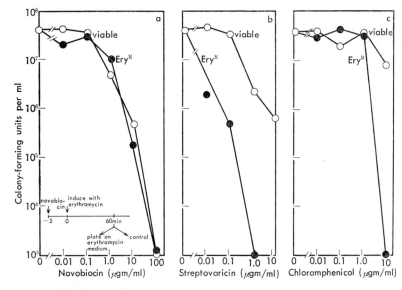

Fig. 10.   a: Effects of novobiocin on viability and erythromycin in-ducibility. Intact cells were preincubated for 5 min with various concen-trations of novobiocin as indicated. Erythromycin was added to a final concentration, 10^{-7} M; and incubation in the presence of erythromycin and novobiocin proceeded for an additional hour, at which time ali-quots were taken and tested for viability and erythromycin resistance. b: Effects of streptovaricin on viability and erythromycin inducibility. Intact cells were preincubated for 5 min with various concentrations of streptovaricin as indicated. Erythromycin was added to a final concen-tration, 10^{-7} M; and incubation in the presence of erythromycin and streptovaricin proceeded for an additional hour, at which time aliquots were taken and tested for viability and erythromycin resistance. c: Effects of chloramphenicol on viability and erythromycin inducibility. Intact cells were preincubated for 5 min with various concentrations of chloramphenicol as indicated. Erythromycin was added to a final con-centration, 10^{-7} M; and incubation in the presence of erythromycin and chloramphenicol proceeded for an additional hour, at which time ali-quots were taken and tested for viability and erythromycin resistance.

Shimizu *et al.* (*17*) have recently isolated a heat-inducible strain. Exposure of this strain at 42°C induced resistance to macrolide antibiotics and to lincomycin, as tested by the turbidimetric method described above. We would expect that upon induction this strain would also be resistant to the streptogramin-B antibiotics as well. In order to rule out a possible direct stoichiometric interaction between erythromycin and the ribosome as the mechanism of the inducible resistance, it would be desirable, as discussed in more detail below, to be able to show that the number of resistant ribosomes present exceeds the number of inducer molecules.

3. Patterns of constitutive expression

Except under unusual circumstances, erythromycin appears to be the only inducer of resistance. By selecting organisms resistant to a lincosamide, streptogramin B, or a macrolide antibiotic (other than erythromycin), one can obtain strains which are constitutively resistant. Erythromycin is not as suitable for selection of such mutants because it can act as an inducer on the selection plate, and indeed all of the colonies so far tested which appear on selective medium containing erythromycin give only inducibly resistant cells. Presumably, such colonies are formed from cells which become induced before they are inhibited by erythromycin. Several patterns of constitutive resistance are shown in Fig. 11. For reference, we show the pattern of resistance of the wild-type parental strain, 1206+ in Fig. 11a. Two constitutive mutants selected with 10 μgm/ml lincomycin are shown in Fig. 11b and c. Three constitutive mutants selected with 20 μgm/ml vernamycin Bα are shown in Fig. 11d, e and f. The two mutants labelled "generalized" show the type of behavior which one would expect of constitutive mutants, *viz.*, resistance to all the antibiotics tested in the upper part of the figure. On the other hand, an unexpected class of constitutive mutants, which we call "variable" constitutive, could also be isolated. Such strains show increased levels of resistance to several but not all antibiotics involved.

Note that there is no marked change in response to antibiotics used in the lower part of the figure for any of the mutants. A more rigorous demonstration that such strains are indeed constitutive, in the same sense that certain mutants of the lac operon are constitutive, will depend on genetic evidence showing that the mutation occurred in a regulatory gene rather than in a structural gene. One unusual strain, not shown, selected for resistance to viridogrisein (10 μgm/ml) was rendered uninducible by erythromycin. In this strain, lincomycin, however, could induce resistance to erythromycin. In another strain described by Hashimoto *et al.* (9), oleandomycin was found to be capable of serving as an inducer in addition to erythromycin.

In general, we can say that the variable pattern is itself variable. The data presently available do not permit us as yet to make any generalization regarding the comparative mechanisms of these two forms of constitutive resistance. However, the very striking specificity of erythromycin-inducible resistance, which only appears to involve three classes of 50S subunit inhibitors, makes it obvious that the streptogramin B family should be included within the framework of future discussions of macrolide and lincosamide antibiotics.

Constitutively resistant selection with lincomycin

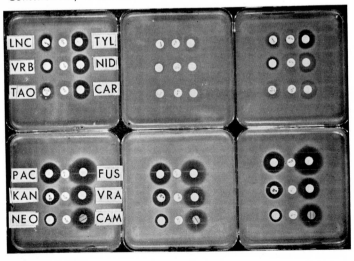

a   b   c

Constitutively resistant selection with vernamycin Bα

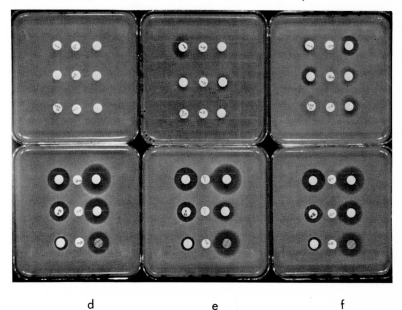

d   e   f

Fig. 11. Patterns of constitutive resistance to lincomycin or vernamycin Bα. Independent isolates from *S. aureus* 1206+, resistant to lincomycin or vernamycin Bα, as indicated, were selected and tested for resistance to various other antibiotics which affect ribosome function. The
sensitive parent strain is included for comparison. The antibiotics used,
their subunit specificity and concentration are given in Table I, except
that VRB denotes vernamycin Bα and VRA denotes vernamycin A. a:
Wild-type parental strain 1206+. b: Generalized constitutive resistant
selected with lincomycin. c: Variable constitutive resistant selected
with lincomycin. d: Generalized constitutive resistant selected with
vernamycin Bα. e: Variable constitutive resistant selected with
vernamycin Bα. f: Variable constitutive resistant selected with
vernamycin Bα.

Structural similarities between erythromycin and lincomycin

The fact that most of the known 50S ribosome subunit inhibitors
compete with each other for binding does not necessarily imply
that they share a common binding site. Their respective binding

sites could merely overlap or be distinct, but functionally coupled. The fact that resistance could only be induced toward three different classes of 50S subunit inhibitors suggested that *these* three classes may have more in common with each other than with other antibiotics which act on this subunit. Structural determinations of erythromycin and lincomycin using X-ray crystallography have recently been performed by Harris *et al.* (8) and by Davis and Parthasarathy (personal communication). We, therefore, constructed the three-dimensional models of these antibiotics based on the crystallographic data and noted several points of coincidence. The three points involve methyl groups as shown schematically in Fig. 12. The coincidence numbered 3 might involve one of the other methyl groups of the cladinose moiety in erythro-

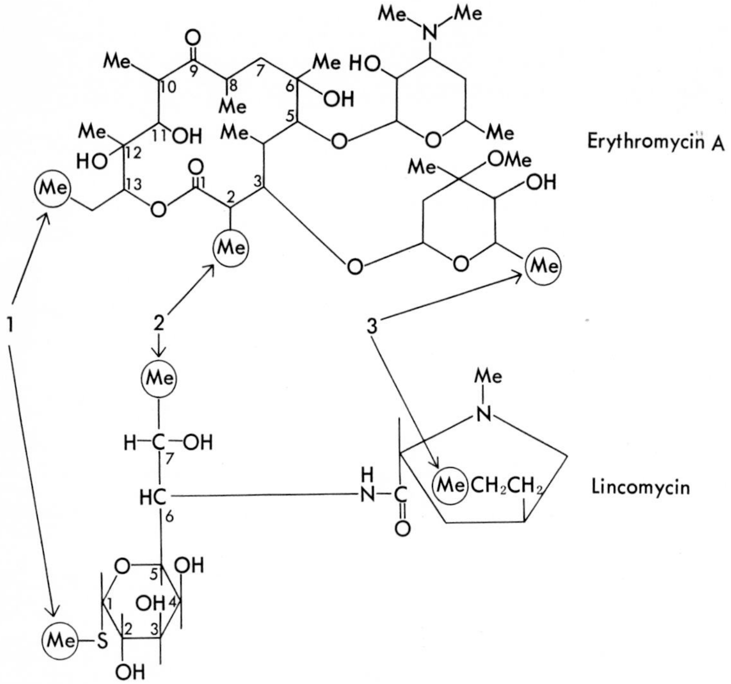

Fig. 12.   Schematic structures of erythromycin A and lincomycin showing three points of similarity deduced from the X-ray crystallographic structures of these two antibiotics.

mycin; it was not possible to decide this unambiguously. In addition, there is coincidence between the 12-OH on the macrolide ring and the 2-OH in lincomycin as numbered in the diagram.

We have no independent evidence that the groups indicated are in fact homologous or that they bind to the same receptor site on the ribosome. It will be interesting to determine the three-dimensional structure of a streptogramin B antibiotic in order to ascertain whether a similar conformation is possible for this molecule as well. It would also be of interest to know in what respects differences between macrolides make it possible for erythromycin to be such an effective inducer of resistance, whereas other macrolides are relatively ineffective.

CRITIQUE

Two main shortcomings of the work on this problem should be mentioned. First, a clear-cut demonstration that the inducible resistance is inducible in the classical sense has not yet been provided. The requirement for RNA and protein synthesis could be explained in terms of the inhibition of the assembly of resistant ribosomes rather than as direct inhibition of some putative mechanism which modifies ribosomes. One might propose that erythromycin "induces" resistance directly by interacting with and modifying the ribosome during its assembly. Even assuming a dense culture from 10^9 to 10^{10} bacteria per ml which would contain 10^{13} to 10^{14} ribosomes per ml (at 10^4 ribosomes per cell), we can see that at the optimum for induction, between 10^{-7} and 10^{-8} M, the medium would still contain between 6×10^{13} and 6×10^{14} erythromycin molecules per ml. It is, therefore, not possible to exclude direct involvement of erythromycin by means of this type of calculation.

This system appears to be more complex than the lac operon of *Escherichia coli*. In addition, the induced change, which we tested for, involves *ribosomes*, which are one step further removed from the gene than is galactosidase, according to the model proposed.

Other than the very remarkable specificity of the "constitutive" strains, which as expected only appear to involve the three classes to which erythromycin induces resistance, there is no independent evidence that this is indeed the case, that is, that the constitutive mutants are affected in a gene which has, or whose product has, a regulatory function. Further genetic studies would be most useful in clarifying these points.

In more recent studies we have noted the appearance of N^6, N^6-dimethyl adenine in 23S ribosomal RNA isolated from purified 50S subunits of erythromycin-induced *S. aureus* 1206; this base is also present in 23S RNA of constitutively resistant cells grown in the absence of erythromycin (*10a*). Dimethyl adenine is otherwise not normally found in the 23S RNA of *S. aureus* 1206. These observations confirm earlier studies of Saito *et al.* (*15*) as well as those from our own laboratory (*23*) in which it was inferred that some alteration of the 50S ribosome subunit was involved in inducible resistance.

Moreover, the methylation reaction not only provides an independent biochemical criterion by which one can characterize erythromycin-resistant strains but also independent support for the presumptive designation of certain strains as constitutively resistant. It is interesting that 23S RNA from constitutively resistant cells is found to contain more dimethyl adenine than 23S RNA from induced cells. This might explain the differences seen in the abilities of 50S subunits from constitutive and induced cells to bind erythromycin, as shown in Fig. 4. It remains to be determined more rigorously whether methylation is the cause of inducible resistance or the result, and whether this is the only significant alteration that occurs.

Acknowledgments
This work was supported by research grants GB-7145 and GB-3080 from the National Science Foundation.

REFERENCES

1   Barber, M., and Waterworth, P. M. 1964. Antibacterial activity of lincomycin and pristinamycin: a comparison with erythromycin. *Brit. Med. J.*, **2**, 603–606.

2 Bourse, R., and Monnier, J. 1968. Effet de l'erythromycin sur la croissance de *Staph. aureus* "resistant dissocie" en bacteriostase par un autre macrolide ou un antibiotique apparente. *Ann. Inst. Pasteur (Paris)*, **110**, 67–79.

3 Chabbert, Y. 1956. Antagonisme *in vitro* entre l'erythromycine et la spiramycine. *Ann. Inst. Pasteur (Paris)*, **90**, 787–790.

4 Chang, F. N., Sih, C. J., and Weisblum, B. 1965. Lincomycin an inhibitor of amino acyl tRNA binding to ribosomes. *Proc. Natl. Acad. Sci. U.S.*, **55**, 431–438.

5 Chang, F. N., and Weisblum, B. 1966. The specificity of lincomycin binding to ribosomes. *Biochemistry*, **8**, 836–843.

6 Garrod, L. P. 1957. The erythromycin group of antibiotics. *Brit. Med. J.*, **2**, 57–63.

7 Griffith, L. J., Ostrander, W. E., Mullins, C. G., and Beswick, D. E. 1965. Drug antagonism between lincomycin and erythromycin. *Science*, **147**, 746–747.

8 Harris, D. R., McGeachin, S. G., and Mills, H. H. 1965. The structure and stereo-chemistry of erythromycin A. *Tetrahedron Letters*, 679–685.

9 Hashimoto, H., Oshima, H., and Mitsuhashi, S. 1968. Drug resistance of staphylococci. IX. Inducible resistance to macrolide antibiotics in *Staphylococcus aureus*. *Japan. J. Microbiol.*, **12**, 321–327.

10 Kono, M., Hashimoto, H., and Mitsuhashi, S. 1966. Drug resistance of staphylococci III. Resistance to some macrolide antibiotics and inducible system. *Japan. J. Microbiol.*, **10**, 59–66.

10a Lai, C. J., and Weisblum, B. 1971. Altered methylation of ribosomal RNA in an erythromycin-resistant strain of *Staphylococcus aureus*. *Proc, Natl. Acad. Sci. U.S.*, **68**, 856–860.

11 Mitsuhashi, S., Hashimoto, J., Kono, M., and Morimura, M. 1965. Drug resistance of staphylococci. II. Joint elimination and joint transduction of the determinants of penicillinase production and resistance to macrolide antibiotics. *J. Bacteriol.*, **89**, 988–992.

12 Nakajima, Y., Inoue, M., Oka, Y., and Yamagishi, S. 1968. A mode of resistance to macrolide antibiotics in *Staphylococcus aureus*. *Japan. J. Microbiol*, **12**, 248–250.

13 Novick, R. P. 1967. Penicillinase plasmids of *Staphylococcus aureus*. *Federation Proc.*, **26**, 29–38.

14 Pattee, P. A., and Baldwin, J. N. 1962. Transduction of resistance to some macrolide antibiotics in *Staphylococcus aureus*. *J. Bacteriol.*, **84**, 1049–1055.

15 Saito, T., Hashimoto, H., and Mitsuhashi, S. 1969. Drug resistance of staphylococci. Decrease in the formation of erythromycin-ribosomes complex in erythromycin-resistant strains. *Japan. J. Microbiol.*, **13**, 119–121.

16 Shimizu, M., Saito, T., Hashimoto, H., and Mitsuhashi, S. 1970. Spira-
    mycin resistance in *Staphylococcus aureus*. Decrease in spiramycin ac-
    cumulation and ribosomal affinity of spiramycin in resistant staphylococ-
    ci. *J. Antibiotics*, **23**, 63–67.

17 Shimizu, M., Saito, T., and Mitsuhashi, S. 1970. Macrolide resistance in
    Staphylococcus aureus. Relationship between spiramycin binding to
    ribosome and inhibition of polypeptide synthesis in a heat-inducible
    mutant. *Japan. J. Microbiol.*, **14**, 155–162.

18 Shimizu, M., Saito, T., and Mitsuhashi, S. 1970. Spiramycin resistance
    in *Staphylococcus aureus*. The stoichiometry of spiramycin-binding to
    ribosomes from spiramycin-sensitive, intermediate- and high- resistant
    strains. *Japan. J. Microbiol.*, **14**, 177–178.

19 Vazquez, D. 1967. The streptogramin family of antibiotics. *In* "Anti-
    biotics," ed. by D. Gottlieb and P. D. Shaw, Springer-Verlag, New
    York, Vol. I, p. 387–403.

20 Weaver, J. R., and Pattee, P. A. 1964. Inducible resistance to erythro-
    mycin in *Staphylococcus aureus*. *J. Bacteriol.*, **88**, 574–580.

21 Weisblum, B., and Davies, J. 1968. Antibiotic inhibitors of the bacterial
    ribosome. *Bacteriol. Rev.*, **32**, 493–528.

22 Weisblum, B., and Demohn, V. 1969. Erythromycin-inducible resistance
    in *Staphylococcus aureus*: survey of antibiotic classes involved. *J. Bacte-
    riol.*, **98**, 447–452.

23 Weisblum, B., Siddhikol, C., Lai, C. J., and Demohn, V. 1971. Erythro-
    mycin-inducible resistance in *Staphylococcus aureus*. Requirements for
    induction. *J. Bacteriol.*, **106**, 835–847.

MACROLIDE RESISTANCE IN STAPHYLOCOCCI

Tetsu Saito, Mikio Shimizu and Susumu Mitsuhashi

Department of Microbiology, School of Medicine, Gunma University, Maebashi, Japan

The strains of *Staphylococcus aureus* which were isolated from clinical specimens showed two types of resistance to macrolide antibiotics (Mac), inducible and constitutive. They acquired high resistance to both Mac and lincomycin (LCM) after prior treatment with subinhibitory concentrations of inducer, but the resistance of cells in the induced population was lost when the cells were grown in broth without inducer (*6*). Such Mac-resistance was first reported by Garrod (*1*) and was termed the dissociated type of resistance, although the resistance mechanisms were not known. The induction of Mac-resistance was reported independently by Weaver and Pattee (*25*) and Kono *et al*. (*5*). Strains carrying the constitutive type of resistance showed cross resistance to all Mac antibiotics and most of them were found to be resistant to LCM (*3, 6*). In strains carrying an inducible type of resistance, erythromycin (EM) was found to be the best inducer examined. When they were grown on plates containing a Mac antibiotic other than EM, we could isolate the mutant carrying the constitutive type of resistance, thereby showing the cross resistance to both Mac and LCM without inducer (3).

1. Genetic analysis of strains carrying inducible Mac-resistance

Staphylococcus aureus MS537 was isolated from a clinical specimen and its resistance was increased by prior treatment with sub-inhibitory concentrations of EM, its Mac-resistance being the inducible type (3, 6). When MS537 was inoculated on plates containing either leucomycin (LM), spiramycin (SP), or LCM, the constitutive types of mutant were isolated and found to be resistant to all Mac antibiotics and LCM, the level of resistance being over 100 μg per ml. Another type of mutant was isolated, and was found to be resistant to both EM and OM but sensitive to other Mac antibiotics and LCM, both EM and OM being active inducers for Mac-resistance (3). One of these mutants was termed MS537–1. Both EM and LM became active inducers for Mac-resistance in another type of mutant and one of them was designated MS537-59. According to the transduction analysis of both MS537 and MS537-1, it was found that the genes governing both inducibility and Mac-resistance were cotransducible and were not separable by transduction with typing phage 52 A so far as examined. In these results, the determinants governing both induc-

TABLE I

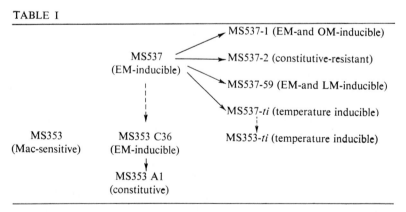

Solid lines represent the relation between parent and mutant strains. Dotted lines indicate the relation between donor of Mac-resistance and transductant.

ibility and Mac-resistance were found to be located close together. MS 537-1 was considered to be the regulator gene(s) mutant in the EM-inducible strains. The relation between parent and mutant strains and their resistance are shown in Tables I and II.

TABLE II
Drug Resistance of *S. aureus* Strains Used

Strain	Drug							
	EM	OM	LM	JM	SP	LCM	PC	CM
MS537	1.6	0.8	0.8	0.8	0.8	0.4	50	—
MS537-*ind*	>100	>100	>100	>100	>100	>100	—	—
MS537-1	>100	50	0.8	0.8	0.8	0.8	—	—
MS537-2	>100	>100	>100	>100	>100	>100	—	—
MS537-59	>100	100	25	25	6.3	25	—	—
MS537-*ti* (30C)[a]	>200	—	25	25	25	25	—	—
MS537-*ti* (42C)[a]	>800	—	>200	>200	>200	>200	—	—
MS353	0.1	0.2	0.2	0.2	0.2	0.2	0.1	3.1
MS353 C36	1.6	0.8	0.8	0.8	0.8	0.8	—	—
MS353 C36-*ind*	>100	>100	>100	>100	>100	>100	—	—
MS353 A1	>100	>100	>100	>100	>100	>100	—	—
MS353-*ti* (30C)[a]	>200	—	25	25	25	25	—	—
MS353-*ti* (42C)[a]	>800	—	>200	>200	>200	>200	—	—
MS642	>100	>100	>100	>100	>100	>100	50	—
MS642-2	0.2	—	0.8	—	0.8	0.4	3.1	—
FS195	3.1	3.1	3.1	3.1	12.5	0.2	50	—
MS353-sp[b]	0.1	1.6	>100	>100	>200	0.4	—	12.5
MS353-sp-O[b]	0.1	1.6	>100	>100	>200	0.4	—	12.5
MS353-er[b]	>200	>200	12.5	12.5	25	25	—	6.3
MS353-lc[b]	>200	>200	12.5	12.5	25	100	—	6.3

MS537 is an inducible-resistant strain and becomes resistant to both Mac and LCM when pretreated with subinhibitory concentrations of EM. MS537-2 is a constitutive-resistant mutant of MS537. MS537-1, MS537-59 and MS537-*ti* are mutants in inducibility of Mac-resistance and were isolated from MS537. MS353 is Mac-sensitive and was used for recipient of transduction. MS353 C36 and MS353-*ti* were obtained by transduction. Relations between these strains are illustrated in Fig. 1. MS642 is constitutive-resistant to Mac antibiotics and resistant to penicillin, and the determinants responsible for resistance to both Mac and penicillin are located on a plasmid (7, 10). MS642-2 is one of the sensitive mutants of MS642, from which the determinants for Mac- and penicillin-resistance were eliminated (7). FS195 is an intermediate-resistant strain to Mac antibiotics. Drug resistance indicated maximum concentration of drug which allowed visible growth of bacteria. [a] Culture temperature. [b] These strains are *in vitro* developed mutants isolated from MS353.

2. Inducible resistance to Mac antibiotics

1) EM-Inducible resistance

Induced populations of Mac-resistance appeared within 10 min of incubation with subinhibitory concentrations of EM, and most of the cells acquired resistance after 1 hr of incubation (*25*). But the resistance of the induced cells was lost when they were grown in the absence of EM. Optimal concentration of EM for induction was demonstrated to be about 1×10^{-7} M at pH 7 at 37° C, and induction was retarded when much higher concentrations of EM were used as inducer because of the inhibitory effect of the drug on protein synthesis (Fig. 1). Similarly, chloramphenicol and actinomycin D were found to inhibit induction of Mac-resistance (*25*).

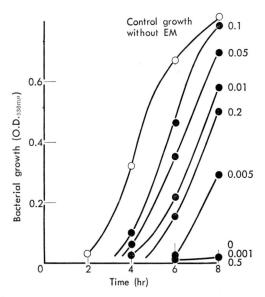

Fig. 1.   Bacterial growth in the presence of 50 mcg of EM/ml after treatment with various concentrations of EM. MS 537 was treated with various concentrations of EM for 30 min. Then an aliquot (0.2 ml) of sample was transferred into 10 ml of BHI containing 50 mcg of EM/ml, and cell growth was measured. Numbers indicate the concentrations of EM in induction mixture (μg/ml).

2) Inducer activities of EM derivatives

Mao and Putterman (8) indicated that the chemical groups in EM essential for binding to ribosome may be 3'-dimethyl amino, 2'-hydroxyl, 9-carbonyl and 3"-methoxy groups, and their binding affinities to ribosomes were related to their antibacterial activities. The inducer activity of EM may correspond to its affinity for binding to the repressor of the structural gene of Mac-resistance, although its antibacterial activity may correspond to its binding affinity for ribosomes. Thus, it is plausible that the inducer activity of EM for Mac-resistance can be separated from its antibacterial activity.

TABLE III
Antibacterial Activity of EM-Derivatives against *S. aureus*

	Drug resistance (mcg/ml)	
	MS537	MS353
EM.A	0.4	0.2
EM.B	0.4	0.2
EM.C	1.6	0.2
2'-O-Benzoyl-EM.A	1.6	0.4
6,9,12-Anhydro-EM.A	6.25	0.4
9-Dihydro-EM.B	12.5	0.8
N-(demethyl)-EM.A	25.0	6.25
EM.A-N-Oxide	25.0	1.6
EM.B-N-Oxide	50.0	6.25
EM.B-Methiodide	50.0	50.0
5-β-Desosaminyl-EM.B	200.0	200.0
3-α-Mycarosyl-EM.B	200.0	200.0
3'-De (dimethylamino) EM.A	200.0	200.0
3'-De (dimethylamino) EM.B	200.0	200.0
Erythronolide B	200.0	200.0
Erythrosamine	200.0	200.0
Desosamine	200.0	200.0

Table III shows the antibacterial activity of EM-derivatives (supplied by Dr. Mao, Abbott Laboratory, U.S.A.). EM-Derivatives may be divided into four groups according to their inducer activity for Mac-resistance, *i.e.*, A, B, C and D (Fig. 2). Group A was found to be the most active inducer and group D was the least, having almost no inducer activity. Both groups B and C were less active inducers than group A. Group A included EM-A, EM-B, EM-C, 6,9,12-anhydro-EM-A and N-(demethyl) EM-A. Group B included 9-dihydro-EM-B, EM-B N-oxide, EM-A N-oxide, EM-B methiodide and 2'-O-benzoyl EM-A. Erythronolide B, 3'-de- (dimethylamino) EM-B and 3'-de- (dimethylamino) EM-A belonged to group C. Group D included erythrosamine, 5-β-desosaminyl EM-B, 3-α-mycarosyl EM-B, 3-α-mycarosyl EM-B and desosamine. It is worth noting that erythronolide B and 3'-de-(demethyl-amino) EM-B have inducer activity in spite of lacking antibacterial activity; 9-carbonyl of lactone ring was not found to be essential for inducer activity, since 6,9,12-anhydro EM-A and 9-dihydro EM-B have inducer activity.

It is difficult to determine the more precise relations in the chemical structure and its inducer activity of EM-derivatives, because

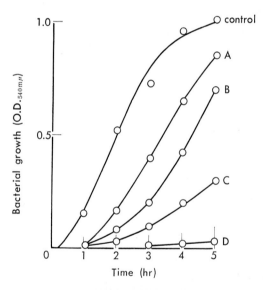

Fig. 2.   Inducer activity of EM-derivatives for Mac-resistance. A log-phase culture of *S. aureus* MS 537 was diluted at one-tenth in BHI broth containing one-tenth of a concentration of each drug resistance (Table III). After incubation with shaking at 37°C for 60 min, each culture was diluted at one-tenth of each drug resistance. Growth of each culture was plotted with shaking at 37°C. A, EM-A; B, 9-dihydro-EM-B; C, erythronolide B; D, non-induction and erythrosamine.

their permeability into bacterial cells may also affect their inducer activity. 5-β-Desosamyl EM-B and 3-α-mycarosyl EM-B contain erythronolide B (lactone ring), but have scarce inducer activity, probably because of their impermeability into bacterial cells.

3) LM-Inducible mutant

Since EM and OM have similar chemical structures, it is possible that OM-inducible mutants could be isolated from an EM-inducible strain MS537. These mutations seem to be located on the regulator gene(s) of Mac-resistance and seem to be the product of altered regulator gene(s), *i.e.*, repressors which may become capable of binding OM. However, LM is slightly different in chemical structure from either EM or OM, since it has a sixteen-member lactone ring and has a side chain of fatty acid and an aldehyde group. From the EM-inducible strain MS537, LM-inducible strains

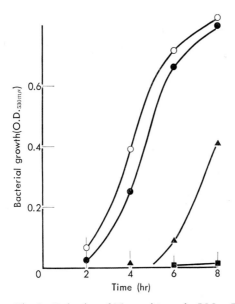

Fig. 3.   Induction of Mac-resistance by LM or EM in mutant MS537-59. For induction of Mac-resistance, cells were pretreated with 0.1 mcg of EM/ml (●), 0.2 mcg of LM/ml (▲) or inoculated without drugs (■). After 2 hr of incubation, the cells (0.2 ml) were inoculated into L tubes containing 9.8 ml of medium with 50 mcg of LM/ml.

were isolated by a one-step mutation (*17*) (Fig. 3). But EM was found to be still a good inducer in such mutants and its optimal concentration was the same as the original strain. The binding site of the repressor for EM in these mutants may remain intact and its acquisition of affinity to LM may be due to the removal of steric hindrance by mutation.

4) Inducer activities of LM derivatives in an LM-inducible mutant
The highest inducer activity of LM was observed in the propyonyl derivative while the deacyl derivative did not show any inducer activity (Fig. 4). The antibacterial activity of deacyl derivative for *S. aureus* was very low (MIC 50 µg/ml), but the inhibition of polyphenylalanine synthesis by this derivative in a cell-free system

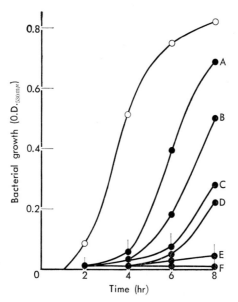

Fig. 4. Comparison between LM-inducing activity and size of acyl-group of LM. Growth curves of MS537-59 in medium in the presence (●) or absence (○) of 50 mcg of LM/ml are shown. Inocula were treated with 1.2×10^{-7}M of LM-A1 (isovaleryl form) or 2.4×10^{-7}M of other LM components for 2 hr at 37°C. Shown are 3-OH series compounds. A, propyonyl; B, butyryl; C, isovaleryl; D, acetyl; E, non-induced; F, deacyl.

was found to be on the same level as that of the isovaleryl form which shows high antibacterial activity (*14*). These results indicate that the acyl group of LM is related to the permeability of LM into bacterial cells and this group may not affect the binding affinity with the repressor. The tetrahydro-derivative had inducer activity but the hexahydro-derivative showed none; therefore, reduction of the conjugate double bond of lactone in LM did not affect inducer activity. It was found that hexahydro-derivative did not show any antibacterial or inhibitory activity in a cell-free system of protein synthesis. However, there still remained the permeability problem to be investigated in the LM derivatives as in the case of EM derivatives.

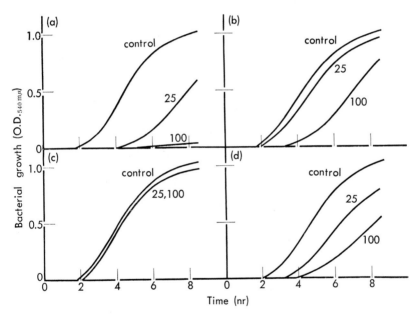

Fig. 5. Effect of temperature on SP-resistance in a temperature-inducible mutant MS353-*ti*. One-half ml of an overnight BHI broth culture of MS353-*ti* at 37°C was inoculated into 10 ml of BHI broth and shaken in a water bath at either 30°C or 42°C. Then 0.5 ml of the exponentially growing culture of MS353-*ti* at either 30°C (upper) or 42°C (lower) was inoculated in 10 ml of BHI broth containing either 25 or 100 mcg/ml of SP. (a), 30°C→30°C; (b), 30°C→42°C; (c), 42°C→42°C; (d), 42°C→30°C.

5) Temperature-inducible mutant

Temperature-inducible (*ti*) mutant MS537-*ti* was isolated from EM-inducible strain MS537 (*18, 19*). Mac-Resistance in this strain was rather low at 30°C. It was induced when inoculated at a higher temperature (42°C), but Mac-resistance of the induced population was decreased when cultured at 30°C (Fig. 5). The determinant(s) for the temperature-inducible resistance in MS537-*ti* was found to be transduced to a Mac-sensitive strain MS353 by typing phage 52A, and the resultant transductant MS353-*ti* showed the same genetic characters as in MS537-*ti* (Table I). Mac-Resistance in MS353-*ti* was also induced by prior treatment with subinhibitory

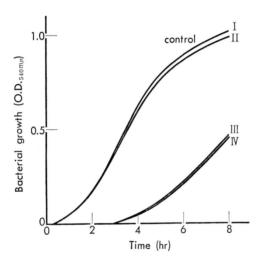

Fig. 6.   Impairment of heat-induction for SP-resistance in phosphate buffer. Cells of MS353-*ti* cultured at either 42°C (a) or 30°C (b) were harvested at mid-exponential growth and washed once with phosphate buffer (pH 7.4). Washed cells of (a) were suspended in phosphate buffer at 42°C (I) or at 30°C (II) for 120 min. Washed cells of (b) were suspended in phosphate buffer at 30°C (III) and (IV) were harvested by centrifugation, suspended in BHI broth containing 100 mcg of SP/ml, respectively and inoculated at 42°C. Control growth without SP. I, 42°C→(42°C)→42°C; II, 42°C→(30°C)→42°C; III, 30°C→(30°C)→ 42°C; IV, 30°C→(42°C)→42°C. (30°C) and (42°C) indicate incubation at 30°C and 42°C in phosphate buffer, and 30°C and 42°C indicate at 30°C and 42°C in BHI broth.

concentrations of EM as well as in the parent strain MS537, but induction of Mac-resistance in MS353-*ti* by either raising the temperature or by EM was inhibited by chloramphenicol. Induction of Mac-resistance in MS353-*ti* by raising the temperature did not take place when the cells were suspended in phosphate buffer, and, conversely, the increased resistance in MS353-*ti* at 42°C was not then decreased even when inoculated at 30°C in phosphate buffer (Fig. 6). These results indicated that some metabolic process, probably turnover of ribosomes, was necessary for the induction of Mac-resistance. It was found that the ribosomal affinity for Mac antibiotics was altered after induction by EM or by elevated temperature, as will be described below.

3. Accumulation of Mac antibiotics in bacterial cells

EM-Uptake by bacterial cells

Nakajima *et al.* (*10*) reported that the accumulation of labeled EM into the EM-inducible strains was decreased after induction with the drug. We observed the same results as shown in Table IV (*16*). The amount of EM accumulated into the non-induced cells, however, was about one-hundredth that of the accumulated tetracycline (TC) in the TC-inducible strain of *S. aureus* reported by Inoue *et al.* (*4*). There, TC-resistance was a result of decrease in the accumulation of the drug into bacterial cells after induction. The small amount of EM accumulated in the non-induced cells

TABLE IV
EM-Uptake by Bacterial Cells before or after Induction

Strain	EM accumulation (cpm/mg dry wt. of cell)
MS353 C36 (non-induced)	17.3
MS353 C36 (induced)	3.7
MS353	20.0

After overnight incubation in broth at 37°C, culture was diluted tenfold with fresh medium and shaken for 1.5 hr at 37°C. EM was added as an inducer to the diluted culture of MS353C36 to a final concentration of 0.1 mcg/ml and the culture was shaken at 37°C. After incubation for 3.5 hr, the culture either with or without induction was placed into a medium containing 50 mcg of ^{14}C-EM/ml. After further shaking for 1.5 hr, EM-uptake was measured.

can be explained by the formation of an EM-ribosome complex in non-induced cells.

The presence or absence of both glucose and Mg^{2+} did not affect SP-uptake nor was uptake inhibited by uncoupling agents such as 2,4-dinitrophenol and sodium azide, even at the concentrations necessary for the inhibition of bacterial growth (Table V). The optimal pH of SP-uptake was 7.0 and the maximal SP-uptake was observed at 20 min after addition of the drug. The SP-uptake increased with increasing amounts of the drug up to a concentration of 1.0 μg per ml (Fig. 7). Mac-Constitutive resistant mutant

TABLE V
Effect of Uncoupling Agents on ^{14}C-SP Uptake by MS537

Agent	Conc. (M)	^{14}C-SP uptake (mcg/mg dry wt. cells)	Inhibition[†] (%)
—	—	0.11	
DNP	2×10^{-4}	0.13	0
NaN₃	2×10^{-2}	0.15	0

DNP: 2,4-Dinitrophenol. ^{14}C-SP and uncoupling agent were added to BHI culture of MS537 at exponential growth. ^{14}C-SP-uptake was determined after incubation for 1 hr at 37°C. For details, see footnote of Table IV. [†] Inhibition was expressed in percent of control without inhibitor.

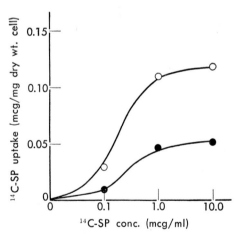

Fig. 7.   Relation between SP-uptake and its concentration in culture medium. SP-Uptake was assayed after 1 hr of incubation. ○, MS537; ●, MS537 induction.

MS537-2 and the induced population of MS537 showed high resistance to Mac antibiotics including SP, and the SP-uptake by these strains was decreased to half that of the non-induced population of the parent strain MS537.

4. *Drug-binding to ribosome*

1) *Formation of EM-ribosome complex*

It is well known that Mac antibiotics bind to bacterial ribosomes and the molar ratio of EM to 70 S ribosome (or 50 S subunit) was found to be about 1:1. Oleinick and Corcoran (*13*) reported that the inhibition of protein synthesis by EM in a cell-free system corresponded to the formation of EM-ribosome complexes. Ribosomes were isolated from either non-induced or induced cells of MS353 C36 and mixed with labeled EM, and then the distribution pattern of EM-ribosome complexes was examined by sucrose density gradient centrifugation. As shown in Fig. 8, EM was found to form a complex with 50 S subunit of ribosome prepared from the non-induced cells of MS353 C36, but the formation of EM-ribo-

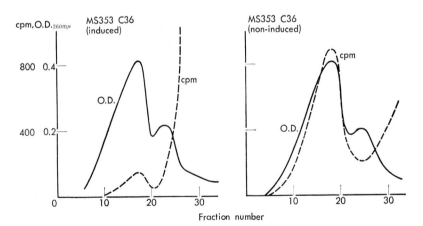

Fig. 8. Sucrose density gradient centrifugation analysis of EM-ribosome complexes. The reaction mixture (0.14 ml) containing 40 A 260 units of dissociated ribosomes and ^{14}C-EM (0.9 mcg in total, 15,600 cpm/mcg) was incubated at 27°C for 30 min. Samples were layered over sucrose gradient (5–20%) and were spun down.

some complexes was greatly decreased in the ribosomes prepared from induced cells. The amounts of EM-ribosome complexes in various strains derived from MS537 were measured by a gel-filtration method using Sephadex G100. As shown in Table VI, the amounts of the EM-ribosome complexes in non-induced cells were the same as those in drug-sensitive cells, but the amount of EM bound to the ribosomes prepared from induced populations was decreased to about one-eighth that of the ribosomes isolated from non-induced populations. Similarly, the affinity of EM with ribosomes prepared from the constitutive mutant from MS353 C36 was greatly decreased. The amounts of EM-binding to the ribosomes prepared from MS537-*ti* cultured at 42°C were decreased, compared with those of the ribosomes of the cells cultured at 30°C (*18*). The amount of EM-binding to the ribosomes prepared from MS537-*ti* cultured at 30°C, however, was found to be still low when compared with that of the non-induced population of MS353 C36, indicating that the partial expression of the inducible resistance took place in MS537-*ti* even at 30°C.

TABLE VI
The Formation of EM-Ribosome Complexes in Staphylococcal Strains

Source of ribosome	EM-Binding (cpm/A260 unit)
MS353 C36 (non-induced)	281
MS353 C36 (induced)	36
MS353 A1	15
MS353	274
MS537-*ti* (30 C)[†]	131
MS537-*ti* (42 C)[†]	9

Ribosomes (30 μl, about 10 A260 units) were mixed with ^{14}C-EM (30 μl, 0.9 γ) in 0.05 M Tris-buffer (pH 7.4) containing both 0.05 M NH$_4$Cl and 0.016 M magnesium acetate and were incubated at 27°C for 30 min. EM-Ribosome complexes were separated by Sephadex G 100 column. † Culture temperature.

2) Time course of induction
To determine the time course of decrease in the affinity of ribosomes with EM, rifampicin was used to stop the induction as reported by Wehrli *et al.* (*26*). Rifampicin was added at various time intervals after induction and then ribosomes were prepared. When both EM and rifampicin were added at zero time, EM-ribosome

complexes were formed, in the control as well, without induction. But the number of EM-ribosome complexes was decreased rapidly even after 5 min of induction, indicating the rapid appearance of the changes in ribosome by induction (Fig. 9).

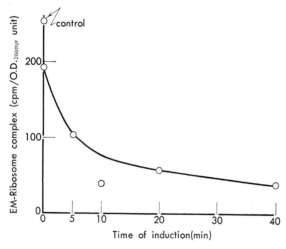

Fig. 9. Time course of induction. EM was added as an inducer to a final concentration of 0.1 mcg/ml. Rifampicin (2 mcg/ml) was used for the interruption of the induction at various time intervals after EM treatment, and induced culture was rapidly chilled by ice. And then ribosomes were isolated.

SP, as well as EM, bound specifically to the 50 S ribosomal sub-unit of the non-induced cells of MS537 at a ratio of about 0.6 molecule per ribosome (Fig. 10). The formation of SP-ribosome complexes was decreased in ribosomes prepared from either induced populations of MS537 or constitutive mutant MS537-2, indicating the reduction of affinity of ribosome with SP (20, 22). As will be described below, there existed a parallel relation between SP-binding to ribosomes and the inhibition of polypeptide synthesis by the drug.

5. *Correlation between Mac-binding to ribosomes and inhibition of polypeptide synthesis*

In Sec. 4, a parallel relation between the level of Mac-resistance

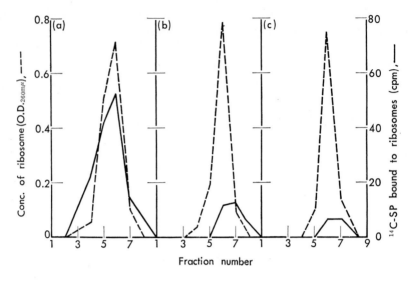

Fig. 10.   Binding of ¹⁴C-SP to ribosomes. ¹⁴C-SP-Ribosome complex was eluted from Sephadex G-100 column. (a) MS537 before induction, (b) MS537 after induction, (c) MS537-2.

and the ribosomal affinity with the drug was discussed. We will next examine the relation between the affinity of ribosomes with Mac antibiotics and the inhibition of polypeptide synthesis by the drugs in a cell-free system. ¹⁴C-Phenylalanine was incorporated into protein in a cell-free system which combined ribosomes from *S. aureus* and the supernatant (S-100) from *Escherichia coli* Q-13 (RNase I⁻). Assay for amino acid incorporation was performed according to the methods of Mao (*7*) and Nierenberg (*11*). As shown in Fig. 11, the rate of incorporation was almost constant for poly-U dependent phenylalanine up to 60 min of incubation, but the incorporation was very low for endogenous *m*-RNA dependent phenylalanine. The incorporation of ¹⁴C-phenylalanine into polypeptide was found to be dependent upon the ribosomes prepared from *S. aureus* and was inhibited by various concentrations of SP ranging from 0.5 to 500 *μ*g per ml (*21*). The results are shown in Table VII.

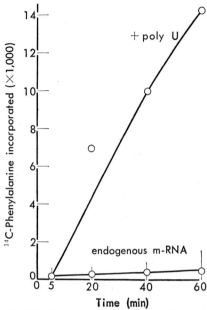

Fig. 11. Time course of polypeptide synthesis. Total volume of the reaction mixture was 2.0 ml containing the following components: 1 mM ATP, 0.05 mM GTP, CTP and UTP, 5 mM creatine phosphate, 0.02 mg of creatine kinase, 1 μCi of ¹⁴C-phenylalanine (297 mCi/mM), 0.06 mM each of the remaining amino acids in Medium A, *E. coli* Q 13 S-100 (67.5 A 260 units) and ribosomes of *S. aureus* MS537 (112 A 260 units). One-half aliquot was sampled up from 2 ml of the reaction mixture at each time. Medium A consists of 0.01 M Tris-acetate (pH 7.5) containing 16 mM magnesium acetate, 50 mM ammonium chloride and 0.1 mM dithioerythritol. The radioactivity was determined by a method described previously (*17*).

TABLE VII

Inhibition of Polypeptide Synthesis by SP

System	¹⁴C-Phenylalanine incorporated	
	cpm	%
Complete system (MS537)	9108	100
− ribosomes	769	8.4
+ SP 0.5 μg/ml	2499	27.0
+ SP 5 μg/ml	1997	21.4
+ SP 50 μg/ml	1398	14.8
+ SP 500 μg/ml	1177	12.5

See the legend of Fig. 14. The reaction mixture was 1.0 ml and was incubated at 37°C for 40 min.

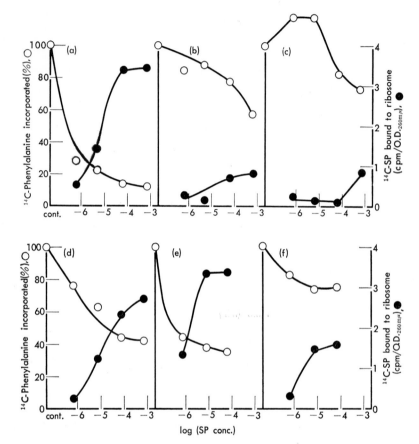

Fig. 12.   Correlation of SP-binding to ribosomes and inhibition of polyphenylalanine synthesis. See footnote, Fig. 11, concerning the reaction mixtures. SP was added to the reaction mixture and radioactivity was assayed after incubation at 37°C for 40 min. Cont.: The radioactivity of ^{14}C-phenylalanine incorporated without SP. (a), MS537; (b), MS537 ind.; (c), MS537-2; (d), FS195; (e), MS642-2; (f), MS642.

As shown in Fig. 12, the SP-binding affinity of ribosomes decreased their affinity for SP in MS642 carrying Mac-constitutive resistance in which the determinant for Mac-resistance was located on a plasmid (2, 9, 12). Accordingly, it was concluded that Mac-resistance in *S. aureus* was related to the decrease in binding of Mac antibiotics to the ribosomes.

As mentioned (*18, 19*), we isolated a temperature-inducible (*ti*) mutant MS353-*ti* in which Mac-resistance was induced when cultivated at a higher temperature (42°C). To eliminate the possibility that pretreatment of a Mac-inducible strain with inducers such as EM and OM caused a decrease in the further binding of Mac antibiotics to ribosomes, we used this mutant. The ribosomes derived from MS353-*ti* cultured at 30°C (30°C ribosome) had a much greater affinity for ^{14}C-SP than those prepared from cells cultured at 42°C (42°C ribosome). The results are shown in Fig. 13. The same results were obtained when ^{14}C-EM was used instead of SP as described in Sec. 4.

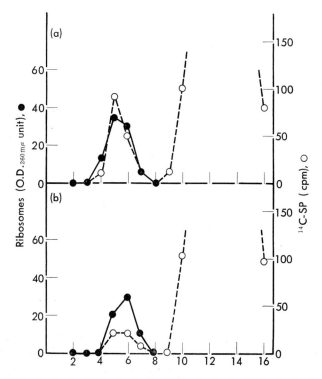

Fig. 13. Binding of ^{14}C-SP to ribosomes of MS353-*ti*. MS353-*ti* was cultured in BHI broth at 30°C (upper) or 42°C (lower), and ribosomes were isolated from these cells, respectively. (a), 30°C ribosomes; (b), 42°C ribosomes.

Incorporation of ¹⁴C-phenylalanine into protein was studied in a cell-free system of the combination of 30°C ribosomes (or 42°C ribosomes) of MS353-*ti* and the supernatant (S-100) of *E. coli* Q-13 (RNase I⁻). The synthesis of ¹⁴C-polyphenylalanine on 30°C ribosome was inhibited by SP, but not on 42°C ribosome (Fig. 14). Accordingly, it was safely concluded that Mac-resistance in *S. aureus* is related to the decrease in Mac-binding to the ribosomes.

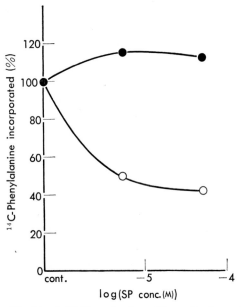

Fig. 14.   Inhibition of polypeptide synthesis on ribosomes prepared from *S. aureus* MS 353-*ti* cultivated at either 30°C or 42°C. ●, 42°C ribosomes; ○, 30°C ribosomes.

6. In vitro developed resistant mutants to Mac antibiotics

As shown in Sec. 5, Mac-resistance in *S. aureus* of clinical origin could be explained by decrease in the affinity of Mac antibiotics for the ribosome. It was reported that there was a ribosomal altera-tion in an EM-resistant mutant of *E. coli* obtained by a one-step mutation after treatment with nitrosoguanidine (*23*). To learn the mechanisms of Mac-resistance in the *in vitro* developed resistant

TABLE VIII

SP-Uptake by *S. aureus* Cells

Strain	^{14}C-SP Uptake	
	cpm/mg dry wt. cell	mcg/mg dry wt. cell
MS353	62.2	0.21
MS353-*sr*	31.5	0.11

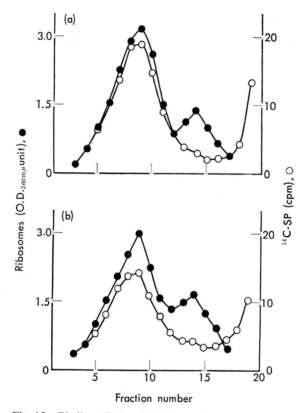

Fig. 15. Binding affinity of ^{14}C-SP to ribosomal subunit of *in vitro* developed resistant mutants. (a), MS353; (b), MS353-*sr*.

mutants in *S. aureus*, we isolated several mutants from a Mac-sensitive strain of *S. aureus* MS353 by successive passages of this strain into a liquid medium containing increased concentrations of each Mac antibiotic. As shown in Table II, MS353-*sr*, a mutant selected by SP, was found to be cross-resistant to SP, LM and josamycin (JM) but still sensitive to both EM and LCM. The resistance in MS353-*sr* was stable even after 15 transfers in SP-free broth, and such resistance patterns were not demonstrated again in more than 10,000 clinical isolates. This was because the Mac-resistant strains of *S. aureus* isolated from clinical specimens always possessed EM-resistance.

MS353-*er* was a mutant selected by EM and was cross-resistant to OM, but resistance to other Mac antibiotics and LCM was found to be intermediate. MS353-*lcr*, a mutant selected by LCM, was found to be cross-resistant to both EM and OM, but showed intermediate resistance to other Mac antibiotics.

It was found that ^{14}C-SP uptake by MS353-*sr* was reduced when compared with that of the parent strain MS353 (Table VIII). But there were no significant differences in the ribosomal affinity to ^{14}C-SP between MS353-*sr* and MS353. Polypeptide synthesis on the ribosomes prepared from MS353-*sr* was inhibited by SP as well as by an SP-sensitive strain MS353, although MS353-*sr* was resistant to SP. The results are shown in Figs. 15 and 16. These

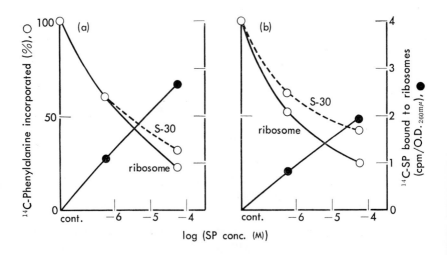

Fig. 16.   SP-Binding to ribosomes and inhibition of polypeptide synthesis in *in vitro* developed resistant mutants. (a), MS353; (b), MS353-*sr*.

results indicated that SP-resistance in MS353-*sr* was not derived from alteration of ribosomes but probably from some other mechanism such as impermeability of the drug into bacterial cells. Further detailed studies remain to be carried out.

7. Discussion

The inducible resistance in *S. aureus* to Mac antibiotics has not yet been clarified in detail because *cis-trans* analysis for the regulator gene(s) could not be applied. Isolation of temperature-inducible mutants (*18, 19*) strongly suggests the existence of a repressor protein for the structural gene(s) of Mac-resistance and of the negative control system. Achievement of inducer activity of Mac antibiotics other than EM, *i.e.*, OM and LM, can be explained as alteration of the repressor protein by mutation, giving it an affinity for such drugs in addition to EM. According to the above conception and results described in this paper, we have presented a tentative model for the inducible resistance to Mac antibiotics in *S. aureus* (Fig. 17). Transduction analysis of the constitutive-resistant mutants did not reveal whether the gene(s) governing resistance to Mac antibiotics and LCM are identical or not. But the isolation of staphylococcal strains resistant to Mac antibiotics but sensitive to LCM suggested that the genes responsible for resistance to both Mac and LCM are separate but closely linked.

The formation of Mac-ribosome complexes was decreased by the acquisition of Mac-resistance through EM induction. The ribosomes prepared from the Mac-constitutive resistant mutants, such as MS537-2 and MS353 A1, lost their affinity with Mac antibiotics. The affinity with Mac antibiotics of ribosomes prepared from the cells of MS537-*ti* cultured at 42°C was decreased as compared with those prepared from cells cultured at 30°C. The inhibition profiles of SP to poly-U directed polyphenylalanine synthesis were found to correspond to the affinity of SP with the ribosomes. These results indicated to us that the 50 S subunits of ribosome were altered in Mac-constitutive resistant strains or by induction in the Mac-inducible resistant strains and that the alteration of ribosome was the most likely mechanism responsible for Mac-resistance. Taubman *et al.* (*24*) and Tanaka *et al.* (*23*) isolated the EM-resistant mutants of *Bacillus subtilis* and *E. coli*, respectively. Tanaka *et al.* (*23*, in this monograph) showed that this resistant mechanism was explained by the alteration of a protein component of the 50 S subunit in ribosome. These resistant strains, however, are *in vitro* developed resistant mutants, and the alteration of a ribosomal protein seems to be caused by the substitution of an amino acid which results from a base exchange by mutation. In the inducible-resistant strain of *S. aureus*, resistance to Mac antibiotics appeared after treatment of the cells with an inducer and this resistance was lost when the cells of induced population were grown in an inducer-free medium. Therefore, it is unlikely that the resistance mechanisms of inducible strains were caused by the substitution of the ribosomal protein of an amino acid. It is more plausible that modification of the 50S subunit components was caused by induction, and the protein or RNA of 50S subunit of ribosome was modified by addition of a group of small molecular weight such as methyl- or acetyl-moiety, *etc.* We assayed

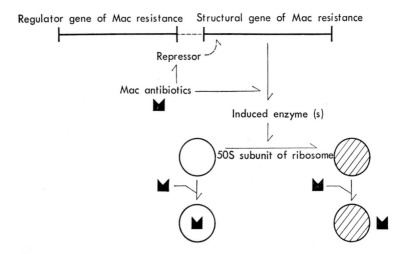

Fig. 17.   Scheme for inducible-resistance to Mac antibiotics.

the 50 S subunit proteins by acrylamide gel electrophoresis and CM-cellulose column. Proteins prepared from either induced or constitutive-resistant cells were labeled by ^{14}C-lysine and those prepared from non-induced cells were labeled by ^{3}H-lysine. The labeled proteins of the 50 S subunit were mixed together and chromatographed by the method described by Otaka *et al.* (*15*). As shown in Fig. 18, the proteins of the 50 S subunit were separated into 15 distinct peaks, but no differences were observed between the induced and non-induced cells or between the non-induced and constitutive-resistant cells.

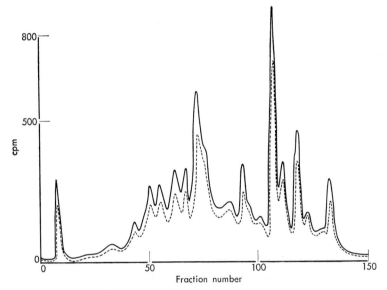

Fig. 18.   CM-Cellulose column chromatography of 50S subunit proteins isolated from constitutive and non-induced cells. Chromatography of ribosomal protein was done according to the method described by Osawa *et al.* (*15*). ---, ^{14}C, MS353 A1 ribosome; —, ^{3}H, MS353 C36 (non-ind.) ribosome.

Induction of Mac-resistance did not take place when the cells were suspended in buffer, suggesting turnover of the ribosome after induction. On the other hand, the experiments on the time course of induction using rifampicin revealed that the affinity of ribosome with EM was greatly decreased within 5 min of incubation with inducer. The possibility that residual protein synthesis may continue during the preparation of ribosomes after the addition of rifampicin cannot be ruled out.

Ribosomes isolated from the non-induced cells were mixed with the supernatant from the induced cells, together with co-factors such as ATP, acetyl CoA, S-adenosyl methionine and GTP, but examination showed no decrease in the ribosomal affinity with EM. Further, the necessity of ribosomal turnover for induction of Mac-resistance remains to be proven.

We could not detect any changes in the ribosomal proteins under the conditions that prevailed, although these results still did not rule out the possibility that the ribosomal protein might be altered. Mao and Putterman (8) suggested the participation of RNA in binding EM to ribosomes in his study of chemical modification methods. A further comparative study of ribosomal RNA may be necessary in order to understand the mechanism of inducible resistance to Mac antibiotics.

SUMMARY

According to genetic and biochemical analyses, it was concluded that increased Mac-resistance after induction in the inducible-resistant strains could be explained by the alteration of 50 S subunit of ribosome and a decreased ribosomal affinity with Mac antibiotics. Acquisition of inducer activity of Mac antibiotics other than EM, including OM and LM, may be explained as an alteration of a repressor protein after mutation, resulting in an acquired affinity for such drugs. On the basis of the above results, we have presented a tentative model for inducible-resistance to Mac antibiotics and we have discussed the possibility of alteration of ribosomes in the inducible strains after induction, or in the constitutive-resistant strains.

REFERENCES

1 Garrod, L. P. 1957. The erythromycin group of antibiotics. *Brit. Med. J.*, **2**, 57–63.

2 Hashimoto, H., Kono, K., and Mitsuhashi, S. 1964. Elimination of penicillin resistance of *Staphylococcus aureus* by treatment with acriflavine. *J. Bacteriol.*, **88**, 261–262.

3 Hashimoto, H., Oshima, H., and Mitsuhashi, S. 1968. Drug resistance of staphylococci. IX. Inducible resistance to macrolide antibiotics in *Staphylococcus aureus. Japan. J. Microbiol.*, **12**, 321–327.

4 Inoue, M., Hashimoto, H., and Mitsuhashi, S. 1970. Mechanism of tetracycline resistance in *S. aureus. In* "Progress in Antimicrobial and Anticancer Chemotherapy (Proc. 6th International Congress of Chemotherapy)," University of Tokyo, Tokyo, Vol. I, p. 433–439.

5 Kono, M., Hashimoto, H., and Mitsuhashi, S. 1964. Drug resistance of staphylococci. Inducible resistance of macrolide antibiotics. Record of the Kanto Branch Meeting of Japan Bacteriol. Assoc., Nov., Tokyo; 1965. *Japan. J. Bacteriol.*, **20**, 122–123.

6 Kono, M., Hashimoto, H., and Mitsuhashi, S. 1966. Drug resistance of staphylococci. III. Resistance to some macrolide antibiotics and inducible system. *Japan. J. Microbiol.*, **10**, 59–66.

7 Mao, J. C.-H. 1967. Protein synthesis in a cell-free extract from *Staphylococcus aureus. J. Bacteriol.*, **94**, 80–86.

8 Mao, J. C.-H., and Putterman, M. 1969. The intermolecular complex of erythromycin and ribosome. *J. Mol. Biol.*, **44**, 347–361.

9 Mitsuhashi, S., Hashimoto, H., Kono, M., and Morimura, M. 1965. Drug resistance of staphylococci. II. Joint elimination and joint transduction of the determinants of penicillinase production and resistance to macrolide antibiotics. *J. Bacteriol.*, **89**, 988–992.

10 Nakajima, Y., Inoue, M., Oka, Y., and Yamagishi, S. 1968. A mode of resistance to macrolide antibiotics in *Staphylococcus aureus. Japan. J. Microbiol.*, **12**, 248–250.

11 Nierenberg, M. W. 1963. Cell-free protein synthesis directed by messenger RNA. "Methods in Enzymology," Academic Press, Vol. VI, p. 17–23.

12 Novik, R. P., and Richmond, M. H. 1965. Nature and interaction of genetic elements governing penicillinase synthesis in *Staphylococcus aureus. J. Bacteriol.*, **90**, 467–480.

13 Oleinick, N. L., and Corcoran, J. W. 1969. Two types of binding of erythromycin to ribosomes from antibiotic-sensitive and resistant *Bacillus subtilis* 168. *J. Biol. Chem.*, **224**, 727–735.

14 Omura, S., Katagiri, M., Umezawa, I., Komiyama, K., Maekawa, T., Sekikawa, K., Matsumae, A., and Hata, T. 1968. Structure-biological

activities relationships among leucomycins and their derivatives. *J. Antibiotics*, **21**, 532–538.

15 Otaka, B., Itoh, T., and Osawa, S. 1968. Ribosomal proteins of bacterial cells: strain- and species-specificity. *J. Mol. Biol.*, **33**, 93–107.

16 Saito, T., Hashimoto, H., and Mitsuhashi, S. 1969. Drug resistance of staphylococci. Decrease in the formation of erythromycin-ribosome complex in erythromycin resistant strain. *Japan. J. Microbiol.*, **13**, 119–121.

17 Saito, T., Hashimoto, H., and Mitsuhashi, S. 1970. Macrolide resistance in *Staphylococcus aureus*. Isolation of a mutant in which leucomycin is an active inducer. *Japan. J. Microbiol.*, **14**, 473–478.

18 Saito, T., Oshima, H., Shimizu, M., Hashimoto, H., and Mitsuhashi, S. 1970. Macrolide resistance in *Staphylococcus aureus*. *In* "Progress in Antimicrobial and Anticancer Chemotherapy (Proc. 6th International Congress of Chemotherapy)," University of Tokyo Press, Vol. II, p. 572–578.

19 Shimizu, M., Saito, T., and Mitsuhashi, S. 1970. Macrolide Resistance in *Staphylococcus aureus*. Relation between spiramycin-binding to ribosome and inhibition of polypeptide synthesis in a heat inducible-resistant mutant. *Japan. J. Microbiol.*, **14**, 155–162.

20 Shimizu, M., Saito, T., and Mitsuhashi, S. 1970. Spiramycin resistance in *Staphylococcus aureus*. The stoichiometry of spiramycin-binding to ribosomes from spiramycin-sensitive, intermediate- and high-resistant strains. *Japan. J. Microbiol.*, **14**, 177–178.

21 Shimizu, M., Saito, T., and Mitsuhashi, S. 1970. Macrolide resistance in *Staphylococcus aureus*. Correlation between spiramycin-binding to ribosomes and inhibition of polypeptide synthesis in cell-free system. *Japan. J. Microbiol.*, **14**, 215–219.

22 Shimizu, M., Saito, T., Hashimoto, H., and Mitsuhashi, S. 1970. Spiramycin resistance in *Staphylococcus aureus*. Decrease in spiramycin-accumulation and the ribosomal affinity of spiramycin in resistant staphylococci. *J. Antibiotics*, **23**, 63–67.

23 Tanaka, K., Teraoka, H., and Tamaki, M. 1968. *Escherichia coli* with altered ribosomal protein component. *Science*, **162**, 576–578.

24 Taubman, S. B., Jones, N. R., Young, F. E., and Corcoran, J. W. 1966. Sensitivity and resistance to erythromycin in *Bacillus subtilis* 168: the ribosomal binding of erythromycin and chloramphenicol. *Biochim. Biophys. Act*, **123**, 438–440.

25 Weaver, J. R., and Pattee, P. A. 1964. Inducible resistance to erythromycin in *Staphylococcus aureus*. *J. Bacteriol.*, **88**, 574–580.

26 Wehrli, W., Knusel, F., and Staehelin, M. 1968. Action of rifamycin on RNA-polymerase from sensitive and resistant bacteria. *Biochem. Biophys. Res. Commun.*, **32**, 284–288.

CHEMICAL AND BIOLOGICAL STUDIES ON
LEUCOMYCINS (KITASAMYCINS)*

Hata Toju and Satoshi Ōmura

The Kitasato Institute, Tokyo, Japan

Leucomycin, a macrolide antibiotic produced from *Streptomyces kitasatoensis* Hata, was discovered by Hata *et al.* in 1953 (*15*). This was 3 years after the discovery of pikromycin (Fig. 1), the first macrolide antibiotic, by Brockmann *et al.* (*7, 34*). Approximately 50 macrolide antibiotics other than the polyene macrolides are known at present, and a few of them are used in current practice.

Leucomycin was recognized as effective in cases of infections caused by gram-positive rods, gram-negative cocci, spirochetae, rickettsia, and larger-sized viruses (*16*). It has been used in practice since 1955. Studies (*3*) on the improvement of a leucomycin-producing strain of *S. kitasatoensis* and its fermentation (*26*) were conducted at the Toyō Jozo Co., Ltd., and methods for the mass production of leucomycin were formulated.

Studies on leucomycin conducted in 1963 are described in a comprehensive review by Watanabe and Takeda (*53*). This review,

---

* Common name of leucomycin was changed to kitasamycin by the International Center of Information on Antibiotics, Liege-Belgium in 1969.

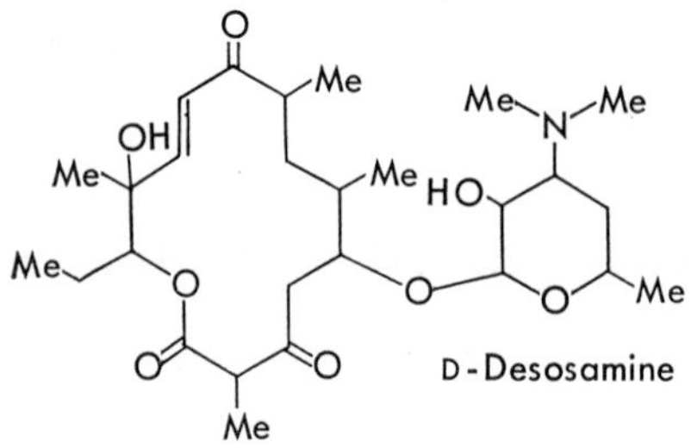

Pikromycin [Brockmann et al. (34)]

Fig. 1.

therefore, will only give their outlines and the emphasis will be placed on the chemical and biological aspects of studies made thereafter.

Extraction and isolation of leucomycin

The fermented broth culture of *S. kitasatoensis* was adjusted to pH 4.0 and filtered. The filtrate was then adjusted to pH 8.0 and extracted with butyl acetate. The butyl acetate layer was then extracted with dilute hydrochloric acid. The extraction procedure was repeated two more times, and the final dilute hydrochloric acid layer was adjusted to pH 8.0 to obtain a white precipitate. Six components were isolated by chromatography on ion-exchange resins (54) and counter-current distribution methods (55). Two components, A_1 and A_2, belonging to the A-group, easily soluble in benzene, and four components, B_1–B_4, from the B-group, hardly soluble in it, were separated. Each component was detected by bioautography of ordinary and reversed phase paper chromatograms of leucomycin using *Bacillus subtilis* as a test organism (*1*). The physicochemical properties of these isolated components are presented in Table I.

With the improvement in productivity of leucomycin, it became necessary to reexamine its components. The reexamination was conducted by the present authors along with studies on the chemical structures of these antibiotics. As shown in Chart 1, the reexa-

TABLE I
Physicochemical Properties of Leucomycins

	A_1	A_2	B_1	B_2	B_3	B_4
Molecular formula	$C_{46}H_{81}O_{17}N$	$C_{65}H_{111}O_{22}N$	$C_{35}H_{59}O_{13}N$	$C_{38}H_{65}O_{16}N$	$C_{34}H_{53}O_{13}N$	$C_{38}H_{59}O_{16}N$
mp	135.0	142.0	214.5	214.0	216.0	221.0
	-138.0	-144.0	-216.0	-216.0	-217.0	-223.8
λ_{max} $^1/_{1000}$ N HCl mμ	233	233	233	233	233	234
ε_{max} ($\times 10^4$)	2.45	1.98	2.24	2.47	2.32	2.45
Antibacterial activity (mcg/mg)	1250	1138	125	269	713	875
pKa'	7.1	7.1	6.6	6.7	6.7	6.8

(Watanabe (55))

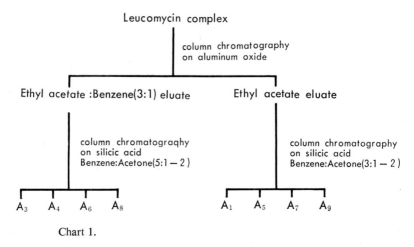

Chart 1.

mination resulted in the isolation of 8 major components by means of chromatography on silica gel and alumina.

In Table II, the physicochemical properties of these components are presented. Leucomycins A_3, A_4, A_6 and A_8 (they belong to the Ac-group) can easily be crystallized from the benzene solution, but crystallization of the remaining components has not been successful so far. All except A_1 have been shown to be new substances by comparing their physicochemical properties with those of the components separated by Watanabe et al. They were named leucomycin A_3 through A_9. Furthermore, A_2 and the B-group components cannot be found in the bulk now produced by an improved strain of S. kitasatoensis.

Chemical structure of leucomycin

Studies on the chemical structure of leucomycin were initiated by Watanabe et al. in 1961 (56, 57). Upon hydrolysis of the components with dilute acid, 4-O-isovaleryl mycarose (2,6-dideoxy-3-C-methyl-L-ribohexose, Lemal et al. (31), Korte et al. (28), and Grisebach et al. (14)) was produced from leucomycins A_1, A_2 and B_1; and 4-O-acetyl mycarose, from leucomycins B_2, B_3 and B_4. Leucomycin A_1 was hydrolyzed with 2N HCl to produce mycaminose (3,6-dideoxy-3-dimethylamino-D-glucose, Foster et al. (11),

TABLE II
Physicochemical Properties of Leucomycins

	Molecular formula (molecular weight)	Anal. C Calcd. Found	H	N%	mp °C	$[\alpha]_D^{25}$ (C, CHCl$_3$)	pK'a in 50% EtOH (equivalent)	UV λ_{max} MeOH (E_{1cm} 1%)
A$_1$	C$_{40}$H$_{67}$O$_{14}$N (785.6)	61.11 61.36	8.60 8.50	1.78 1.70		−66.0 (1.0)	6.69 (800±15)	232.0 (400)
A$_3$	C$_{42}$H$_{69}$O$_{15}$N (828.0)	60.92 60.57	8.40 8.19	1.69 1.75	120–121	−55.4 (1.8)	6.70 (835±10)	231.5 (351)
A$_4$	C$_{41}$H$_{67}$O$_{15}$N (814.0)	60.50 60.80	8.30 8.13	1.72 1.69	126–127	−50.0 (1.0)	6.70 (820±10)	231.5 (375)
A$_5$	C$_{39}$H$_{65}$O$_{14}$N (774.0)	60.52 60.61	8.74 8.75	1.81 1.85		−52.0 (1.0)	6.69 (780±10)	232.0 (380)
A$_6$	C$_{40}$H$_{65}$O$_{15}$N (799.9)	60.06 60.15	8.19 8.10	1.75 1.71	135–137	−56.0 (1.0)	6.72 (801±15)	231.5 (375)
A$_7$	C$_{38}$H$_{63}$O$_{14}$N (757.9)	60.22 60.10	8.38 8.40	1.85 1.90		−65.0 (1.3)	6.73 (770±15)	232.0 (405)
A$_8$	C$_{39}$H$_{63}$O$_{15}$N (785.9)	59.60 59.71	8.08 8.12	1.78 1.80	147–149	−58.3 (1.8)	6.75 (790±15)	232.0 (380)
A$_9$	C$_{37}$H$_{61}$O$_{14}$N (743.9)	59.74 59.65	8.27 8.31	1.88 1.91		−65.1 (1.3)	6.75 (750±15)	232.0 (396)

(Ōmura et al. (41))

Richardson (*48*), and Hofheinz and Grisebach (*17*)), which had been obtained from carbomycin.

Based on spectrometric analysis, color reaction and decomposition reaction, an estimated chemical structure of A_1 having a 21-membered lactone ring was presented by Watanabe *et al.* (*58*). The present authors commenced studies on the isolation and chemical structure of the components of leucomycin and found that the above-mentioned chromatography on silica gel and

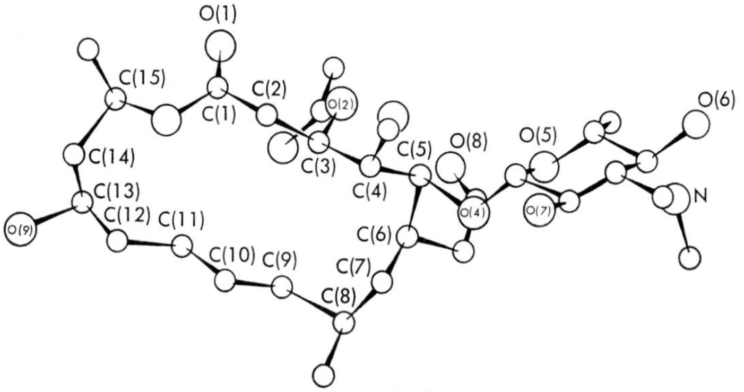

Molecular structure projected along the c axis. [Hiramatsu *et al.*, (*23*)]

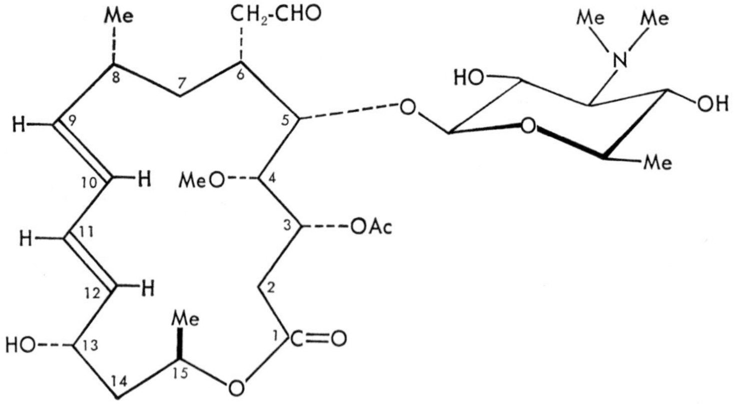

Fig. 2. Absolute configuration of demycarosyl iso-leucomycin A_3 (VI).

alumina made it possible to separate the components effectively. Then, studies on the chemical structure were focused especially on leucomycin A_3, which was comparatively easy to separate (36–38). IR and NMR of leucomycin were studied in detail, and then the products obtained by its decomposition with acids and ozone were examined to disclose their structural resemblance to carbomycin (29, 59, 60). Leucomycin A_3 was successfully converted to carbomycin B with activated MnO_2, and its planar structural formula was derived. Hiramatsu et al. (23) determined its absolute configuration based on an X-ray analysis of a crystal of demycarosyl-leucomycin A_3 (VI) hydrobromide obtained by its decomposition with acids (Fig. 2). The relationship between demycarosyl-leucomycin A_3 and leucomycin A_3 of its parent substance became clear. Furthermore, the chirality of the asymmetric carbon atom in the 9-position of the lactone was demonstrated by the present authors (38).

Iso-leucomycin A_3 was also obtained by treating leucomycin A_3 with dilute acids at conditions of pH 2.0 and 60°C. This is a compound, whose hydroxyl group had made an allylic rearrangement to the same position as that of the compound presented for X-ray analysis (38). Based on a series of the above-mentioned studies on the chemical structure of leucomycin A_3, including those conducted by Celmer (9), carbomycins A and B were found to have the absolute configurations shown in Fig. 3.

Afterwards, Paul and Tchelitcheff (47), Kuehne and Benson (29) and Ōmura et al. (39) conducted studies to demonstrate that the chemical structure of spiramycin was related to that of leucomycin. The main reactions indicating the relationship among leucomycin, carbomycin and spiramycin are summarized in Chart 2. To prevent the rearrangement of the allylic hydroxyl group during decomposition with acid, the acid hydrolyzation reaction was conducted with tetrahydro-leucomycin or spiramycin. Spiramycin is different from leucomycin in that the former does not have an acyl group on mycarose, and forosamine (deoxyamino sugar, 2,3,6-trideoxy-4-dimethylamino-D-erythroaldohexose, Paul and Tchelitcheff (46) and Stevens et al. (50)) combines with the lactone at its 9-position by a β-glucosidic bond. The mutually related constitu-

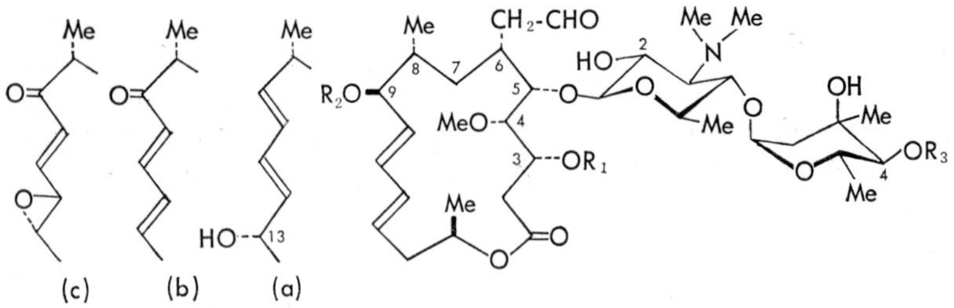

			R_1	R_2	R_3
Leucomycin	A_1(Ia)	(as shown)	H	H	CO·CH$_2$·CH(CH$_3$)$_2$
"	A_3(Ib)	"	CO·CH$_3$	H	"
"	A_4(Ic)	"	CO·CH$_3$	H	CO·CH$_2$·CH$_2$·CH$_3$
"	A_5(Id)	"	H	H	"
"	A_6(Ie)	"	CO·CH$_3$	H	CO·CH$_2$·CH$_3$
"	A_7(If)	"	H	H	"
"	A_8(Ig)	"	CO·CH$_3$	H	CO·CH$_3$
"	A_9(Ih)	"	H	H	"
"	u (Ii)	"	CO·CH$_3$	H	H
"	v (Ij)	"	H	H	H
Iso-leucomycin	A_3(II)	(cf. offset a)	CO·CH$_3$	—	CO·CH$_2$·CH(CH$_3$)$_2$
Spiramycin	A (IIIa)	(as shown)	H	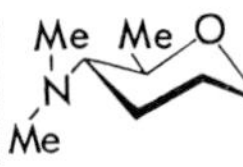 [Me Me O N Me sugar]	H
"	B (IIIb)	"	CO·CH$_3$		H
"	C (IIIc)	"	CO·CH$_2$·CH$_3$		H
Niddamycin	(IV)	(cf. offset c)	H	—	CO·CH$_2$·CH(CH$_3$)$_2$
Magnamycin	A (Va)	(cf. offset c)	CO·CH$_3$	—	"
"	B (Vb)	(cf. offset b)	CO·CH$_3$	—	"

Fig. 3.

tional formulas of spiramycin, carbomycin and leucomycin were finally established after several revisions. At that time, Celmer (*10*) pointed out abnormalities in the old constitutional formulas from the standpoint of macrolide biogenetic theory. These new formulas, however, have been normalized.

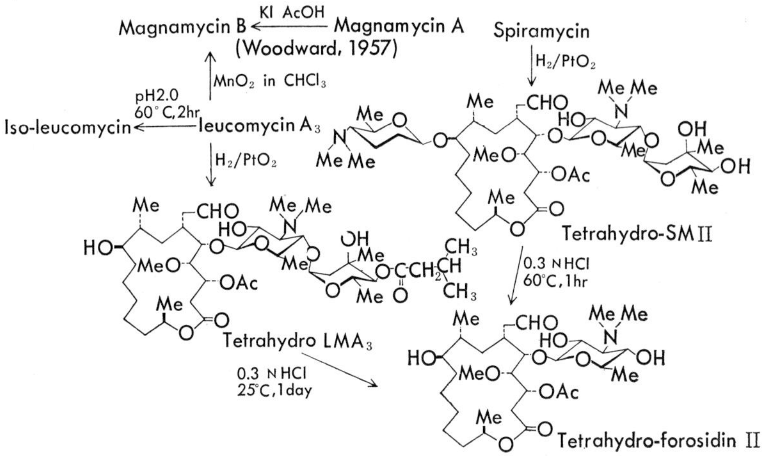

Chart 2.

The chemical structure of leucomycin A_1 was established in comparative studies on leucomycins A_1 and A_3 *(40)*; and then, those of leucomycins A_4–A_7 were determined by the present authors *(41)*. In Fig. 3, their relationship is presented. Of them, leucomycins A_1, A_5, A_7 and A_9 were named as Fr-group components, because they had free hydroxyl groups at the 3-position of the lactone. On the other hand, leucomycins A_3, A_4, A_6 and A_8, had hydroxyl groups which were acetylated, and were named Ac-group components. Afterwards, components U and V were obtained upon selective deacylation of the acyl group of the mycarose of leucomycin by the enzyme esterase produced by the fungi of the genus *Diaporthe*, *Cercospora* and *Colletorichum* (Abe *et al.* *(2)*). These components were also obtained by alkaline hydrolysis of leucomycins belonging to the Fr- and Ac-groups, and were found to exist naturally as well.

Now that the structural relationships among the leucomycin components, carbomycin and spiramycin, are clear, it is interesting to note where they are located in the classification table of macrolide antibiotics. Table III is presented as a classification of the macrolides. Though it might be the simplest one, it is made with respect to the number of ring atoms of the large lactone (Ōmura

TABLE III
Classification of Macrolide Antibiotics with Respect to the Number (*n*) of Member Atoms of the Lactone Ring

n	Macrolide	*n*	Polyene macrolide
12	methymycin neomethymycin	26	lucensomycin pimaricin
14	narbomycin	27	trichomycin
	pikromycin oleandomycin erythromycin A,B,C megalomicin	28	fungichromin filipin rimocidin tetrin A
	landamycin	30	
	albocycline	32	mycoticin A,B
	kujimycin	34	
16	carbomycin A,B	36	
	chalcomycin leucomycin A_1-A_9 cirramycin A	38	amphotericin B nystatin DJ-400
	spiramycin I-III	40	
18	borrelidine		
20			
22			
24			

(Ōmura (*42*))

(*42*)). Polyene macrolides are included in the table. In view of their common characteristic that they have antibacterial activity on gram-positive bacteria, compounds with $n=12$–16 are considered to belong to one group. Next comes borrelidine which shows an activity on *Borrelina* and *Tetrahymena geleii* (*49*). This is followed by the polyene macrolides ranging from leucensomycin with a 26-membered ring to nystatin (Fig. 4) with a 38-membered ring, all having antifungal effects (*32*). Except for chalcomycin, 16-membered ring compounds including leucomycin, carbomycin, spiramycin and cirramycin A characteristically have a formyl group ($-CH_2CHO$) in the 6-position of the lactone ring. Furthermore, many macrolide antibiotics have from 1 to 3 deoxy sugars; but the macrolide having a disaccharide (4-O-α-D-mycarosyl-D-

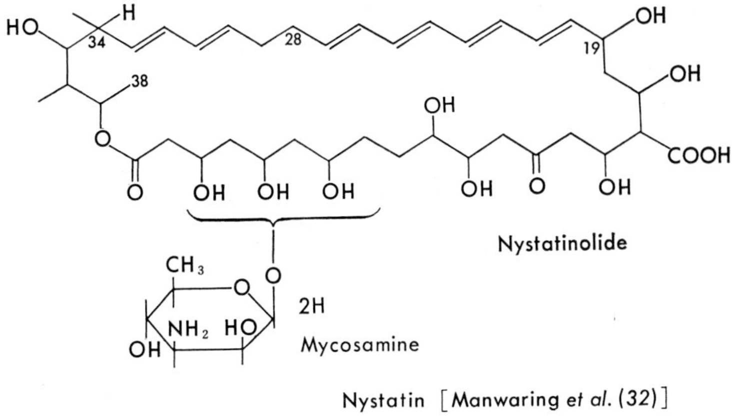
HO
H
34
28
19
OH
38
OH
OH
O
COOH
O
OH
OH
OH
OH
O
OH
Nystatinolide
CH3
O
O
2H
NH2
HO
OH
Mycosamine
Nystatin [Manwaring et al. (32)]

Fig. 4.

mycaminoside) moiety is only a 16-membered ring group. Besides, the relationships of β-D and α-L (Klyne's rule (*25*)) hold also for the glycoside bond, as well as for the sugars in the other glycosides (Table IV).

The stabilities of leucomycin A_3, spiramycin, erythromycin and oleandomycin against acids were compared (*43*). In Fig. 5, their stabilities in a hydrochloric acid-sodium citrate buffer at room temperature are shown. It is indicated that leucomycin is the most stable of the 4 macrolide antibiotics. Acetyl spiramycin is reported to be more stable than spiramycin (*52*). This stabilization resulting from acetylation in the 4″-position is worth noticing, because its acid stability can be supposed from the fact that naturally existing leucomycin, in which the 4-position of its mycarose was acylated, and spiramycin, in which the corresponding position, remained free.

Biological activity of leucomycin

As for the biological activity of leucomycin, many fundamental facts and much clinical data have already been published. Generally speaking, leucomycin is known to have a biological activity similar to that of other macrolide antibiotics. Below are given some

TABLE IV
Configurations of Sugars of Macrolide Antibiotics

Sugar	Glycoside bond	R_1	R_2	R_3	R_4	R_5	R_6	R_7	R_8	Antibiotic
D-Mycosamine	β	OH	H	NH_2	H	H	OH	Me	H	pimaricin
D-Desosamine	β	H	OH	$N(Me)_2$	H	H	H	Me	H	oleandomycin, erythromycin A, B, C, narbomycin, PA 133A, B
D-Mycaminose	β	H	OH	$N(Me)_2$	H	H	OH	Me	H	carbomycin, tylosin, spiramycin, leucomycins, nidamycin, cirramycin
D-Rodosamine	β	H	OH	$N(Me)_2$	H	H	OH	H	MeH	megalomycin
D-Chalcose	β	H	OH	OMe	H	H	H	Me	H	chalcomycin, lankamycin, kujimycin
D-Mycinose	β	H	OMe	H	OMe	H	OH	Me	H	chalcomycin, tylosin
D-Forosamine	β	H	H	H	H	H	$N(Me)_2$	Me	H	spiramycins
L-Oleandrose	α	H	H	H	OMe	OH	H	H	Me	oleandomycin
L-Cladinose	α	H	H	OMe	Me	OH	H	H	Me	erythromycin A, B
L-Mycarose	α	H	H	OH	Me	OH	H	H	Me	carbomycin A, B, tylosin, nidamycin, spiramycins, leucomycins
L-Arcanose	α	H	H	OMe	Me	H	OAc	H	Me	lankamycin, kujimycin

(Celmer (10))

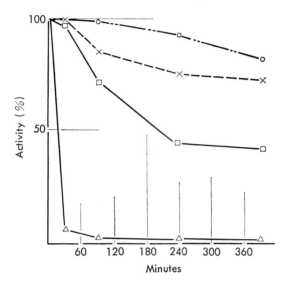

Fig. 5. Stability tests of macrolide antibiotics in acidic medium of pH 1.75. ○, leucomycin A; ×, oleandomycin; □, spiramycin; △, erythromycin A (Ōmura (43))

of the latest results. Bruehil (8), Francesco *et al.* (12) and the present author (18) reconfirmed the effectiveness of leucomycin on gram-positive bacteria and gram-negative cocci. The MIC of leucomycin against staphylococci isolated from patients was less than 1.6 mcg/ml in 80–97% of the cases. Table V shows the antibacterial spectra of LM-A$_1$ and the erythromycin tested by the author. The antibacterial activity of LM-A$_1$ was the same or higher than erythromycin on gram-positive bacteria other than *B. subtilis*.

LM-A$_1$ has a low toxicity and its LD$_{50}$ in mice is 650 mg/kg by I. V. administration, 2,000 mg/kg by P. O. administration and >800 mg/kg by S. C. administration. Furthermore, its distribution in tissues was very high in the bile. In the experiment conducted by Giulio and Ravagnan (13), it was demonstrated that when leucomycin was administered orally it reached levels in various tissues as high as or higher than their serum levels. Consequently, its effect *in vivo* is expected to surpass its *in vitro* effects.

TABLE V

Minimum Inhibitory Concentrations (mcg/ml) of Leucomycin A_1 and Erythromycin (agar streak dilution method)

Test organism	LM-A_1 free base (1260 mcg/mg)		EM free base (960 mcg/mg)	
	24hr	48hr	24hr	48hr
B. subtilis PCI 219	0.2	0.2	0.1	0.1
B. anthracis	0.2	0.2	0.8	0.8
Staph. aureus FDA 209P	0.2	0.2	0.2	0.2
Staph. albus	0.8	1.56	0.2	0.4
Staph. citreus	0.05	0.1	0.05	0.2
Sarcina lutea	0.0125	0.0125	0.0125	0.0125
Micrococcus flavus	0.025	0.025	0.05	0.05
Mycobact. ATCC 607		0.8		3.12
Staph. aureus Yoshioka	100	100	100	100
Staph. aureus Shinozaki	100	100	100	100
Staph. aureus Yonemoto	0.4	0.8	100	100
Staph. aureus Asano	0.2	0.4	0.1	0.2
E. coli NIHJ	25	50	6.25	12.5
Shigella flexneri E 20	25	25	50	50
Shigella sonnei E 33	50	50	50	50
Salm. typhosa H 901 w	50	50	50	100
Salm. paratyphi A	3.125	3.125	1.56	3.125
Kleb. pneumoniae PCI 602	3.125	3.125	3.125	3.125
Vibrio comma Inaba	0.8	0.8	3.125	3.125
Salm. enteritidis	12.5	25	12.5	50

(Hoshino *et al.* (*18*))

Table VI indicates that the median curative doses of leucomycin A_1 (CD_{50}) by I. V., P. O. and P. R. (per rectal) administrations against streptococcal, pneumococcal and staphylococcal infections in mice were equivalent to or greater than those of erythromycin (*21*).

The treatment of animals infected with various microorganisms similar to those that afflict humans has been improved in recent years. However, infection with mycoplasma (PPLO) is one of the most serious diseases in the animal field. Fortunately, macrolide antibiotics are reported to be effective *in vitro* against mycoplasma (Hoshino *et al.* (*20*), Arai *et al.* (*5*), Ōmura *et al.* (*35*)). Furthermore, the macrolide substances, leucomycin, tylosin and spiramycin were more effective *in vivo* and *in vitro* than erythromycin and oleandomycin. The results of experiments performed by Arai *et al.* (*6*) are presented in Table VII. In his experiments, the *in vitro* effects of a total of 27 antibiotics, including 11 macrolides, on *Mycoplasma pneumoniae* and 3 oropharyngeal mycoplasmas of human origin were investigated. Of all the antibiotics studied, leucomycin was the most effective.

Concerning the mode of action of macrolides, it is known that leucomycin, like other macrolide antibiotics, combines specifically with the 50S fraction of the bacterial ribosome to inhibit the biosynthesis of protein (Tago and Nagano (*51*)).

On the other hand, Mao and Wiegand (*33*) pointed out that low-pK macrolides (spiramycin, *etc.*) inhibit both aminoacyl-tRNA and peptidyl-tRNA binding to ribosomes. The high-pK macrolides (erythromycin, *etc.*) probably inhibit only peptidyl-tRNA binding.

In this connection the pKa of leucomycin was 7.5 and that of erythromycin was 8.6 when tested by the authors. Therefore, the action of the erythromycin group might be different from that of the leucomycin group.

Mitsuhashi *et al.* (*27, 30*) classified the resistance patterns of *Streptococcus aureus* to macrolide antibiotics into 3 groups. They are the A-group, which showed resistance to all macrolide antibiotics, the B-group, which is resistant to erythromycin and oleandomycin; and the C-group, which is induced by erythromycin and oleandomycin to produce resistance. Erythromycin can be an inducer to produce resistance of staphylococci (C-group), but leucomycin cannot be the inducer. Leucomycin was demonstrated to be effective against strains of the B- and C-groups of staphylococcus, which can be induced by erythromycin.

The mixed preparation of leucomycin and chloramphenicol (Kasuga (*24*)) seemed to increase the antibacterial activity of leucomycin, and to decrease the resistance of the B- or C-group of the staphylococcus. On the other hand, Hoshino *et al.* (*22*) found that the blood level of leucomycin could be increased by using it in combination with various sulfa drugs and fatty acids.

TABLE VI
Therapeutic Effect of LM-A₁ and Erythromycin on Streptococcal, Diplococcal and Staphylococcal Infections in Mice

Administration route	Streptococcal infection Median curative dose (CD_{50}) (mg/kg)		Diplococcal infection Median curative dose (CD_{50}) (mg/kg)		Staphylococcal infection Median curative dose (CD_{50}) (mg/kg)	
	LM-A₁ tartrate	EM-glucoheptonate	LM-A₁ tartrate	EM-glucoheptonate	LM-A₁ base	EM-base
I.V.	12	16	440–500	250		
I.P.	16	22	80–110	66.5	1.7	6–16
P.O.	210	155	495	100	40–80	40
P.R.	585	400–570	275	650	65	98

(Hoshino et al. (21))

TABLE VII

Activities of 27 Antibiotics on the Growth of *M. pneumoniae* and 3 Oropharyngeal Mycoplasmas Tested on Agar Medium by Diffusion Assay

Antibiotics		Minimum inhibitory concentration (mcg/ml)			
		M. pneumoniae Mac	*M. hominis*	*M. solivarium*	*M. orale*
Macrolides	Leucomycin	0.3	0.3	0.3	1.5
	Tylosin	0.3	12.5	6	6
	Magnanycin	0.3	6	25	25
	Angolamycin	1.25	12.5	25	100
	Relomycin	1.6	12.5	>50	50
	Oleandomycin	0.6	>100	>100	50
	Shincomycin A	2.5	12.5	>100	25
	Shincomycin B	0.6	25	>50	100
	Spiramycin	0.6	>50	>50	25
	Neutramycin	5.0	6	>50	100
	Erythromycin	0.1	>50	>50	25
Tetracyclines	Tetracycline	1.25	50	25	25
	Oxytetracycline	0.6	6	50	25
	Chlortetracycline	6.2	>50	>50	100
Other antibiotics	Lincomycin	50	0.6	1.25	6
	Streptomycin	100	>100	>100	>100
	Kanamycin	100	12.5	50	50
	Penicillin	>500	>500	>500	>500
	Cephaloridine	100	50	100	100
	Chloramphenicol	>50	50	100	100
Antitumor antibiotics	Mitomycin C	0.6	0.7	0.7	0.3
	Quinomycin	<1.6	12.5	12.5	6
	Puromycin	3.1	50	50	25
	Cycloheximide	>100	>100	100	>50
	Chromomycin A₃	3.1	100	100	25
	Aureothricin	<1.6	25	>50	12.5
	Actinomycin D	0.3	0.3	0.3	0.3

(Arai *et al.* (6))

Chemical modification of leucomycin

After the chemical structures of the leucomycins were determined, various derivatives were synthesized and their biological properties were studied to increase their blood levels and antibacterial activities. The MICs of leucomycin components and their related compounds against *S. aureus*, *B. subtilis* and *Klebsiella pneumoniae* were compared by the authors (*44*, *45*). However, there is no distinct difference in the activities of leucomycin A_3 and its derivatives whose allyl alcohol system (C_9–C_{13}) on the lactone ring were modified as shown in Table VIII. In this connection, it is reported that the tetrahydro derivative of spiramycin, which has a structure similar to leucomycin, has only a slightly more effective than spiramycin itself against *Staphylococcus epidermidis* and *Escheri-*

TABLE VIII
Minimum Inhibitory Concentrations (MIC) of Leucomycins and Their Related Compounds

Compounds			MIC (mcg/ml)		
			S. aureus	*B. subtilis*	*K. pneumoniae*
Leucomycin A_3			0.2–0.78	0.1–0.78	6.25
10,11,12,13 Tetrahydro leucomycin A_3			0.2	0.2	12.5
Magnamycin A			0.4	0.1	25
Magnamycin B			0.1	0.2	25
Iso-leucomycin A_3			1.56	0.78	25
9,10,11,12 Tetrahydro iso-leucomycin A_3			0.78	0.78	12.5
Spiramycin			0.78	0.78	25
Leucomycins	Ac group	A_3	0.04	0.60	10
		A_4	0.15	1.25	10
		A_6	0.30	1.25	10
		A_8	0.60	2.50	10
		U	3.12	6.25	25
	Fr group	A_1	0.04	0.30	5
		A_5	0.80	0.30	5
		A_7	0.15	0.30	10
		A_9	0.30	1.25	10
		V	3.12		25

(Ōmura *et al.* (*44*))

TABLE IX

Minimum Inhibitory Concentrations (MIC) of Leucomycin and Its Related Compounds

Compounds ($\begin{smallmatrix}Me & -X\\ 8 & 6\\ 7\end{smallmatrix}$)	MIC (mcg/ml)		
	S. aureus	B. subtilis	K. pneumoniae
–CHO (Leucomycin Ac)	0.39	0.39	6.25
–CH$_2$OH	25	25	50
=CH–N–NH·C–NH$_2$ (with S below)	6.25	12.5	100
–CH=N–NH–⟨⟩	1.56	1.56	6.25
–CH=N·N (CH$_3$)$_2$	0.78	6.25	12.5
–CH=N–N⟨ ⟩N–CH$_3$	0.78	0.78	12.5

(Ōmura et al. (45))

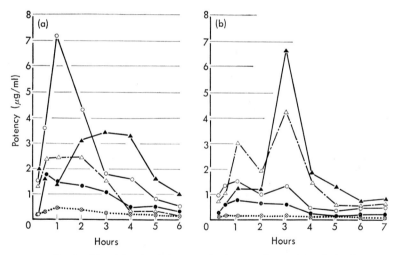

Fig. 6.   Blood levels of leucomycin-Ac complex and its derivatives (in rabbits). (a): Intraduodenal administration [300 mg (potency)/kg]. (b): Oral administration [300 mg (potency)/kg].   ●, –CHO; ⊗, –CH=N–NH·CNH$_2$ (with S above); ▲, –CH=N–NH–⟨⟩; △, –CH=N–N (CH$_3$)$_2$; ○, –CH=N=N⟨ ⟩N–Me (Ōmura et al. (45)).

chia coli (*4*). As for the hydroxyl group in the 4-position of mycarose, its activity is low when it remains free as in leucomycins U
and V, but the activity increases when the hydroxyl group is
acetylated. Of all the leucomycin components, A_1 has the highest
activity.

In Table IX are listed some derivatives for modifying the aldehyde group, which indicated that compounds are active if the π
electron remains there. The blood levels of the compounds listed in
Table IX, whose aldehyde groups were modified, were compared
to find some compounds indicating a high blood level, such as the

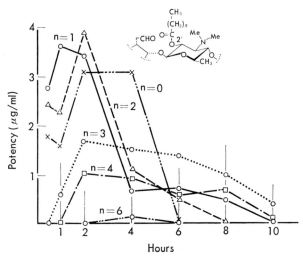

n	Compounds	Potency (mcg/mg)	3×10^{-4} mole/kg (mg/kg)
0	2′ Acetyl LMA$_3$	1440	251.0
1	2′ Propionyl LMA$_3$	1200	275.2
2	2′ Butyryl LMA$_3$	288	269.4
3	2′-*n*-Valeryl LMA$_3$	475	273.6
4	2′-*n*-Caproyl LMA$_3$	520	277.8
6	2′-*n*-Caprylyl LMA$_3$	490	286.2

Fig. 7.   Blood level and potency of 2′-acyl derivatives of leucomycins.
Blood levels were assayed after oral administration (3×10^{-4} mole/kg)
of compounds in mice by cup method (Ōmura *et al.* (*44*)).

hydrozone of N-methyl piperazine (Fig. 6). Furthermore, the antibacterial activities and blood levels of the derivatives, obtained by introducing various aliphatic acyl groups into the 2-position of mycaminose, were compared (Ōmura et al. (39)). In general, when the number of carbon atoms of the acyl group increases, the potency of the compound and its maximal blood levels decrease. However, some compounds (n=3, valeryl derivative) remained the same (Fig. 7).

An outline of recent chemical and biological research carried out on leucomycin was given. As mentioned, leucomycin is effective in cases of infections due to bacteria of the B- and C-groups. Moreover, leucomycin, characteristically, is not an inducer of macrolide resistance to the C-group of staphylococcus. In addition to the fact that it produces remarkable clinical effects in combined use with chloramphenicol, its action to inhibit the appearance of resistant strains of staphylococcus seems to be worthy of special mention. Furthermore, in animal husbandry, leucomycin has been successfully used for the treatment of infections in animals infected with mycoplasmas. It is believed that its applications will increase in the future.

REFERENCES

1 Abe, J., Suzuki, Y., Watanabe, T., and Satake, S. 1960. Studies on leucomycin. I. Paper chromatography of leucomycin and related antibiotics. *Nippon Kagaku Zasshi*, **81**, 969–971 (in Japanese).

2 Abe, J., Watanabe, T., Take, T., Sato, Y., Yamaguchi, T., Asano, K., Hata, T., and Ōmura, S. 1969. Unpublished data.

3 Abe, J., Iida, Y., Fukumura, M., Takeda, T., Satake, K., and Watanabe, T. 1963. Selective production of leucomycin main components with a mutant of *Streptomyces kitasatoensis*. *J. Antibiotics*, **16**, 214–215.

4 Adamski, R. J., Heymann, H., Geftic, S. G., and Barkulis, S. S. 1966. Preparation and antibacterial activity of some spiramycin derivatives. *J. Med. Chem.*, **9**, 932–934.

5 Arai, S., Yoshida, K., Izawa, A., Kumagai, K., and Ishida, N. 1966. Effect of antibiotics on growth of *Mycoplasma pneumoniae* Mac. *J. Antibiotics*, **19**, 118–120.

6 Arai, S., Yoshida, K., Kudō, A., and Kikuchi, M. 1967. Effect of antibiotics on the growth of various strains of mycoplasma. *J. Antibiotics*, **20**, 246–253.

288   H. TOJU and S. ŌMURA

7   Brockmann, H., and Henkel, W. 1950. Pikromycin, ein Neues Antibiotikum aus Actinomyceten. *Naturwiss*, **37**, 138–139 (in German).

8   Bruehil, P. 1966. Antibacterial activity of kitasamycin *in vitro*. *Therapiewoche*, **16**, 329–331.

9   Celmer, W. D. 1966. Macrolide stereochemistry. IV. On the total absolute configuration of carbomycin (magnamycin). *J. Am. Chem. Soc.*, **88**, 5028–5030.

10   Celmer, W. D. 1966. Biogenetic constitutional and stereochemical unitary principles in macrolide antibiotics. *Antimicrobial Agents and Chemotherapy—1965*, 144–156.

11   Foster, A. B., Inch, T. D., Lehmann, J., Stacey, M., and Webber, J. M. 1962. Carbohydrate components of antibiotics. Part III. Synthesis of 3,6-dideoxy-3-dimethyl-amino-β-D-glucose hydrochloride monohydrate. The absolute configuration of mycaminose. *J. Chem. Soc. (London)*, 2116–2118.

12   Francesco, F., Cipriani, P., and Ravagnan, L. 1968. *In vitro* and *in vivo* antibacterial effect of kitasamycin. *Antibiotica*, **6**, 5–23.

13   Giulio, R., and Ravagnan, G. 1968. Serum and tissue levels after oral administration of kitasamycin in man. *Antibiotica*, **6**(2), 61–71.

14   Grisebach, H., Hofheinz, W., and Doerr, N. U. 1963. Eine synthesis der DL-mycarose und DL-Epi-mycarose. *Chem. Ber.*, **96**, 1823–1826.

15   Hata, T., Sano, Y., Ohki, N., Yokoyama, Y., Matsumae, A., and Ito, S. 1953. Leucomycin, a new antibiotic. *J. Antibiotic*, **6**, 87–89.

16   Hata, T., Sano, Y., Yokoyama, Y., Itō, S., Okazaki, S., Takano, K., Itō, H., Owada, Y., Saitō, Y., and Soekawa, M. 1953. Studies on leucomycin. III. Experimental treatment in animals with leucomycin. *J. Antibiotics*, **6**(4), 163–171.

17   Hofheinz, W., and Grisebach, H. 1962. Die Stereochemie der Mycaminose. *Z. Naturforsch*, **176**, 355–356 (in German).

18   Hoshino, Y., Matsumae, A., Yamamoto, H., and Hata, T. 1966. Studies on leucomycin A_1, biological studies. *J. Antibiotics*, **19**, 23–29.

19   Hoshino, Y., Umezawa, I., Yamamoto, H., Matsumae, A., and Hata, T. 1966. Studies on leucomycin A_1. II. Studies on blood and tissue levels, and toxicities. *J. Antibiotics*, **19**, 30–36.

20   Hoshino, Y., Maekawa, T., Umezawa, I., Yamamoto, H., Matsumae, A., and Hata, T. 1966. Studies on leucomycin. Some effects of leucomycin on PPLO. 39th Annual Meeting of the Japan Bacteriological Society. Abstract, 86.

21   Hoshino, Y., Umezawa, I., Yoshida, T., Matsumae, A., Yamamoto, H., and Hata, T. 1966. Studies on leucomycin A_1. Experimental treatments of animal infected with several pathogene bacteria. *J. Antibiotics*, **19**, 37–41.

22   Hoshino, Y., Matsumae, A., Yamamoto, H., and Hata, T. 1966. Studies

on leucomycin A_1. IV. Combined effects of leucomycin with sulfa drugs. *J. Antibiotics*, **19**, 42–48.

23 Hiramatsu, M., Fukusaki, A., Noda, T., Naya, K., Tomiie, Y., Nitta, I., Watanabe, T., Take, T., Abe, J., Ōmura, S., and Hata, T. 1967. The crystal and molecular structure of demycarosyl leucomycin A_3 hydrobromide. *Bull. Chem. Soc. Japan*, **43**, 1966–1975.

24 Kasuga, T. 1967. Combined effects with leucomycin and chloramphenicol. *Toyō Yakujihō*, **8**, 8–9 (in Japanese).

25 Klyne, W. 1950. The configuration of the anomeric carbon atoms in some cardiac glycosides. *Biochem. J.*, **47**, xli–xlii.

26 Kooama, A., Chika, T., Yamaguchi, J., and Aizawa, M. 1968. Studies on the leucomycin fermentation. *J. Ferment. Technol.*, **46**, 225–232.

27 Konno, M., Hashimoto, H., and Mitsuhashi, S. 1966. Drug resistance of staphylococci. III. Resistance to some macrolide antibiotics and inducible system. *Japan. J. Microbiol.*, **10**, 59–66.

28 Korte, F., Claussen, U., and Gohring, U. K. 1962. Synthesis der D,L-Epimycarose und der D,L-Mycarose. *Tetrahedron*, **18**, 1257–1264 (in German).

29 Kuehne, M. E., and Benson. 1965. The structures of the spiramycin and magnamycin. *J. Am. Chem. Soc.*, **87**, 4660–4662.

30 Kono, M., Kasuga, T., and Mitsuhashi, S. 1966. Drug resistance of staphylococci. IV. Resistance patterns to some macrolide antibiotics in *Staphylococcus aureus* isolated in the United States. *Japan. J. Microbiol.*, **10**, 109–113.

31 Lemal, D. M., Pacht, P. D., and Woodward, R. B. 1962. The synthesis of L-(−)mycarose and L-(−)cladinose. *Tetrahedron*, **18**, 1275–1293.

32 Manwaring, D. G., Rickards, R. W., and Giding, T. 1969. The structure of the aglycone of the macrolide antibiotic nystatin. *Tetrahedron Letters* (60), 5319–5322.

33 Mao, J. C., and Wiegand, R. G. 1968. Mode of action of macrolide. *Biochim. Biophy. Acta*, **157**, 404–413.

34 Muxfeldt, H., Shrader, S., Handen, H., and Brockmann, H. 1968. The structure of pikromycin. *J. Am. Chem. Soc. (London)*, **90** (17), 4748–4749.

35 Ōmura, S., Lin, Y. C., Yajima, T., Nakamura, S., Tanaka, N., Umezawa, H., Yokoyama, S., Homma, Y., and Hamada, M. 1967. Screening of antimycoplasma antibiotics. *J. Antibiotics*, **20**, 241–245.

36 Ōmura, S. 1967. Studies on leucomycins. Ph. D. Thesis, University of Tokyo Press, Tokyo.

37 Ōmura, S., Katagiri, M., Ogura, H., and Hata, T. 1968. The chemistry of leucomycin. III. Structure and stereochemistry of leucomycin A_3. *Chem. Pharm. Bull.*, **16**, 1181–1186.

38 Ōmura, S., Katagiri, M., Hata, T., Hiramatsu, M., Kimura, T., and Naya, K. 1968. The allylic rearrangement of the hydroxyl group from

C-9 to C-13 and the absolute configuration at C-9 of leucomycin A$_3$. *Chem. Pharm. Bull.*, **16**, 1402–1404.

39 Ōmura, S., Nakagawa, A., Ohtani, M., Hata, T., Ogura, H., and Furuhata, K. 1969. Structure of the spiramycins (foromacidines) and their relationship with the leucomycins and carbomycins (magnamycins). *J. Am. Chem. Soc.*, **91**, 3401–3404.

40 Ōmura, S., Katagiri, M., and Hata, T. 1968. The chemistry of leucomycin. IV. Structure of leucomycin A$_1$. *J. Antibiotics*, **21**(3), 199–203.

41 Ōmura, S., Katagiri, M., and Hata, T. 1968. The chemistry of leucomycin. VI. Structures of leucomycin A$_4$, A$_5$, A$_6$, A$_7$, A$_8$, and A$_9$. *J. Antibiotics*, **21**, 272–276.

42 Ōmura, S. 1970. Large lactone compounds produced by microorganism, macrolide. *Chemistry and Biology*, **8**, 139–150.

43 Ōmura, S. 1966. Unpublished data.

44 Ōmura, S., Katagiri, M., Nakagawa, A., Yamada, H., Umezawa, I., Komiyama, K., and Hata, T. 1970. Studies on the chemical structure and some biological properties of leucomycin (kitasamycins) and their related antibiotics. *In* "Progress in antimicrobial and anticancer chemotherapy (Proceedings of the 6th international congress of chemotherapy)," University of Tokyo Press, Tokyo, 1043–1049.

45 Ōmura, S., Yamada, H., Nakagawa, A., Katagiri, M., and Hata, T. 1970. Structure-biological activities relationship among leucomycin and their derivatives. III. Derivatives on aldehyde. 90th Annual Meeting of the Pharmaceutical Society of Japan Abstracts.

46 Paul, R., and Tchelitcheff, S. 1957. Structure de la spiramycin. II. Etude des produits de degradation caracterisation du dimethylamino-5-methyl-6-hydroxy-2-tetrahydropyrane. *Bull. Soc. Chim. France*, 734–737 (in French).

47 Paul, R., and Tchelitcheff, S. 1965. Structure de la spiramycin. VI. Establissement de la formule developpee. *Bull. Coc. Chim. France*, 650–656 (in French).

48 Richardson, A. C. 1962. The synthesis of D- and L-mycaminose hydrochloride. *J. Chem. Soc. (London)*, 2758–2760.

49 Schierlein, W. K. 1966. Die konstitution des borrelidins. *Experimentia*, **22** (6), 355–359 (in German).

50 Stevens, C. L., Gutowski, G. E., Taylor, K. G., and Bryant, C. P. 1966. The stereochemistry and synthesis of forosamine. A deoxyamino sugar moiety of the spiramycin antibiotics. *Tetrahedron Letters*, 5717–5721.

51 Tago, K., and Nagano, M. 1970. Mechanism of inhibition of protein synthesis by leucomycin. *In* "Progress in Antimicrobial and Anticancer Chemotherapy (Proceedings of the 6th International Congress of Chemotherapy)," University of Tokyo Press, Tokyo, 199–201.

52 Takahira, H., Kata, H., Sugiyama, N., Ishii, S., Haneda, T., Uzu, K.,

Kumake, K., and Kojima, R. 1966. Fundamental studies on acetyl spiramycin. *J. Antibiotics*, **19**, 95–100.

53 Watanabe, T., and Takeda, K. 1962. Leucomycin. *J. Antibiotics, Ser. B*, **9**(4), 237–248.

54 Watanabe, T. 1960. Studies on leucomycin. II. Preparative chromatography of macrolides on amberlite IRC-50. *Bull. Chem. Soc., Japan*, **33** (8), 1100–1104.

55 Watanabe, T. 1960. Studies on leucomycin. III. Isolation and properties of six antibacterial components in leucomycin complex. *Bull. Chem. Soc. Japan*, **33**, 1104–1108.

56 Watanabe, T., Nishida, H., and Satake, K. 1961. Studies on leucomycin. V. Isolation of mycarose-4-isovalerate from leucomycin A_1. *Bull. Chem. Soc. Japan*, **34**(9), 1285–1288.

57 Watanabe, T., Fujii, T., and Satake, K. 1961. 4-O-acetyl mycarose, a new O-acetyl sugar obtained from leucomycin minor components. *J. Biochem.*, **50**(3), 197–201.

58 Watanabe, T., Fujii, T., Sakurai, H., Abe, J., and Satake, K. 1964. Structure of leucomycin. IUPAC Symposium of the Chemistry of Natural Products. Abstract, 145.

59 Woodward, R. B., Weiler, L. S., and Dutta, P. C. 1965. The structure of magnamycin. *J. Am. Soc.*, **87**, 4662–4664.

60 Woodward, R. B. 1957. Struktur und Biogenese der Makrolide. Eine Neue Klasse von Naturstoffen. *Angew. Chem.*, **69**, 50–58 (in German).

STRUCTURE-ACTIVITY RELATIONSHIP OF SPIRAMYCIN DERIVATIVES

Keizo Uzu and Hiroshi Takahira

Tokyo Research Laboratory, Kyowa Hakko Kogyo Co., Ltd., Tokyo, Japan

Spiramycin and its derivatives

Spiramycin is one of the macrolide antibiotics produced from *Streptomyces ambofaciens* (5), isolated by Pinnert-Sindico of the Rhône-Poulenc Laboratory. This antibiotic is as effective against gram-positive and gram-negative bacteria as erythromycin and oleandomycin. The chemical structure of spiramycin was first presented by Paul and Tchelitcheff (4), Kuehne and Benson (2) and recently by Omura *et al.* (3) as shown in Fig. 1.

As seen in this formula, spiramycin is a macrolide antibiotic with a 16-membered lactone as an aglycon and three different sugar moieties-mycaminose, forosamine and mycarose. The derivatives of spiramycin have been studied by Paul and Tchelitcheff (4), by Adamski *et al.* (1) and by the authors. Chart 1 shows the derivatives prepared by them.

Spiramycin (I) was hydrogenated catalytically in the presence of Pd-C (10% Pd) to produce a tetrahydro derivative (II). Reduction

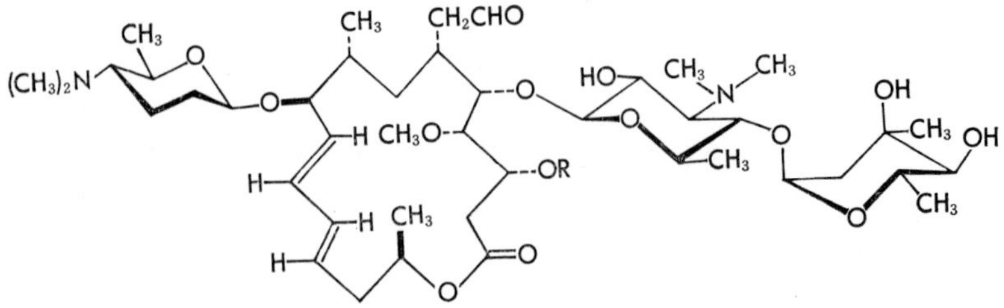

Fig. 1.   The structure of spiramycin. R=H: spiramycin I (I-a), R= CH₃CO: spiramycin II (I-b), R=C₂H₅CO: spiramycin III (I-c).

of I with NaBH₄ gave a dihydrospiramycin (III), which had no aldehyde. II was hydrogenated catalytically in the presence of PtO₂ to give a hexahydro derivative (IV), which had no proton signal for an aldehyde group, like III. Acid hydrolysis of spiramycin (I) gave neospiramycin (V), which had no mycarose. Catalytic hydrogenation gave tetrahydro (VI) and hexahydro derivatives (VII) by the same procedure as that of I. More drastic acid hydrolysis of neospiramycin (V) resulted in forocidine (XVIII) which lost both mycarose and forosamine. I was acylated with acyl chloride in the presence of a weak alkali to produce monoacyl derivatives (VIII) which showed two different pKa values, 5.35 and 8.05, from those of the original spiramycin (I), which were 7.1 and 8.40.

The change of pKa values indicated that the hydroxy group adjacent to the dimethylamino group in mycaminose was acylated. I was acylated with acid anhydride in pyridine at a low temperature to give a diacyl derivative (IX). When I was acylated with acid anhydride in pyridine at a higher temperature, new acyl derivatives (X) were obtained, which were almost equivalent in pKa, 5.2 and 8.25, to those of IX but different in NMR spectrum from IX. When X was partially hydrolyzed by refluxing in methanol, new monoacyl compounds (XI) were obtained, which showed pKa values of 6.9 and 8.20, which are almost equivalent to I. These pKa values indicated that the acyl group attached to the hydroxy group adjacent to the dimethylamino group in mycaminose was removed. The structure of the new diacyl (X) and monoacyl deriv-

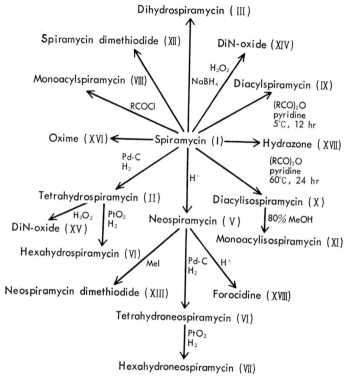

Chart 1.   Preparation of spiramycin derivatives.

atives (XI) has not yet been elucidated. Since these compounds may be derivatives of a stereoisomer of I, they are designated tentatively as derivatives of isospiramycin.* When spiramycin (I) and neospiramycin (V) were treated with methyl iodide, quarternary dimethiodides (XII and XIII) were obtained. Di-N-oxides (XIV and XV) were obtained by treatment of I and II with hydrogen peroxide. Oxime and hydrazone derivatives (XVI and XVII) were prepared as usual.

* Monoacetylspiramycin and diacetylspiramycin in previous reports (6a, b) are derivatives of isospiramycin.

TABLE I
Antibacterial Activity of Spiramycin Derivatives

	1000 mcg/mg
Spiramycin	1210
Tetrahydrospiramycin	276
Hexahydrospiramycin	817
Neospiramycin	432
Tetrahydroneospiramycin	t
Hexahydroneospiramycin	t
Dihydrospiramycin	460
Diacetylisospiramycin	451
Dipropionylisospiramycin	487
Monoacetylisospiramycin	522
Monopropionylisospiramycin	518
Monoacetylspiramycin	532
Monopropionylspiramycin	347
Monobutyrylspiramycin	332
Monovalerylspiramycin	229
Monocaproylspiramycin	113
Monoheptanoylspiramycin	

TABLE II
Antibacterial Activity of Spiramycin Derivatives

Number	Compound	MIC† (μg/ml) S. epidermidis	E. coli
1	Spiramycin dimethiodide	62.5	150.0
2	Spiramycin oxime	250.0	500.0
3	Spiramycin thiosemicarbazone	25.0	500.0
4	Spiramycin di-N-oxide	>150.0	>150.0
5	Tetrahydrospiramycin di-N-oxide	>250.0	>500.0
6	Triacetylspiramycin	22.0	62.5
7	Dibenzoylspiramycin	100.0	250.0
8	Spiramycin maleate	11.2	62.5
9	Triacetyl tetrahydrospiramycin	25.0	250.0
10	Spiramycin hydrazone	18.75	>75.0
11	Spiramycin phenylhydrazone	>25.0	>75.0
12	Spiramycin-2-benzothiazolyl hydrazone	>25.0	>75.0
13	Spiramycin-2-quinolylhydrazone	>25.0	>75.0
14	Dihydrospiramycin	>25.0	>75.0
15	Neospiramycin dimethiodide	>250.0	100.0
16	Tetrahydroneospiramycin	12.0	21.5
17	Hexahydroneospiramycin	>25.0	20.0
18	Hexahydrospiramycin	6.1	22.5
19	Spiramycin	13.4	42.2
20	Tetrahydrospiramycin	5.48	25.0
21	Neospiramycin	6.2	19.6
22	Forocidine	>25.0	>75.0

† Minimum inhibitory concentration.

Structure-activity relationship

1. In vitro antibacterial activity (1, 6)

Table I shows the *in vitro* antibacterial activity against *Bacillus subtilis* ATCC 6633 by the cup method. Table II shows the MIC against *Staphylococcus epidermidis* and *Escherichia coli* (*1*). Neospiramycin and tetrahydrospiramycin showed almost the same activity as spiramycin. But hexahydrospiramycin and dihydrospiramycin, in which the aldehyde group changes into the hydroxymethyl group, showed only slight activity. Forocidine, which lost mycarose and forosamine, showed no antibacterial activity. From these results, it can be presumed that mycarose and the conjugated double bond are not so closely related to the antibacterial activity, but that the aldehyde group has a very great influence on activity.

2. Acid stability (6)

Table III shows the acid stability of the above described derivatives. The derivatives of isospiramycin had remarkable resistance against acid hydrolysis. They showed no change in antibacterial activity for 300 min in 0.1 N hydrochloric acid. However, spiramycin (I) and its derivatives were decomposed to substances having no antibacterial activity.

TABLE III
Acid Stability of Spiramycin Derivatives

	0	30	60	180	300 min
Spiramycin	100	73	61	31	22
Diacetylspiramycin	100	85	63	40	11
Monoacetylspiramycin	100	94	89	61	38
Monopropionylspiramycin	100	97	93	53	40
Monobutyrylspiramycin	100	111	112	70	43
Monovalerylspiramycin	100	109	92	74	51
Tetrahydrospiramycin	100	70	53	36	23
Neospiramycin	100	87	71	41	30
Diacetylisospiramycin	100	136	116	117	120
Monoacetylisospiramycin	100	114	133	110	138

3. Acute toxicity (6)

Table IV shows the acute toxicity of spiramycin derivatives. In general, the toxicity of monoacylspiramycin increases in propor-

TABLE IV
Acute Toxicity of Spiramycin Derivatives (LD$_{50}$)

Intravenus		Subcutaneous	
Spiramycin	185 mg/kg	Spiramycin	1470 mg/kg
Diacetylisospiramycin	144	Tetrahydrospiramycin	1350
Dipropionylisospiramycin	120	Neospiramycin	1187
Monoacetylisospiramycin	313		
Monoacetylspiramycin	206		
Monopropionylisospiramycin	242		
Monopropionylspiramycin	135		
Monobutyrylspiramycin	94		
Monovalerylspiramycin	84		
Monocaproylspiramycin	75		
Monoheptanoylspiramycin	94		
Tetrahydrospiramycin	181		
Neospiramycin	168		

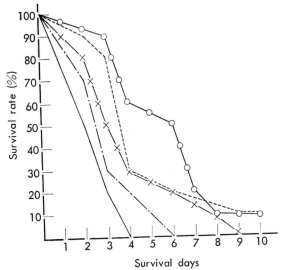

Fig. 2. Protective effect of spiramycin, reduced spiramycin and neo-spiramycin on intravenous staphylococcal infection of mice. —, control; ---, spiramycin, 5mg/mouse; ○, tetrahydrospiramycin, 5mg/mouse; ---, hexahydrospiramycin, 5mg/mouse; ×, neospiramycin, 5mg/mouse.

tion to the increase of numbers of carbon. LD_{50} values of diacylisospiramycin and monoacylspiramycin were low, where the OH-group adjacent to the $(CH_3)_2N$ of mycaminose is acylated. However, the LD_{50} value of monoacylisospiramycin which was acylated only on the secondary OH-group of mycarose was higher; the toxicity of this derivative was half that of the former two.

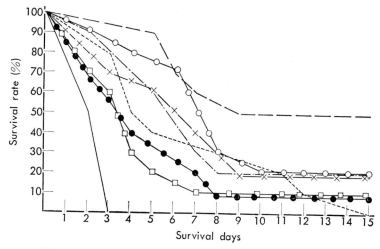

Fig. 3. Protective effect of spiramycin and various esters on intravenous staphylococcal infection of mice. —, control; ⋯, spiramycin, 5mg/mouse; - -, monoacetylisospiramycin, 2.5mg/mouse; - - -, monoacetylspiramycin, 5mg/mouse; ○, diacetylisospiramycin, 5mg/mouse; ×, monopropionylspiramycin, 5mg/mouse; □, monobutyrylspiramycin, 5mg/mouse; ●, monovalerylspiramycin, 5mg/mouse.

4. In vivo chemotherapeutic effect (6)

Mouse protection tests were carried out in order to examine the chemotherapeutic effect *in vivo* of various derivatives of spiramycin. The chemotherapeutic effects of tetrahydrospiramycin, hexahydrospiramycin and neospiramycin are shown in Fig. 2. Tetrahydrospiramycin and neospiramycin were as effective as spiramycin, while hexahydrospiramycin was considerably inferior. A comparison of the chemotherapeutic effects of diacetylisospiramycin, monoacetylisospiramycin, monoacylspiramycin and spira-

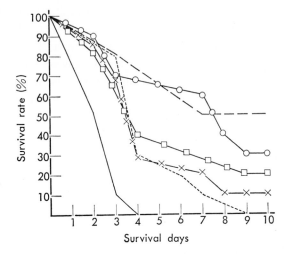

Fig. 4. Protective effect of spiramycin, monoacylisospiramycin and diacylisospiramycin on intravenous staphylococcal infection of mice. —, control; ---, spiramycin, 5mg/mouse; - -, monoacetylisospiramycin, 2.5mg/mouse; ○, monopropionylisospiramycin, 2.5mg/mouse; ×, diacetylisospiramycin, 2.5mg/mouse; □, dipropionylisospiramycin, 2.5mg/mouse.

TABLE V
Concentration of Spiramycin and Its Derivatives in the Serum Following Oral Administration to Rats of 500 mg/kg

Compound \ Time	1	3	5	10	20 hr
Spiramycin	6.5 mcg/ml	5.4	3.4	trace	trace
Diacetyl-isospiramycin	12.4	10.9	10.0	1.8	1.1
Monoacetyl-spiramycin	15.2	8.3	5.9	trace	trace
Monoacetyl-isospiramycin	4.1	4.6	6.0	1.2	1.3

mycin is shown in Fig. 3. Monoacetylisospiramycin had a remarkable effect, diacetylisospiramycin was inferior to monoacetylisospiramycin but superior to spiramycin, and monoacylspiramycin was as effective as spiramycin. Then, a comparative test among

monoacetylisospiramycin,diacylisospiramycin,monopropionyliso-
spiramycin and spiramycin was conducted in order to reconfirm
the effect of the first. The results are shown in Fig. 4. As shown in

TABLE VI
Concentration of Spiramycin and Its Derivatives in the Liver Following Oral Administration to Rats of 500 mg/kg

Compound	Time 1	3	5	10	20 hr
Spiramycin	75 mcg/g	120	143	302	224
Diacetyl- isospiramycin	83	113	154	645	122
Monoacetyl- spiramycin	152	108	87	171	55
Monoacetyl- isospiramycin	45	163	298	1430	570

TABLE VII
Concentration of Spiramycin and Its Derivatives in the Lung Following Oral Administration to Rats of 500 mg/kg

Compound	Time 1	3	5	10	20 hr
Spiramycin	52 mcg/g	98	126	70	67
Diacetyl- isospiramycin	166	176	217	226	120
Monoacetyl- spiramycin	217	187	148	61	46
Monoacetyl- isospiramycin	47	121	154	161	99

TABLE VIII
Concentration of Spiramycin and Its Derivatives in the Spleen Following Oral Administration to Rats of 500 mg/kg

Compound	Time 1	3	5	10	20 hr
Spiramycin	72 mcg/g	91	116	89	86
Diacetyl- isospiramycin	97	143	183	171	135
Monoacetyl- spiramycin	202	193	142	64	38
Monoacetyl- isospiramycin	23	124	147	170	119

302   K. UZU and H. TAKAHIRA

this figure, the chemotherapeutic effect of monoacetylisospiramycin was remarkable when compared with that of spiramycin.

TABLE IX
Concentration of Spiramycin and Its Derivatives in the Kidney Following Oral Administration to Rats of 500 mg/kg

Compound ＼ Time	1	3	5	10	20 hr
Spiramycin	21 mcg/g	48	71	62	39
Diacetyl-isospiramycin	37	59	80	59	40
Monoacetyl-spiramycin	63	90	55	59	53
Monoacetyl-isospiramycin	17	64	90	102	46

5. Absorption and excretion (6)

Tests on the blood level, tissue level and urine excretion of spiramycin derivatives were made. The results are shown in Tables V, VI, VII, VIII and IX. As shown in Table V, diacetylisospiramycin and monoacetylspiramycin, whose hydroxy group adjacent to the $(CH_3)_2N$ of mycaminose was acetylated, are so rapidly absorbed in the intestinal tract that the blood level reaches its maximum point in a short time and falls rapidly after 5 hr, as in the case of erythromycin. Only the blood level of monoacetylisospiramycin reaches a peak somewhat later and is maintained longer. The tissue level of diacetylisospiramycin and monoacetylisospiramycin reached a peak approximately 10 hr after administration. These two derivatives had a strong affinity for organs and remained longer, especially in the liver. The excretion in the urine in 24 hr was 6.2% for spiramycin and 3.5% for monoacetylisospiramycin.

REFERENCES

1   Adamski, R. J., Heymann, H., Geftic, S. G., and Barkulis, S. S. 1965. Preparation and antibacterial activity of some spiramycin derivatives. *J. Med. Chem.*, **9**, 932.
2   Kuehne, M. E., and Benson, B. W. 1965. The structures of the spiramycin and magnamycin. *J. Am. Chem. Soc.*, **87**, 20, 4660–4662.

3   Omura, S., Nakagawa, A., Otani, M., and Hata, T. 1965. Structure of the spiramycins (foromacidines) and their relationship with the leucomycins and carbomycins (magnamycins). *J. Am. Chem. Soc.*, **91**, 12, 3401.

4   a   Paul, R., and Tchelitcheff, S. 1957. Structure de la spiramycine. I. Etude des produits de dégradation: caractérisation du mycarose. *Bull. Soc. Chim. France*, 443;   b   II. Etude des produits de dégradation: caractérisation du diméthylamino-5 méthyl-6 hydroxy-2 tetrahydropyranne. *Bull. Soc. Chim. France*, 734;   c   III. Etude des produits de dégradation: caractérisation du mycaminose. *Bull. Soc. Chim. France*, 1059;   d   1959. IV. Présence d'une lactone macrocyclique: étude de ses produits d'oxydation. *Bull. Soc. Chim. France*, 150;   e   1965. V. Mode d'enchaînement des divers produits d'hydrolyse. *Bull. Soc. Chim. France*, 189;   f   1965. VI. Establissement de la formule développée. *Bull. Soc. Chim. France*, 650.

5   Pinnert-Sindico, S., Ninet, L., Preud'homme, J., and Cosar, C. 1955. A new antibiotic—spiramycin. *Antibiotics Annual 1954–1955*, 724.

6   a   Takahira, H., Kato, H., Sugiyama, N., Ishii, S., and Uzu, K. 1965. Monoacetyl-spiramycin, a new derivative of spiramycin. *J. Antibiot., Ser. A*, **18** (6), 269;   b   Uzu, K., Takahira, H., Kato, H., Sugiyama, N., and Ishii, S. 1970. The studies on spiramycin derivatives. New spiramycin ester, acetylspiramycin. *In* "Progress in Antimicrobial and Anticancer Chemotherapy (Proceedings of the 6th International Congress of Chemotherapy)," University of Tokyo Press, Tokyo, Vol. I, p. 49;   c   Takahira, H. 1970. The studies on spiramycin derivatives. *J. Antibiot., Ser. B*, in press.

MODE OF ACTION OF LINCOMYCIN AND RELATED ANTIBIOTICS

R. E. Monro, R. Fernandez-Muñoz, M. L. Celma and
D. Vazquez

Instituto de Biologiá Celular, Velázquez 144, Madrid, Spain

1. Discovery, structure

In 1962 the isolation of a new antibiotic, lincomycin, was reported
(*27*). The antibiotic was obtained from fermenting cultures of
Streptomyces lincolnensis, var. lincolnensis. The structure of lincomycin was soon elucidated (*17*), and a number of related compounds were also obtained. The most important members of the
group are shown in Fig. 1. 4′-Depropyl-4′-ethyllincomycin (Fig.
1 B) was produced along with lincomycin during fermentations
(*17*). Prolongation of the fermentations led to the transformation
of lincomycin to lincomycin sulphoxide and 1-demethyl-thio-1-
hydroxylincomycin (*3*) (Fig. 1 C, D). Several analogues were also
obtained by chemical modification of lincomycin. Some of these
with variations at C-7, C-4′ and N-1 (Fig. 1 E–P) are of particular
interest because they are more active than lincomycin against
intact cells (*59*).

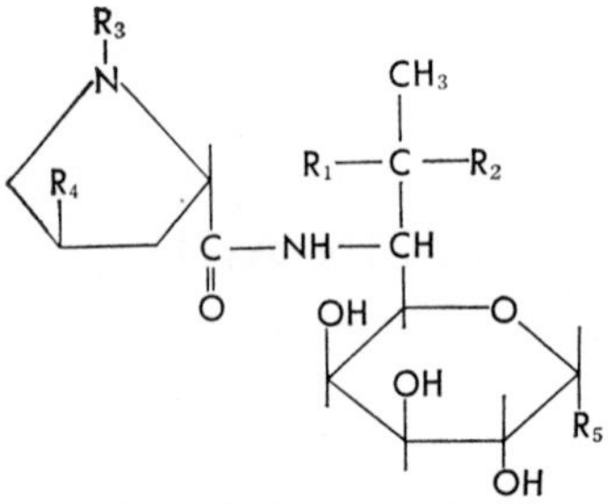

Compound	R$_1$	R$_2$	R$_3$	R$_4$	R$_5$
A Lincomycin	OH	H	CH$_3$	C$_3$H$_7$	SCH$_3$
B 4'-Depropyl-4'-ethyllincomycin (U 21,699)	OH	H	CH$_3$	C$_2$H$_5$	SCH$_3$
C Lincomycin sulfoxide	OH	H	CH$_3$	C$_3$H$_7$	S-CH$_3$ ($\overset{\uparrow}{O}$)
D 1-Demethylthio-1-hydroxylincomycin	OH	H	H	C$_3$H$_7$	OH
E 7-Chloro-7-deoxy-N-demethyl-4'-depropyl-4'-pentyllincomycin	H	Cl	H	C$_5$H$_{11}$	SCH$_3$
F 7-Chloro-7-deoxy-N-demethyl-4'-depropyl-4'-hexyllincomycin	H	Cl	H	C$_6$H$_{13}$	SCH$_3$
G 7-Chloro-7-deoxy-N-demethyl-lincomycin	H	Cl	H	C$_3$H$_7$	SCH$_3$
H 7-Chloro-7-deoxy-N-demethyl-N-ethyl-4'-depropyl-4'-butyllincomycin	H	Cl	C$_2$H$_5$	C$_4$H$_9$	SCH$_3$
J 7-Chloro-7-deoxylincomycin (clinimycin or clindamycin)	H	Cl	CH$_3$	C$_3$H$_7$	SCH$_3$
K 7-Chloro-7-deoxylincomycin (epi-clinimycin or epi-clindamycin)	Cl	H	CH$_3$	C$_3$H$_7$	SCH$_3$
L 7-Chloro-7-deoxy-4'-depropyl-4'-ethyl lincomycin	H	Cl	CH$_3$	C$_2$H$_5$	SCH$_3$
M 4'-Depropyl-4'-pentyl-N-demethyllincomycin	OH	H	H	C$_5$H$_{11}$	SCH$_3$
N N-Demethyllincomycin	OH	H	H	C$_3$H$_7$	SCH$_3$
P 7-O-Acetatelincomycin	OH	C$_2$H$_3$O	CH$_3$	C$_3$H$_7$	SCH$_3$
Q Celesticetin	OCH$_3$	H	CH$_3$	H	SC$_2$H$_4$-O-C(=O)-(phenyl-OH) 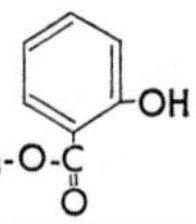

Fig. 1.   The lincomycin group of antibiotics. Except for epi-clindamycin, all of the lincomycin analogues with a Cl in the 7 position had the L-*threo* configuration as opposed to the D-*erythro* configuration found in lincomycin. Epi-clindamycin was less active than clindamycin (*23, 24*).

Long before lincomycin was known, the antibiotic celesticetin had been obtained and purified from cultures of *Streptomyces caelestis* (*10, 15*). Its chemical structure (Fig. 1 Q) was released (*16*) at the same time as that of lincomycin; and because of similarities in structure and function, celesticetin is considered to be a member of the lincomycin family. Not much work has been carried out with celesticetin, owing to its low activity in intact cells.

2. Specificity

The lincomycin antibiotics are active against gram-positive bacteria, blue-green algae, and to a lesser extent gram-negative bacteria (*10, 27*). They have no known effect on the cytoplasm of Eukaryotic organisms but inhibit the growth of chloroplasts (*43*) and in certain cases mitochondria (*13*).

Recent evidence indicates that lincomycin is active against mitochondria in yeasts but not in mammals (*13*). In this respect, lincomycin contrasts with chloramphenicol, which, though having a

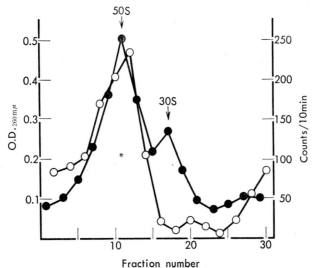

Fig. 2.   Profile of ribosomes from *A. montana* after treatment with ^{14}C-lincomycin and zonal centrifugation on a sucrose gradient at a low Mg^{2+} concentration (*42*). ●, O.D.; ○, counts/10 min.

closely related mode of action, is active against mitochondria in both types of organisms (*13*). Antibiotics of the lincomycin family thus have the advantage of being less toxic to humans and animals than chloramphenicol.

A number of lincomycin analogues, such as 7-chloro-7-deoxy-lincomycin (also known as clindamycin or clinimycin) (Fig. 1 J), and 7-chloro-7-deoxy-N-demethyl-4′-depropyl-4′-pentyllincomy-cin (Fig. 1 E) possess antiplasmodial activity and are also more active than lincomycin against both gram-positive and gram-negative bacteria (*23, 24*). The antiplasmodial activity is presumably due to the sensitivity of the protozoal mitochondria to the analogues.

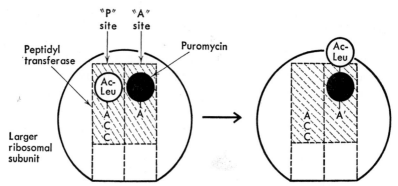

Fig. 3.   Diagrammatic representation of the fragment reaction (*29, 31, 33, 35*). Acetyl-leucine was transferred from CCA to puromycin, giving acetyl-leucyl-puromycin and CCA. Other substrates could also be used, such as CACCA-Met-f. The reaction was catalyzed by preparations of the 50S ribosomal subunit (as shown) or of complete ribosomes. Only the first three nucleotides (C_p C_p A) interacted with the peptidyl trans-ferase center. The fragment reaction assay had the advantage over other assays for peptide bond formation in that interactions between sub-strates and ribosomes were confined to the immediate vicinity of the peptidyl transferase centre. Properties of the catalytic centre could thus be specifically examined.

3. Mode of action

1) Inhibition of protein synthesis

Soon after the first reports on lincomycin appeared, Josten and Allen examined the effects of the antibiotic on the biochemistry of intact bacteria (20). Its addition to growing cultures led to an immediate and complete cessation of protein synthesis, but had little or no effect for several minutes on the synthesis of DNA or RNA. It was concluded that the primary action of lincomycin is to inhibit protein synthesis.

This conclusion was confirmed by the demonstration that lincomycin inhibits amino acid incorporation in cell-free systems from the bacteria Escherichia coli (51) and Bacillus stearothermophilus (7) and the blue-green alga, Anacystis montana (41). The relative sensitivities of the two bacterial cell-free systems correspond to those of gram-negative and gram-positive bacteria, respectively; the former being much less sensitive than the latter.

In the E. coli cell-free system, celesticetin was also shown to be inhibitory (51). The effects of antibiotics on the synthesis of three different polypeptides were examined: poly U-directed polyphenylalanine synthesis, poly A-directed polylysine synthesis and poly C-directed polyproline synthesis. Sensitivities to lincomycin were in the order polyPro>polyLys>polyPhe; while with celesticetin, they were polyPro>polyPhe>polyLys. This difference between the action of lincomycin and celesticetin has yet to be explained.

2) Site of action

In the same year that Josten and Allen reported the inhibition of protein synthesis by lincomycin, Barber and Waterworth demonstrated the antagonism between lincomycin and erythromycin in their action on intact bacteria (4). We already knew that chloramphenicol bound specifically to the 50S subunit of bacterial ribosomes (50, 52) and that its binding was inhibited by erythromycin (49, 62). This prompted us to test the effect of lincomycin and celesticetin on the binding to ribosomes of ^{14}C-chloramphenicol. In both cases, strong inhibition was observed (53). It was concluded that lincomycin and celesticetin act on the 50S subunit at positions closely related to the chloramphenicol binding site.

At about the same time as the above study, Chang et al. (7) independently arrived at the conclusion that lincomycin acts on the 50S ribosomal subunit. Their approach was to test the effects of lincomycin on hybrid ribosomes obtained by mixing 50S and

30S subunits from sensitive and resistant organisms (*B. stearo-thermophilus* and *E. coli*).

Direct evidence for the specific interaction of lincomycin with the 50S ribosomal subunit was obtained when ^{14}C-lincomycin became available. The labelled lincomycin bound strongly to 70S ribosomes from a gram-positive bacteria (*8*) and from blue-green algae (*42*); and when the ribosomes were subsequently resolved into subunits by zonal centrifugation at a low Mg^{2+} concentration, the label was coincident with the 50S but not the 30S peak (Fig. 2). When lincomycin was added to isolated subunits, it bound to 50S but not to 30S subunits (*8*). Lincomycin binding required K^+ or NH_4^+ (*8*) and was inhibited by erythromycin (*8*), chloramphenicol (*42*), and spiramycin III (*42*), but not by tetracycline (*8*).

Early experiments failed to detect any binding of lincomycin to ribosomes from a gram-negative organism (*E. coli*) (*8*). Subsequent work, using more sensitive techniques, has shown that interaction does take place, but that the affinity of *E. coli* ribosomes for lincomycin is much less than that of ribosomes from gram-positive organisms (*11*) (Sec. *6)*).

3) Genetics

Genetic studies also implicate the 50S ribosomal subunit as the site of action of lincomycin. Thus, a change in this subunit was shown by Apirion to be responsible for the enhanced sensitivity of lincomycin-sensitive mutants (*lir* mutants) isolated from *E. coli* (*1*). Further analysis of the *lir* mutants by polyacrylamide gel ionphoresis tentatively implicated one of the 50S proteins as the site of the change (*22*).

4) Binding of aminoacyl-tRNA

Chang *et al.* showed that lincomycin weakly inhibits the poly U-directed binding of Phe-tRNA to ribosomes from *B. stearother-mophilus* (*7*). However, there was less than 50% inhibition even at lincomycin concentrations two orders of magnitude greater than those necessary for a comparable inhibition of polyphenylalanine synthesis. Lincomycin had no effect on the binding of poly U to ribosomes.

We examined the effects of a number of antibiotics on the poly-nucleotide-directed binding of aminoacyl-tRNA to ribosomes from *E. coli* (*57*). Lincomycin and celesticetin weakly inhibited poly U-directed binding of Phe-tRNA, but had no effect on poly A-directed Lys-tRNA binding or poly C-directed Pro-tRNA binding. Lincomycin and celesticetin had little effect on the initial rate of Phe-tRNA binding but gave progressively more inhibition as the incubation time was extended. There was no inhibitory effect on the poly U-directed binding of Phe-tRNA to 30S subunits, but the stimulation of this binding which occurs upon addition of 50S subunits was partially inhibited.

These studies on aminoacyl-tRNA binding support the other evidence that lincomycin and celesticetin act on the 50S subunit, but they do not indicate that the antibiotics directly inhibit amino-acyl-tRNA binding. Indeed, the small inhibitions which were ob-served may well have been due to blockage of the formation of di- and tripeptides of phenylalanine, which we observed to be formed in appreciable quantities under the conditions employed (*57*).

It is not possible to equate the above binding studies with the step of protein synthesis in which aminoacyl-tRNA enters the mRNA . . . ribosome . . . nascent polypeptide complex, since it is now known that the step does not take place with free aminoacyl-tRNA but involves a complex of aminoacyl-tRNA with a super-natant factor and GTP (*48*). The effects of lincomycin and celesti-cetin in a system involving these factors have not yet been reported. Nevertheless, the failure of lincomycin and celesticetin to inhibit effectively aminoacyl-tRNA binding in the system without these factors is of interest, because, in the light of later studies (Sec. *9)*), it suggests that there are sites on the 50S subunit, in addition to the peptidyl transferase centre, which are important for interaction of tRNA with the ribosome.

5) Inhibition of peptide bond formation
In parallel with the studies on lincomycin, work was in progress on the mechanism of peptide bond formation in protein synthesis. We had obtained evidence that the reaction is catalyzed by an

active centre on the 50S ribosomal subunit, and that it is specifically inhibited by chloramphenicol (*30, 47*). Complementary evidence was obtained by Rychlik (*44*). Moreover, we had just developed a highly resolved system, known as the "fragment reaction," for studying the catalysis of the peptidyl transfer reaction using iso-lated 50S subunits (Fig. 3). Chloramphenicol was an effective inhibitor, thus confirming its specific action on peptide bond for-mation (*31*).

The demonstration that chloramphenicol inhibits the 50S-catalyzed peptidyl transfer reaction correlated very well with the demonstration that it binds to the 50S subunit, and suggested that the binding site might be at the catalytic centre. Moreover, the observation that lincomycin and celesticetin competed with chloramphenicol for binding to the 50S subunit suggested that they might also be inhibitors of peptide bond formation. We, therefore, tested them in our new system. Table I shows that lincomycin and celesticetin, as well as a number of other anti-biotics, are excellent inhibitors of the fragment reaction catalyzed by *E. coli* ribosomes. Lincomycin and celesticetin were, in fact, even better inhibitors in this system than in the cell-free system for synthesis of polypeptides (*51*). We concluded that chloram-phenicol, lincomycin, celesticetin, carbomycin, spiramycin III, streptogramin A, and a number of other antibiotics interact with the 50S ribosomal subunit at closely related sites, and by so doing interfere with the peptide bond-forming step of protein synthesis (*32*).

A puzzling aspect of these studies is the observation that ery-thromycin and certain other macrolides do not inhibit the frag-ment reaction (Table I), even though they are good inhibitors of chloramphenicol (*53, 62*) and lincomycin (Sec. *11)*) binding to ribosomes. It was conceivable that erythromycin could not interact with ribosomes in the conditions of the fragment reaction. The experiments in Table II strikingly eliminate such a possibility. Thus, a nearly complete inhibition of the fragment reaction by chloramphenicol or lincomycin is fully reversed by the addition of erythromycin. Similar observations in different systems have been obtained by other workers (*8, 60*).

TABLE I

Effects of Inhibitors on the Fragment Reaction

	Formyl-methionyl-puromycin formation (as % of control) in presence of inhibitor at conc. of		Conc. giving 50% inhibition
	10^{-3} M	10^{-4} M	(mM)
Chloramphenicol	6	12	8 to 26
Angolamycin	52	54	—
Carbomycin	7	1	3 to 3.6
Spiramycin III	28	30	10 to 20
Lancamycin	75	86	—
Streptogramin A	—	5	2.5 to 4
Lincomycin	3	18	1.8 to 3.7
Celesticetin	5	34	35 to 49
Gougerotin	−5	9	27 to 31
Sparsomycin	9	35	42 to 67
Amicetin	−6	25	33 to 44
Tetracycline	25	87	>100

The data were reproduced from Ref. (32) by kind permission of the editor.

A study on the effects of antibiotics on poly A-directed poly-lysine synthesis in an *E. coli* cell-free system (46) supports the proposition that lincomycin and chloramphenicol inhibit peptide bond formation, while erythromycin, though binding at a related site, acts on a different step of protein synthesis. Thus, lincomycin and chloramphenicol inhibited the synthesis of di- and trilysine as well as larger peptides, whereas erythromycin inhibited the synthesis of only larger lysine peptides and allowed the accumulation of dilysine, trilysine, and small amounts of tetralysine. At the concentrations employed, the action of erythromycin was dominant over the action of lincomycin and chloramphenicol. There have been other reports (21) that chloramphenicol, like erythromycin, allows the synthesis of small peptides; but the results of Teraoka *et al.* (46) suggest that chloramphenicol does, in fact, inhibit the formation of all peptide bonds. Variable effects on dipeptide formation have also been observed with spiramycin and carbomycin (26, 40). But taking all of the factors into consideration, especially pre-incubation and kinetic effects, it does appear that these two macrolides also inhibit the formation of all peptide

TABLE II
Reversal by Erythromycin of the Chloramphenicol and Lincomycin Effect on the
Fragment Reaction

	% Fragment reacted
Exp. 1	98
Control	
+chloramphenicol (0.1 mM)	11
+erythromycin (1 mM)	98
+erythromycin (1 mM)+chloramphenicol (0.1 mM)	100
Exp. 2	89
Control	
+lincomycin (0.1 mM)	2
+erythromycin (1 mM)	92
+erythromycin (1 mM)+lincomycin (0.1 mM)	100

The data were reproduced from Ref. (*36*) by kind permission of the editor.

bonds. On the other hand, oleandomycin, like erythromycin (to
which it it structurally related), allows the synthesis of small peptides (*26, 40, 46*). These conclusions are in agreement with the results of the fragment reaction assays for the action of antibiotics
on peptide bond formation (Table I). Results from other systems
(*18*) also support the conclusion that chloramphenicol and lincomycin act on peptide bond formation, while erythromycin acts
on a different step, possibly translocation.

6) The lincomycin binding site
The fragment reaction (Fig. 3) can only take place if methanol or
ethanol is present (*31, 35*). Alcohol appears to induce a conformational change in the 50S subunit, which exposes the P-site
on the peptidyl transferase centre (*35*). We were, therefore, very
interested to observe that alcohol also greatly enhances the binding
of lincomycin to *E. coli* ribosomes (*11*), the binding constant being
lowered by a factor of nearly 1/200 by the addition of 33 % ethanol
(Table III). The binding of erythromycin and a number of other
antibiotics responds to alcohol in a similar manner (*12*), but
chloramphenicol binding is hardly affected (Table III).

The discovery of conditions in which lincomycin binds more
strongly to *E. coli* ribosomes opened the way to a more thorough

TABLE III
Effect of Ethanol on the Affinity of Ribosomes for Lincomycin and Chloramphenicol

| | Dissociation constant | |
	No ethanol	33% (v/v) ethanol
Lincomycin	$(3.4\pm1)\times 10^{-5}$	$(1.7\pm0.2)\times 10^{-6}$
Chloramphenicol	$(0.6\pm0.15)\times 10^{-6}$	$(2.2\pm0.2)\times 10^{-6}$

Data were taken from Ref. (*11*) by kind permission of the editor.

investigation of its action. Preliminary evidence was already available, indicating that there is one site available for chloramphenicol binding per 50S ribosomal subunit (*50, 62*). We developed more quantitative methods for the study of antibiotic binding and confirmed the existence of one chloramphenicol site per ribosome (*11, 35*). When the same methods were applied to the binding of lincomycin in the presence of ethanol, a single binding site per 50S subunit was also found (Fig. 4). A close relationship between the chloramphenicol and lincomycin binding sites is indicated by the observation that their binding is mutually exclusive: both cannot bind to the same ribosome simultaneously (*35, 42, 53*).

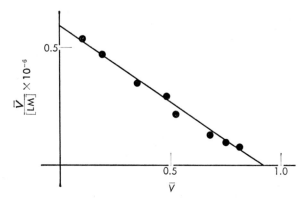

Fig. 4.   Scatchard plot for the binding of ^{14}C-lincomycin to *E. coli* ribosomes in the presence of 33% (v/v) ethanol.

7) Effect of lincomycin on sparsomycin action

Substrate binding at the P-site on the peptidyl transferase centre is stimulated by sparsomycin (*14, 19, 34*). In the fragment reaction

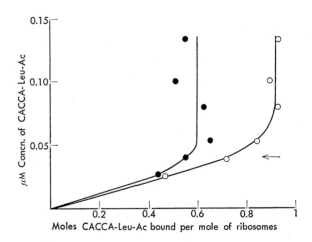

Fig. 5.   Sparsomycin-induced complex formation (^{3}H) CACCA-Leu-Ac and 50S ribosomal subunits (○) or β-cores therefrom (●). The graph shows moles of substrate bound per mole of ribosomes at varied substrate concentrations and 0.055 μM ribosomes (arrow indicates ribosome or core concentration).

TABLE IV

Effects of Various Antibiotics on Sparsomycin-induced Binding of CACCA-Leu-Ac to Ribosomes

Addition	Final conc. (mM)	Percentage of control sparsomycin-stimulated binding
None	—	100
Chloramphenicol	1	3
Carbomycin	0.1	0
Spiramycin III	0.1	0
Streptogramin A	0.1	2
Lincomycin	1	5
Amicetin	1	27
Gougerotin	1	42

Data were reproduced from Ref. (*34*) by kind permission of the editor.

system, a remarkably stable complex is formed (*34*). The complex contains a substrate, a 50S subunit, and presumably sparsomycin, bound together by non-covalent bonds. The substrate, once bound, cannot react with puromycin. At saturating substrate concentrations, sparsomycin induces the binding of about one molecule of fragment per 50S subunit (Fig. 5), thus providing evidence for the existence of one peptidyl transferase centre per ribosome (*35*). Formation of the sparsomycin complex is strongly inhibited by lincomycin, chloramphenicol and a number of related antibiotics (Table IV) (*14, 19, 34*). The hypothetical scheme in Fig. 6 provides possible explanations for some of the characteristics of sparsomycin action.

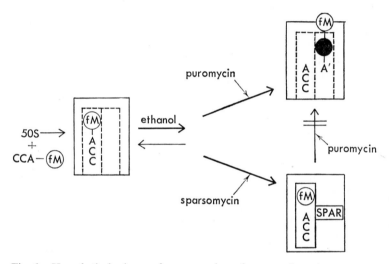

Fig. 6. Hypothetical scheme of sparsomycin and puromycin action. Initially a CCA-peptidyl group bound at the P-site on the peptidyl transferase center of the 50S subunit in a step probably requiring Mg^{2+} and K^+ and probably promoted by ethanol. In a second step, the bound fragment either interacted with sparsomycin or reacted with puromycin to give, respectively, the sparsomycin complex or peptidyl-puromycin. Under our conditions, both reactions were essentially irreversible and the products were non-interconvertible. Sparsomycin or puromycin might interact with the ribosome either after or before the binding of the CCA-peptidyl group.

8) Structure and function of the 50S ribosomal subunit

All of the results considered above support the proposition that there is one peptidyl transferase centre on every 50S subunit and that lincomycin, chloramphenicol, sparsomycin and a number of other antibiotics act on protein synthesis by binding at the centre or at allosterically linked sites. In order to investigate the relationships of these sites to the ribosome structure, we have made use of a system developed by Staehelin and co-workers for the dissociation and reconstitution of 50S ribosomal subunits *(45)*. A series of discreet cores (α, β, γ) can be prepared from 50S subunits by isopycnic centrifugation in CsCl-Mg^{2+} solutions. The cores contain intact 23S and 5S RNA, but lack increasing numbers of the 30 odd proteins which go to make up the 50S subunit. The β-cores lack all of the acidic proteins (about five) and at least one of the basic proteins. The γ-cores lack, in addition, approximately six more of the basic proteins. Sedimentation analysis suggests that the conformation of the core particles is much the same as that of native 50S subunits *(45)*.

TABLE V

Activities of Protein-deficient Cores from 50S Subunits

		Activity		
		β-Cores	γ-Cores	Split protein
(a)	Chloramphenicol binding	+	−	0
(b)	Lincomycin binding	+	−	0
(c)	Sparsomycin action	+	−	0
(d)	Fragment reaction	+	−	0

Data (a), (b) and (c) were estimated in terms of number of binding sites available, and (d) in terms of initial rate using CACCA-Leu-Ac as a substrate *(35, 58)*.

Beta- and γ-core preparations were tested for activity in four different assays *(35)*. The results (Table V) show that the β-cores possess good activity for catalysis of the fragment reaction, for the binding of chloramphenicol and lincomycin, and for the sparsomycin-induced binding of CACCA-Leu-Ac. In contrast, the γ-cores were devoid of all these activities. The split protein fractions obtained in preparation of the cores were also inactive. Other experiments *(45)* have shown that restoration of activity can be achieved by readdition of split proteins to the γ-cores. The proteins required for such a restoration are confined to the split proteins obtained in the conversion of β- to γ-cores.

The results of this study provide further support for the model in which lincomycin, chloramphenicol and sparsomycin act directly on the peptidyl transferase centre of 50S subunits, since all four activities are lost simultaneously upon removal of about six proteins from the β-cores without a major conformational change. The study is also a step toward the correlation of the structure and function of the 50S subunit. The observation that β-cores are fully active clearly eliminates the acidic proteins and certain basic proteins from being possible components of the peptidyl transferase centre. The reversible loss of activity in going from β- to γ-cores makes further identification of the active component(s) difficult. It seems probable that the split protein obtained in the conversion of β- to γ-cores contains the component(s) responsible for the catalysis of the peptidyl transfer and the binding of substrates and antibiotics, but that in order for this component to be active it must be situated in the special environment provided by the ribonucleoprotein particle. Alternatively, it is possible a) that the centre is still intact on the γ-cores but the split proteins are required for its active conformation, or b) that the core and split protein fractions contain complementary components of the centre, more than one of which is needed for activity. At present we have no evidence as to whether the centre is composed of one or more protein molecules or, indeed, whether the 23S or 5S RNA might not also take an active part in the functioning of the centre.

9) Substrate binding at the peptidyl transferase centre
It is possible to visualize several mechanisms by which antibiotics could interfere with the function of the peptidyl transferase centre. The simplest of these is direct competition with the substrate for binding at the A- or P-site on the peptidyl transferase centre. In order to investigate such a possibility, we developed assays for substrate binding at these two sites (5, 6).

There is evidence that only the CpCpA moiety of tRNA interacts with the peptidyl transferase centre, and that other parts of the tRNA molecules interact with other parts of the ribosome (33). In order to obtain a specific assay for binding at the peptidyl transferase centre, it is, therefore, necessary to use substrates containing only the terminal portion of tRNA. CACCA-Leu-Ac and CACCA-

Leu were found to be suitable. Although no binding of these "fragments" to isolated 50S subunits could be detected in normal conditions of protein synthesis, a weak binding was observed to take place in the conditions of the fragment reaction. This could be enhanced by raising the concentrations of ribosomes and alcohol. As expected for a simple non-covalent type of interaction, the binding under such conditions is rapid and reversible; and the substrate can be recovered intact after formation and dissociation of the complex. We have no direct evidence that the fragments bind . at the A- and P-sites, but our knowledge of their specificities in the peptidyl transfer reaction (33) makes it reasonable to suppose that the leucyl fragment would tend to bind at the A-site, while the acetylated leucyl fragment would tend to bind at the P-site. The differential responses to antibiotics, described below, provide strong evidence that the two fragments do, in fact, bind at distinct sites it this assay system.

Table VI shows that the binding of CACCA-Leu-Ac to 50S subunits is inhibited by lincomycin, carbomycin, spiramycin III and streptogramin A, but is stimulated by celesticetin, chloramphenicol, oleandomycin and erythromycin. Responses with CACCA-Leu were qualitatively similar with the notable differences being that chloramphenicol and oleandomycin were inhibitory while erythromycin had no effect. The inhibitory action of carbomycin, spiramycin and streptogramin A on the binding of CACCA-Leu-Ac would probably be close to 100% if it were possible to make allowance for blanks due to nonspecific interaction between fragment and ribosome. In comparison, the inhibition by lincomycin was only partial. The concentrations of antibiotics employed in these assays were sufficient to give nearly complete inhibition of the fragment reaction with puromycin (except in the cases of erythromycin and oleandomycin).

Pestka has also developed an assay for fragment binding to ribosomes at what is presumed to be the A-site (39). He reports that the binding of CACCA-Phe can occur in the absence of alcohol if 70S ribosomes but not 50S subunits are employed. The system has an advantage over the one described above in that it employs more natural conditions (no alcohol). On the other hand,

TABLE VI
Binding of CACCA-Leu-Ac and CACCA-Leu to 50S Subunits: Effects of Antibiotics

Antibiotic	Conc. (mM)	Binding of CACCA-Leu-Ac (% of control)	Binding of CACCA-Leu (% of control)
Streptogramin A	0.1	7.6	11
Spiramycin III	0.1	12	24
Carbomycin	0.1	12	10
Lincomycin	1	36	4
Chloramphenicol	1	126	0
Celesticetin	1	123	120
Oleandomycin	1	125	64
Erythromycin	1	156	106
Viridogrisein	1	160	120

Reproduced from Refs. (5), (6) and (36) by kind permission of the editor.

the requirement for 70S ribosomes, which has not yet been explained, clearly lowers the specificity of the system, since binding at the peptidyl transferase centre might be affected not only by direct action on the centre but also by factors affecting interaction between the 50S and 30S subunits.

Table VII shows some of Pestka's data on the action of antibiotics. The binding of CACCA-Phe to 70S ribosomes is inhibited by chloramphenicol, vernamycin A (equivalent to streptogramin A) and, less effectively, by spiramycin III. Erythromycin is weakly stimulating. In a footnote, lincomycin is recorded as being inhibitory but no data are given. The results obtained in Pestka's system and in our alcohol system are thus in essential agreement and provide evidence that the binding of the terminus of aminoacyl-tRNA at the A-site on the peptidyl transferase centre is inhibited by lincomycin, chloramphenicol, streptogramin A, and spiramycin III, but not by erythromycin or celesticetin.

Inhibition of fragment binding by an antibiotic in these assays does not necessarily imply that the substrate and antibiotic compete directly for binding at overlapping sites. The substrate and antibiotic binding sites might be spatially separated but allosterically linked. We are inclined to think that the allostery model is closer to reality in cases where inhibition is only partial, such as the action of lincomycin on the P-site and of spiramycin III on the

322   R. E. MONRO *et al.*

TABLE VII
Binding of CACCA-Phe to 70S Ribosomes

Antibiotic	Conc. (mM)	Binding of CACCA-Phe (% of control)
Vernamycin A	0.1	9
PA 114 A	0.1	9
Spiramycin III	0.1	36
Chloramphenicol	0.1	19
Erythromycin	0.1	120
PA 114 B	0.1	133

Lincomycin was also found to inhibit Phe-oligonucleotide binding to ribosomes. Data were reproduced from Ref. (*39*) by kind permission of the author and editor. Antibiotics vernamycin A and PA 114 A are similar to streptogramin A, whereas PA 114 B, like viridogrisein, belongs to the streptogramin B group (*56*).

A-site. The allostery model may also hold in certain cases of nearly complete inhibition. Thus, studies with puromycin suggest that lincomycin and chloramphenicol do not bind directly at the A-site (*11*), even though they effectively inhibit CACCA-Leu and CACCA-Phe binding. A more quantitative analysis of competition between substrates and antibiotics will probably be necessary before relations between their binding sites can be adequately understood.

10) Competition between antibiotics for binding to the ribosome
We have already noted that 50S ribosomal subunits can bind stoichiometric amounts of lincomycin or chloramphenicol, and that the binding of these two antibiotics is mutually exclusive. Other works indicate that erythromycin (*11, 25, 38, 61*), spiramycin and streptogramin A (*54, 55*) also interact specifically with 50S subunits. In several cases, competition between antibiotics for binding to 50S subunits has been demonstrated (*9, 11, 12, 49, 53, 55, 60–62*). Our own available data on such effects are summarized in Table VIII. All of the antibiotics in the table, with the possible exception of berninamycin, are known to act on the 50S subunit.

The data (Table VIII) confirm that there is a close relationship between the sites for lincomycin and chloramphenicol action. Thus, the binding of these two antibiotics is not only mutually

TABLE VIII
Effects of Antibiotics on the Binding to Ribosomes of Chloramphenicol, Erythromycin and Spiramycin I

Added antibiotic	Conc. (mM)	Inhibition of binding of			
		CM	Linco	Ery	Spira I (ξ)
Chloramphenicol	0.1	+($\neq$)	+	—	33%
	5			30%	
Lincomycin	0.1	+($\neq$)	+	—	50%
	10			52%	
Celesticetin	0.1	57%*	—	—	
	1	+*	+	25%	
Macrolides					
Erythromycin	0.1	+($\neq$)	+	+	+
Spiramycin III	0.1	+($\neq$)	+	70%	+
Neospiramycin III	0.1	+($\neq$)	+	+	+
Forodicin III	0.1	+($\neq$)	+	35%	+
Carbomycin	0.1	+($\neq$)	+	80%	+
Oleandomycin	0.1	+*	+	33%	+
Angolamycin	0.1	+($\neq$)	+	12%	22%
Lancamycin	0.1	+*	+	—	
Methymycin	0.1	+*	46%	18%	—
Chalcomycin	0.1	75%	80%	—	
Other compounds					
Streptogramin A	0.1	+($\neq$)	+	+	+
Streptogramin B	0.1	63%*	+	+	
Viridogrisein	0.1	42%*	+	+	+
Amicetin	0.1	—*	—	—	
	1	−12% (estim.)*	—	—	
Sparsomycin	0.1	14%*	—	—	
	0.5	18%*	—	—	
Gougerotin	0.1	−($\neq$)	—	—	
	1	—*	—	—	
Puromycin	1	—*	20%	25%	
	5	54%*	40%		
Siomycin	0.1	—*	—	—	
Thiostrepton	0.01	—*	—	—	
Bottromycin	0.01	—*	—	—	
	0.1	—*	—	—	
Berninamycin	5 μg/ml	—*	—	—	
	45 μg/ml	—*	—	—	

In this table "+" indicates inhibition greater than 80% and "−" indicates inhibition less than 20%. The concentrations of the labelled antibiotics, whose binding was estimated, were in the range from 1 to 5 M. *E. coli* ribosomes were used in all cases except those marked "$\neq$" or "ξ" in which ribosomes from *B. megaterium* or *B. subtilis* were used, respectively. The binding of lincomycin and in certain cases (indicated by *) of chloramphenicol was assayed in the presence of 33% (v/v) ethanol (conditions of the fragment reaction). The data were taken from the following references: chloramphenicol (CM) (*11, 12, 49, 53*), lincomycin (Linco) (*11*), spiramycin (Spira I) (*55*) and erythromycin (Ery) (*11*).

exclusive, but is inhibited by the same range of other antibiotics. The binding of both lincomycin and chloramphenicol is blocked by celesticetin, streptogramins A and B (equivalent to the vernamycins, synergistins, and PA114 compounds), and by several macrolides, including erythromycin. The binding of both lincomycin and chloramphenicol is only weakly and partially blocked by sparsomycin, gougerotin and puromycin, and is unaffected by amicetin, siomycin, thiostrepton (bryamycin), bottromycin and berninamycin.

Not only is the binding of lincomycin and chloramphenicol inhibited by erythromycin and spiramycin, but complementary assays (Table VIII) show that the binding of erythromycin and spiramycin is inhibited by lincomycin and chloramphenicol. At 0.1 mM lincomycin, the inhibition of erythromycin and spiramycin binding is only partial; but raising the concentration to 5 mM gives a nearly complete inhibition of erythromycin binding (11). It follows that the binding of lincomycin and erythromycin and probably also spiramycin is mutually exclusive, but that the affinity of the ribosome for lincomycin is much less than that for erythromycin. This conclusion is in agreement with direct measurements of the binding constants for lincomycin and erythromycin (11, 25, 38). On the other hand, erythromycin binding cannot be completely reversed by chloramphenicol and reaches a plateau value of about 30–50 % inhibition either in the presence or in the absence of ethanol as the chloramphenicol concentration is raised (11). Incomplete competition between chloramphenicol and erythromycin for binding to B. subtilis ribosomes has been claimed by Corcoran and co-workers (37). However, in view of the very effective inhibition of chloramphenicol binding by erythromycin in Bacillus megaterium and in E. coli (11, 53, 62), it is clear that there is a close relationship between the binding sites for chloramphenicol and erythromycin, even though the two sites may not actually overlap (11).

Most, but not all, of the antibiotics which compete with lincomycin for binding to the 50S subunit are inhibitors of peptide bond formation, as determined in fragment reaction assays (Table I). The notable exceptions are erythromycin, oleandomycin, neospiramycin III, forocidin III, streptogramin B, and viridogrisein, all of which are excellent inhibitors of lincomycin binding but have little effect on the fragment reaction. Among these, neospiramycin III is of particular interest: it has the same structure as spiramycin III but lacks one of the sugar residues (Fig. 7). It is, therefore, highly probable that it binds at the same site as spiramycin III, and that it is the extra sugar residue of spiramycin III which interferes with substrate binding at the peptidyl transferase centre. Since lincomycin has an effect similar to that of spiramycin III on substrate binding, it is reasonable to suppose that the binding site for lincomycin overlaps the binding site of this sugar. The competition of neospiramycin III for lincomycin indicates that the lincomycin binding site probably also overlaps other parts of the spiramycin binding site. It is probable that the binding site for lincomycin also overlaps the binding sites for the other macrolides, and that the variable effects of the macrolides on the peptidyl transferase centre are due to differences in extension of the molecules, as illustrated by the spiramycin-neospiramycin example.

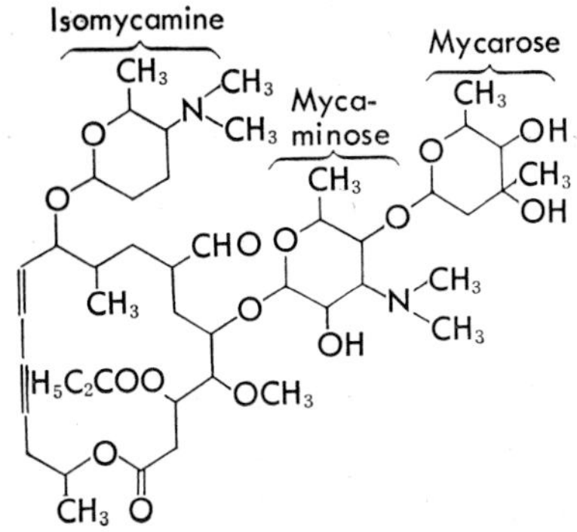

Fig. 7. Structure of spiramycin III. The mycarose could be removed chemically from spiramycin III to form neospiramycin III. From neospiramycin III the antibiotic forocidin III was formed by removing the isomycamine residue.

11) Relations between antibiotic binding sites: genetic studies
Corcoran and co-workers (*61*) tested an erythromycin-resistant strain of *B. subtilis* for sensitivity to other antibiotics. Cross-resistance was observed with several other macrolides but not with

lincomycin or methymycin (a macrolide monoglycoside). To explain these results, it was suggested that the genetic mutation leading to erythromycin resistance affected the binding site for the neutral sugar, which is present in erythromycin but not in lincomycin or methymycin.

Weisblum and Demohn (60) studied a class of erythromycin-resistant mutants of *Staphylococcus aureus*, which in normal conditions are sensitive to other macrolide antibiotics, but in the presence of erythromycin become resistant to them. The phenomenon of erythromycin-induced resistance was observed with lincomycin, the macrolides and the streptogramin B group compounds, but not with chloramphenicol, amicetin and streptogramin A. The phenomenon is analogous to the reversal of lincomycin action by erythromycin in the fragment reaction system (Table II), and although not fully understood, presumably indicates that the binding of erythromycin excludes, or at least disfavours, the binding of lincomycin and the other sensitive antibiotics. The results of Weisblum and Demohn can, therefore, be taken as *in vivo* evidence to complement the *in vitro* studies on competition between lincomycin and other antibiotics. The only inconsistency between the two types of study is that the antagonism between erythromycin and chloramphenicol was observed in the *in vitro* but not the *in vivo* system. This discrepancy may have been due to the use of different organisms in the different studies.

12) Specificity reconsidered

The knowledge which has been aquired about the mode of action of the lincomycin antibiotics helps to explain their specificity toward different organisms (Part 2). In general, the activity of lincomycin in cell-free protein synthesizing systems correlates with its *in vivo* activity. Thus lincomycin inhibits cell-free protein synthesis in systems from bacteria (7, 51), blue-green algae (41) and from yeast mitochondria (13), but has no effect on cell-free protein synthesis systems from the cytoplasm of Eukaryotes, or from mammalian mitochondria (13). Lincomycin is more active against cell-free systems from gram-positive than from gram-negative bacteria (7, 51).

TABLE IX

Binding of Lincomycin and Clindamycin to Ribosomes from *E. coli*, *A. montana* and from the Cytoplasm of Yeast

Source of ribosomes	Antibiotic	Binding
Bacteria (*E. coli*)	Lincomycin	+
	Clindamycin	+
Yeast (*S. cerevisiae*)	Lincomycin	−
	Clindamycin	−
Blue-green algae (*A. montana*)	Lincomycin	+

Experimental conditions as indicated in Ref. (*11*).

The sensitivity of protein synthesis to lincomycin in different systems correlates with the capacity of the ribosomes to bind lincomycin; ribosomes from bacteria and blue-green algae bind lincomycin, whereas ribosomes from the cytoplasm of Eukaryotes do not (Table IX). Ribosomes from gram-positive bacteria have a greater affinity for lincomycin than ribosomes from gram-negative bacteria (*7, 11*).

Recent data also provide information on the basis for the different relative activities of the lincomycin analogues. It has been reported that clindamycin is about 15 times more active than lincomycin against *in vitro* growth of *E. coli* (*24*). However, the results in Tables X and XI show that the two antibiotics have

TABLE X

Effects of Lincomycin and Its Analogues on Polyphenylalanine Synthesis

Added antibiotic	Phenylalanine incorporation (% of control)
Lincomycin	22
Clindamycin	14
Epi-clindamycin	46
U-24729 A	10
Celesticetin	52

[14]C-Phenylalanine incorporation in a cell-free system from *E. coli* MRE 600 was studied as previously described (*51*). Ribosomes were preincubated for 15 min at 37°C with the required antibiotic at concentration 5×10^{-4} M prior to addition of ^{14}C-phenylalanil-tRNA to start incorporation.

TABLE XI

Effects of Lincomycin and Its Analogues on the Fragment Reaction

Added antibiotic	Ac-Leucil-puromycin formation (% of control)
Lincomycin	33
Clindamycin	54
Epi-clindamycin	88
U 24729 A	33

E. coli MRE 600 ribosomes were used. Conditions were similar to those previously described, but CACCA-Leu-Ac was employed as the substrate (*32*). Required antibiotics were added at a concentration of 6.6×10^{-6} M.

TABLE XII

Binding of ^{14}C-Lincomycin and ^{14}C-Clindamycin to *E. coli* Ribosomes: Effects of Antibiotics of the Lincomycin Group

Added antibiotic	Conc. (*μ*M)	Binding of ^{14}C-Lincomycin (% of control)	Binding of ^{14}C-Clindamycin (% of control)
Lincomycin	5	—	30
	500	—	0
Clindamycin	1	90	—
	300	0	—
Epi-clindamycin	1	100	—
	5	—	65
	300	0	—
	500	—	0
U 24729 A	1	85	—
	5	—	50
	300	0	—
	500	—	0
Celesticetin	1	80	—
	300	13	—

^{14}C-Lincomycin (1 *μ*M) and ^{14}C-clindamycin (5 *μ*M) were added when required. Binding experiments were carried out in presence of 33% (v/v) ethanol in the conditions of the fragment reaction (*11*). ("—" indicates that the experiment was not performed.)

similar levels of activity when tested against cell-free polypeptide synthesis in *E. coli* extracts, or against the fragment reaction catalyzed by *E. coli* ribosomes. Moreover, studies on the binding of labelled clindamycin to ribosomes and on the inhibition of labelled lincomycin binding by clindamycin (Table XII) show that the two antibiotics have about the same affinity for *E. coli* ribosomes. It is difficult to escape the conclusion that the different activities of clindamycin and lincomycin against protein synthesis in intact bacteria is due to permeability factors rather than different affinities for the ribosomes. The relevance of permeability effects is suggested by clinical studies which show that clindamycin is taken up more effectively than lincomycin after oral administration into the blood stream. The basis for the greater activity of 7-chloro-7-deoxy-N-demethyl-4'-depropyl-4' pentyllincomycin appears to be the same as that for clindamycin (Tables X–XII). On the other hand, the reduced activity of epi-clindamycin as compared to clindamycin is clearly due to a lowered affinity for the ribosome (Tables X–XII). The low activity of celesticetin, as compared to lincomycin, is due, at least in part, to its lower affinity for the ribosome (Table XII). Celesticetin also has qualitatively different effects on substrate binding (Sec. 9)). These conclusions were strengthened by the results obtained in studies on the effect of antibiotics of the lincomycin group on the binding of ^{14}C-labelled chloramphenicol (Table XIII) in the absence of ethanol.

TABLE XIII
Binding of ^{14}C-Chloramphenicol: Effects of Antibiotics of the Lincomycin Group

Added antibiotic	Conc. (μM)	Binding of ^{14}C-chloramphenicol (% of control)
Lincomycin	250	59
Clindamycin	250	65
Epi-clindamycin	250	97
U 24729 A	250	32
Celesticetin	250	100

^{14}C-Chloramphenicol was added to a final concentration of 1 μM. Conditions for the assay were as reported elsewhere without ethanol (11, 53).

4. Discussion

Much clearly remains to be understood about structure-function relationships of lincomycin, chloramphenicol, the macrolides, and other related antibiotics. The functional studies surveyed in this paper show that all of these antibiotics bind to the 50S ribosomal subunit at related sites. The antibiotics have variable effects on the catalysis of peptide bond formation, and on the binding of substrates at the P- and A-sites on the peptidyl transferase catalytic centre.

We consider it probable that the lincomycin antibiotics and the macrolides all bind at sites which spatially overlap at one or more positions. Clues as to where the overlaps take place are provided by the detailed binding studies, as illustrated by the spiramycin-neospiramycin-lincomycin example (Sec. *10)*).

There is some evidence that interference with substrate binding at the A-site by lincomycin and chloramphenicol is due to an allosteric mechanism rather than direct competition (Sec. *10)*). It might even be thought that allosteric mechanisms are responsible for the actions of all of the antibiotics under consideration. However, it is difficult to visualize how there could be a sufficient variety of distinct conformational states to account for the variety of qualitatively distinct effects of the different antibiotics. It is probable that at least some of the antibiotics, possibly including lincomycin, bind in such a way as to interfere directly with substrate binding. Other antibiotics, such as erythromycin, clearly do not compete with substrate binding, as evidenced by their failure to inhibit the fragment reaction and the resolved substrate binding assays. Nevertheless, erythromycin presumably acts at a closely related site, in view of its competition with other antibiotics.

There is some evidence that erythromycin inhibits translocation (*18*). However, neither erythromycin nor any of the other antibiotics which compete with lincomycin and chloramphenicol, interfere with the G-factor ("translocase")-ribosome linked hydrolysis of GTP (*26, 28*). It is, therefore, improbable that erythromycin interferes with the primary step leading to translocation, though it might interfere with the actual movement of the CCA-peptidyl group from the A- to the P-site.

Any comprehensive explanation for the structural basis of the activity of lincomycin will have to take into account the different relative activities of the lincomycin analogues. Of particular interest is the recent observation that phosphorylation of the 3-hydroxyl group of lincomycin (by microbial transformation) leads to inactivation (*2*). The sulphur atom of lincomycin is clearly not essential for activity, since 1-demethylthio-1-hydroxylincomycin has a biological spectrum similar to that of lincomycin (3).

SUMMARY

Lincomycin, chloramphenicol, the macrolides, and the strepto-gramin type antibiotics inhibit protein synthesis by interacting strongly and specifically with the 50S ribosomal subunit at mutually related sites. One molecule of antibiotic binds per 50S subunit. Most, but not all, of these antibiotics inhibit peptide bond formation, a reaction of protein synthesis which is catalyzed by a peptidyl transferase centre on the 50S subunit. Several, but not all, of these peptidyl transferase-active antibiotics interfere with substrate binding at the P- or the A-site on the catalytic centre. All of these antibiotics, including those which do not inhibit peptide bond formation, probably bind to the ribosome in positions at or close to the peptidyl transferase centre, but their detailed mechanisms of action are not yet fully understood.

Acknowledgments

This work was supported by grants from the United States National Institutes of Health (AI 08598) and Lilly Indiana de España. One of us (R.E.M.) has been supported by a European Molecular Biology Organization fellowship. Two of us (R.F.M. and M.L.C.) are fellows of the "Formación de Personal Investigador." The work was carried out with the technical assistance of Miss Rosario Gutierrez and Miss Pilar Ochoa. Antibiotics were gifts from different sources as indicated in previous publications (5, 53).

REFERENCES

1 Apirion, D. 1967. Three genes that affect *Escherichia coli* ribosomes. *J. Mol. Biol.*, **30**, 255.

2 Argoudelis, A. D., and Coats, J. H. 1969. Microbial transformation of antibiotics. II. Phosphorylation of lincomycin by streptomycin species. *J. Antibiotics*, **22**, 341.

3 Argoudelis, A. D., and Mason, D. J. 1969. Microbial transformation of antibiotics. I. Production of lincomycin sulfoxide and demethylthio-

1-hydroxylincomycin by *S. lincolnensis. J. Antibiotics*, **22**, 289.

4   Barber, M., and Waterworth, P. M. 1964. Antibacterial activity of lincomycin and pristinamycin: a comparison with erythromycin. *Brit. Med. J.*, II, 603.

5   Celma, M. L., Monro, R. E., and Vazquez, D. 1970. Substrate and antibiotic binding sites at the peptidyl transferase centre of *E. coli* ribosomes. *FEBS Letters*, **6**, 273.

6   Celma, M. L., Monro, R. E., and Vazquez, D. Substrate and antibiotic binding sites at the peptidyl transferase center of *E. coli* ribosomes: binding of UACCA-Leu to 50S subunits. *FEBS Letters*, **13**, 247.

7   Chang, F., Shih, C., and Weisblum, B. 1966. Lincomycin, an inhibitor of amino acyl sRNA binding to ribosomes. *Proc. Natl. Acad. Sci. U.S.*, **55**, 431.

8   Chang, F. N., and Weisblum, B. 1967. The specificity of lincomycin binding to ribosomes. *Biochemistry*, **6**, 836.

9   Chang, F. N., Siddhikol, C., and Weisblum, B. 1969. Subunit localization studies of antibiotic inhibitors of protein synthesis. *Biochim. Biophys. Acta*, **186**, 396.

10   DeBoer, C., Dietz, A., Wilkins, J. R., Lewis, C. N., and Savage, G. M. 1955. Celesticetin- a new, crystalline antibiotic. I. Biologic studies of celesticetin. *Antibiotics Annual 1954–1955*, 832.

11   Fernandez-Muñoz, R., Monro, R. E., Torres-Pinedo, R., and Vazquez, D. Substrate and antibiotic binding sites at the peptidyl transferase center of *E. coli* ribosomes: studies on the chloramphenicol, lincomycin and erythromycin sites. *European J. Biochem.*, in press.

12   Fernandez-Muñoz, R., Monro, R. E., and Vazquez, D. 1971. Ribosomal peptidyl transferase: binding of inhibitors. *Methods in Enzymology*, **20**, 481.

13   Firkin, F. C., and Linnane, A. W. 1969. Phylogenetic differences in the sensitivity of mitochondrial protein synthesizing systems to antibiotics. *FEBS Letters*, **2**, 330.

14   Herner, A. E., Goldberg, I. H., and Cohen, L. B. 1969. Stabilization of N-acetylphenylalanyl transfer ribonucleic acid binding to ribosomes by sparsomycin. *Biochemistry*, **8**, 1335.

15   Hoeksema, H., Crum, G. F., and DeVries, W. H. 1955. Isolation and purification of celesticetin. *Antibiotics Annual 1954—1955*, 837.

16   Hoeksema, H. 1964. Celesticetin, IV. The structure of celesticetin. *J. Am. Chem. Soc.*, **86**, 4224.

17   Hoeksema, H., Bannister, B., Birkenmeyer, R. D., Kagan, F., Magerlein, B. J., Mackeller, F. A., Schroeder, W., Slomp, G., and Herr, R. R. 1964. Chemical studies on lincomycin. I. The structure of lincomycin. *J. Am. Chem. Soc.*, **86**, 4223.

18   Igarashi, K., Ishitsuka, H., and Kaji, A. 1969. Comparative studies on

the mechanisms of action of lincomycin, streptomycin and erythromycin. *Biochem. Biophys. Res. Commun.*, **37**, 499.

19   Jiménez, A., Monro, R. E., and Vazquez, D. 1970. Interaction of Ac-Phe-tRNA with *E. coli* ribosomal subunits. 1. Sparsomycin-induced formation of a complex containing 50S and 30S subunits but not mRNA. 2. Resistance of the sparsomycin-induced complex to hydroxylamine action. *FEBS Letters*, **7**, 103 and 109.

20   Josten, J. J., and Allen, P. M. 1964. The mode of action of lincomycin. *Biochem. Biophys. Res. Commun.*, **14**, 241.

21   Julian, G. R. 1965. [14]C Lysine peptides synthesized in an *in vitro Escherichia coli* system in the presence of chloramphenicol. *J. Mol. Biol.*, **12**, 9.

22   Krembel, J., and Apirion, D. 1968. Changes in ribosomal proteins associated with mutants in a locus that affects *Escherichia coli* ribosomes. *J. Mol. Biol.*, **33**, 363.

23   Lewis, C. 1968. Antiplasmodial activity of 7-halogenated lincomycins, *J. Parasitology*, **54**, 169; Antiplasmodial activity of halogenated lincomycin analogues in Plasmodium berghei-infected mice. *Antimicrobial Agents and Chemotherapy—1967*, 537.

24   Magerlein, B. J., Birkenmeyer, R. D., and Kagan, F. 1967. Chemical modification of lincomycin. *Antimicrobial Agents and Chemotherapy— 1966*, 727; Lincomycin. VI. 4′ Alkyl analogs of lincomycin. Relationship between structure and antibacterial activity. *J. Med. Chem.*, **10**, 355.

25   Mao, J. C. -H., and Putterman, M. 1969. The intermolecular complex of erythromycin and ribosome. *J. Mol. Biol.*, **44**, 347.

26   Mao, J. C.-H., and Robishaw, E. E. 1971. Effects of macrolides on peptide bond formation and translocation. *Biochemistry*, **10**, 2054.

27   a   Mason, D. J., Dietz, A., and Deboer, C. 1963. Lincomycin, a new antibiotic. I. Discovery and biological properties. *Antimicrobial Agents and Chemotherapy—1962*, 554;   b   Herr, R. R., and Bergy, M. E. 1963. Lincomycin, a new antibiotic. II. Isolation and characterization. *Antimicrobial Agents and Chemotherapy—1962*, 560; c Hanke, L. J., Mason, D. J., Burch, M. R., and Treick, R. W. 1963 Lincomycin, a new antibiotic. III. Microbiological assay. *Antimicrobial Agents and Chemotherapy—1962*, 565;   d Lewis, C., Clapp, H. W., and Grady, J. E. 1963. *In vitro* and *in vivo* evaluation of lincomycin, a new antibiotic. *Antimicrobial Agents and Chemotherapy—1962*, 570.

28   Modolell, J., Vazquez, D., and Monro, R. E. 1971. Ribosomes, G-factor and siomycin. *Nature New Biology*, **230**, 109.

29   Monro, R. E. 1967. Catalysis of peptide bond formation by 50S ribosomal subunits from *Escherichia coli*. *J. Mol. Biol.*, **26**, 147.

30   Monro, R. E., Maden, B. E. H., and Traut, R. R. 1967. The mechanism of peptide bond formation in protein synthesis. *In* "Symp. Fed. European

Biochem. Soc.—1966," ed. by D. Shugar. Academic Press, London, p. 179.

31 Monro, R. E., and Marcker, K. A. 1967. Ribosome-catalyzed reaction of puromycin with formyl-methionine-containing oligonucleotide. *J. Mol. Biol.*, **25**, 347.

32 Monro, R. E., and Vazquez, D. 1967. Ribosome-catalyzed peptidyl transfer: effects of some inhibitors of protein synthesis. *J. Mol. Biol.*, **28**, 161.

33 Monro, R. E., Cerna, J., and Marcker, K. A. 1968. Ribosome-catalyzed peptidyl transfer: substrate specificity at the P-site. *Proc. Natl. Acad. Sci. U.S.*, **61**, 1042.

34 Monro, R. E., Celma, M. L., and Vazquez, D. 1969. Action of sparsomycin on ribosome-catalyzed peptidyl transfer. *Nature*, **222**, 356.

35 Monro, R. E., Staehelin, T., Celma, M. L., and Vazquez, D. 1969. The peptidyl transferase activity of ribosomes. *Cold Spring Harbor Symp. Quant. Biol.*, XXXIV, 357.

36 Monro, R. E., Fernández-Muñoz, R., Celma, M. L., Jiménez, A., Battaner, E., and Vazquez, D. 1970. Antibiotics acting on the peptidyl transferase centre of ribosomes. *In* "Progress in antimicrobial and anticancer chemotherapy (Proceedings Sixth International Congress of Chemotherapy)," University of Tokyo Press, Tokyo, Vol. II, p. 473.

37 Oleinick, N. L., Wilhelm, J. M., and Corcoran, J. W. 1968. Non-identity of the site of action of erythromycin A and chloramphenicol on *Bacillus subtilis* ribosomes. *Biochim. Biophys. Acta*, **155**, 290.

38 Oleinick, N. L., and Corcoran, J. W. 1969. Two types of binding of erythromycin to ribosomes from antibiotic-sensitive and -resistant *Bacillus subtilis* 168. *J. Biol. Chem.*, **244**, 727.

39 Pestka, S. 1969. Studies on the formation of transfer ribonucleic acid-ribosome complexes, XI. Antibiotic effects on phenylalanyl-oligonucleotide binding to ribosomes. *Proc. Natl. Acad. Sci. U.S.*, **64**, 709.

40 Pulkrábek, P., Cerna, J., and Rychlik, I. Synthesis of tRNA-bound peptides in the presence of puromycin or of antibiotics inhibiting ribosomal transpeptidization. *Collection Czech. Chem. Commun.*, in press.

41 Rodriguez-Lopez, M., and Vazquez, D. 1970. The effects of the rifamycin antibiotics on algae. *FEBS Letters*, **9**, 171.

42 Rodriguez-Lopez, M., Celma, M. L., Fernandez-Muñoz, R., and Vazquez, D. 1968. Atti VII Simposio Internazionale di Agrochimica su "La sintesi biologica delle proteine," p. 63.

43 Rodriguez-Lopez, M., and Vazquez, D. 1968. Comparative studies on cytoplasmic ribosomes from algae. *Life Sciences*, **7**, 327.

44 Rychlik, I. 1966. Release of lysine peptides by puromycin from polylysyl-transfer RNA in presence of ribosomes. *Biochim. Biophys. Acta*, **114**, 425.

45 Staehelin, T., Maglott, D., and Monro, R. E. 1969. On the catalytic centre of peptidyl transfer: a part of the 50S ribosome structure. *Cold Spring Harbor Symp. Quant. Biol.*, XXXIV, 39.

46   Teraoka, H., Tanaka, K., and Tamaki, M. 1969. A comparative study on the effects of chloramphenicol, erythromycin and lincomycin on polylysine synthesis. *Biochim. Biophys. Acta*, **174**, 776.

47   Traut, R. R., and Monro, R. E. 1964. The puromycin reaction and its relation to protein synthesis. *J. Mol. Biol.*, **10**, 63.

48   Various contributions in *Cold Spring Harbor Symp. Quant. Biol.*, XXXIV, (1969).

49   Vazquez, D. 1963. Antibiotics which affect protein synthesis: the uptake of ^{14}C-chloramphenicol by bacteria. *Biochem. Biophys. Res. Commun.*, **12**, 409.

50   Vazquez, D. 1964. The binding of chloramphenicol by ribosomes from *Bacillus megaterium*. *Biochem. Biophys. Res. Commun.*, **15**, 464.

51   Vazquez D. 1966. Antibiotics affecting chloramphenicol uptake by bacteria. Their effect on amino acid incorporation in a cell-free system. *Biochim. Biophys. Acta*, **114**, 289.

52   Vazquez, D. 1966. Mode of action of chloramphenicol and related antibiotics. *Symp. Soc. Gen. Microbiol.*, **16**, 169.

53   Vazquez, D. 1966. Binding of chloramphenicol to ribosomes. The effect of a number of antibiotics. *Biochim. Biophys. Acta*, **114**, 277.

54   Vazquez, D. 1967. Inhibitors of protein synthesis at the ribosome level. Studies on their site of action. *Life Sciences*, **6**, 381.

55   Vazquez, D. 1967. Binding to ribosomes and inhibitory effect in protein synthesis of the spiramycin antibiotics. *Life Sciences*, **6**, 845.

56   Vazquez, D. 1967. The streptogramin family of antibiotics. *In* "Antibiotics," ed. by D. Gottlieb and P. D. Shaw, Springer-Verlag, Berlin-Heidelberg-New York, Vol. I, p. 387.

57   Vazquez, D., and Monro, R. E. 1967. Effects of some inhibitors of protein synthesis on the binding of aminoacyl sRNA to ribosomal subunits. *Biochim. Biophys. Acta*, **142**, 155.

58   Vazquez, D., Staehelin, T., Celma, M. L., Battaner, E., Fernandez-Muñoz, R., and Monro, R. E. 1969. Inhibitors as tools in elucidating ribosomal function. *In* "Inhibitors tools in cell research," ed. by Th. Bücher and H. Sies, Springer-Verlag, Berlin-Heidelberg- New York, p.100.

59   a Wagner, J. G., Novak, E., Patel, N. C., Chichester, C. G., and Lummis, W. L. 1968. Absorption, excretion and half-life of clinimycin in normal adult males. *Am. J. Med. Sciences*, **256**, 25; b Brodasky, T. F., Argoudelis, A. D., and Eble, T. E. 1968. The characterization and thin-layer chromatographic quantitation of the human metabolite of 7-deoxy-7 (S)-chlorolincomycin (U-21, 251 F). *J. Antibiotics*, **21**, 327.

60   Weisblum, B., and Demohn, V. 1969. Erythromycin-inducible resistance in *Staphylococcus aureus*: survey of antibiotic classes involved. *J. Bact.*, **98**, 447.

61   Wilhelm, J. M., Oleinick, N. L., and Corcoran, J. W. 1968. Interaction

of antibiotics with ribosomes: structure—function relationships and a possible common mechanism for the antibacterial action of the macrolides and lincomycin. *Antimicrobial Agents and Chemotherapy—1967*, 236.

62   Wolfe, A. D., and Hahn, F. E. 1965. Mode of action of chloramphenicol. IX. Effects of chloramphenicol upon a ribosomal amino acid polymerization system and its binding to bacterial ribosome. *Biochim. Biophys. Acta*, **95**, 146.

NAME INDEX

SUBJECT INDEX

341